THE **Language** OF **Mental Health**

A Glossary OF Psychiatric Terms

THE Language OF Mental Health

A Glossary OF Psychiatric Terms

By

Narriman C. Shahrokh
Chief Administrative Officer,
Department of Psychiatry and Behavioral Sciences
University of California, Davis School of Medicine
Sacramento, California

Robert E. Hales, M.D., M.B.A.
Joe P. Tupin Chair, and Professor and Chair,
Department of Psychiatry and Behavioral Sciences
University of California, Davis School of Medicine
Editor-in-Chief, Books, American Psychiatric Publishing, Inc.

Katharine A. Phillips, M.D.
Professor of Psychiatry and Human Behavior,
Brown University School of Medicine
Director, Body Dysmorphic Disorder Program, Rhode Island Hospital
Providence, Rhode Island

Stuart C. Yudofsky, M.D.
D.C. and Irene Ellwood Professor and Chairman,
Menninger Department of Psychiatry and Behavioral Sciences
Baylor College of Medicine
Houston, Texas

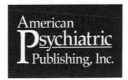

American Psychiatric Publishing, Inc.

Washington, DC
London, England

Manufactured in Canada on acid-free paper
15 14 13 12 11   5 4 3 2 1
First Edition

Typeset in Adobe's Baskerville Book and Veljovic Book

American Psychiatric Publishing, Inc.
1000 Wilson Boulevard
Arlington, VA 22209
www.appi.org

Library of Congress Cataloging-in-Publication Data
The language of mental health : a glossary of psychiatric terms / Narriman C. Shahrokh...[et al.]. — 1st ed.
    p. ; cm.
  Includes bibliographical references.
  ISBN 978-1-58562-345-7 (pbk. : alk. paper) 1. Psychiatry—Dictionaries.
I. Shahrokh, Narriman C.
  [DNLM: 1. Psychiatry—Dictionary—English.   WM 13]
  RC437.L28 2011
  616.89003—dc22

                                                    2010051728

British Library Cataloguing in Publication Data
A CIP record is available from the British Library.

Contents

Preface

Verba volant, scripta manent. ("Spoken words fly away, written words remain.")

—Caius Titus to the Roman Senate

This book concerns itself with terms currently relevant to the mental health field. Like any glossary, it seeks to elucidate the meanings of its terms through definitions, examples, and qualifications. It is impossible to imagine a glossary of mental health terms without "schizophrenia," "psychosis," "depression," and myriads of others that deal with the need to classify and qualify conditions central to the mental health field. In addition, there is a need to define the many psychosocial and pharmacological treatments for these disorders and many others.

This volume is meant to be a resource for anyone who needs concise but thorough explanations of terms that have pertinence to the practice and study of mental health. There is a new awareness that psychiatric concepts must be understood to comprehend not only the actions of individuals but also the greater trends in social and economic developments. Psychiatry is at its core a medical science, but there is an essential need for the greater world to understand its tenets: hence the importance of a volume that presents "the language of mental health."

This is a compact presentation of the current state of psychiatry and is intended for the widening audience concerned with its workings. Whereas the standard terms still form this glossary's foundation, many of the definitions and examples have been edited to allow those outside the field to grasp the meanings more easily. The book's scope has grown to include the influences that other disciplines and new technologies have brought to its already complex composition, and Web site addresses have been included, where pertinent, as still further sources of reference. In the end, this reference expresses what must be a transient consideration of this field. This is because psychiatry, with its continuing efforts to classify and understand the depths and processes of the human mind, remains ultimately an evolving brain science whose subject continues to be elusive.

We have put in SMALL CAPS type those terms within definitions that have their own entries. We have also attempted to include for each term a brief definition if the term can be better explained in the context of a more encompassing or general subject that is referenced as well (e.g., *triskaidekaphobia* and *phobia*). Thus, every term has at least a brief explanation, even if a reference follows to a more thorough, generic definition. We hope that you find this reference book useful and informative.

Narriman C. Shahrokh
Robert E. Hales, M.D., M.B.A.
Katharine A. Phillips, M.D.
Stuart C. Yudofsky, M.D.

A

AA See ALCOHOLICS ANONYMOUS (AA).

AAAP See AMERICAN ACADEMY OF ADDICTION PSYCHIATRY (AAAP).

AACAP See AMERICAN ACADEMY OF CHILD AND ADOLESCENT PSYCHIATRY (AACAP).

AAMI See AGE-ASSOCIATED MEMORY IMPAIRMENT (AAMI).

AAPL See AMERICAN ACADEMY OF PSYCHIATRY AND THE LAW (AAPL).

AASM See AMERICAN ACADEMY OF SLEEP MEDICINE (AASM).

aberrant behavior A behavior that deviates from what is normal and expected.

Abilify Brand name for the ATYPICAL ANTIPSYCHOTIC drug ARIPIPRAZOLE.

Abnormal Involuntary Movement Scale (AIMS) A widely used ASSESSMENT screening scale for TARDIVE DYSKINESIA, a chronic, involuntary MOVEMENT DISORDER that may develop in patients who have been treated for long periods with ANTIPSYCHOTICS, especially CONVENTIONAL ANTIPSYCHOTIC medications such as HALOPERIDOL (HALDOL).

abnormality In psychological terms, any mental, emotional, or behavioral activity that deviates from culturally or scientifically accepted norms.

ABPN See AMERICAN BOARD OF PSYCHIATRY AND NEUROLOGY (ABPN).

abreaction Emotional release or discharge after recalling a painful experience that has been repressed because it was not consciously tolerable (see CONSCIOUS). A therapeutic effect sometimes occurs through partial or repeated discharge of the painful AFFECT. See also SYSTEMATIC DESENSITIZATION.

absolutistic thinking A belief in absolutes, a "black and white" way of thinking, with no middle ground or gray areas.

abstinence Forgoing some kind of gratification, such as not engaging in sex. In the area of alcohol or drug DEPENDENCE, being without the substance on which the subject had been dependent.

abstract attitude (categorical attitude) A type of COGNITIVE functioning that includes assuming a mental set voluntarily; shifting voluntarily from a specific aspect of a situation to the general; keeping

SMALL CAPS type indicates terms defined as main entries elsewhere in this glossary.

1

in mind simultaneously various aspects of a situation; grasping the essentials of a whole, breaking it into its parts, and isolating them voluntarily; and/or thinking or performing symbolically. A characteristic of many psychiatric disorders is the person's inability to assume the abstract attitude or to shift readily from the concrete to the abstract and back again as demanded by circumstances.

abstract thinking A thinking that is removed from the facts of the "here and now," is characterized by the ability to use facts to develop generalizations. Often it is tested by asking patients to interpret proverbs.

abulia Lack of will or motivation, often expressed as inability to make decisions or set goals.

abuse (child, elder, spouse) To misuse, attack, or injure. The abuse may be sexual, physical, or emotional. See ABUSED CHILD.

abuse (of psychoactive substances) Impairment in social and occupational functioning resulting from the pathological and "COMPULSIVE" use of a substance. The concept is closely related to the definition of substance DEPENDENCE, which has similar SYMPTOMS of impairment but may also include evidence of physiological TOLERANCE or WITHDRAWAL. Typical symptoms of substance abuse include inability to fulfill major ROLE obligations at work, school, or home; recurrent use of the substance in situations in which such use is physically hazardous; substance-related legal problems; and continued use even though it causes or exaggerates interpersonal problems.

abused child A child or an infant who has suffered repeated injuries, which may include bone fractures, neurological and psychological damage, or sexual ABUSE at the hands of a parent, parents, or parent surrogate(s). The physical abuse is often precipitated by the child's normal and age-appropriate mildly irritating behavior. Child abuse also includes child neglect.

academic problem School difficulty that is not due to a MENTAL DISORDER. Examples are failing grades or significant underachievement in a person with adequate intellectual capacity.

academic skills disorders See LEARNING DISORDERS.

acalculia Loss of previously possessed facility with arithmetic calculation.

acamprosate A medication used in ALCOHOL DEPENDENCE to help control RELAPSE and maintain ABSTINENCE. Acamprosate's therapeutic effects are thought to be due to actions on **GABA** (GAMMA-AMINOBUTYRIC

ACID) RECEPTORS. Marketed under the brand name CAMPRAL. See "Medications Used in Psychiatry."

accident proneness Susceptibility to accidents based on psychological causes or motivations, usually UNCONSCIOUS.

accreditation Official certification (by an organization that has responsibility for reviewing the standards) that established standards have been met, such as the process by which hospitals and health facilities are surveyed and approved by THE JOINT COMMISSION (TJC) (formerly Joint Commission on Accreditation of Healthcare Organizations [JCAHO]).

acculturation The SOCIALIZATION process by which minority groups gradually learn and adopt various elements of the dominant CULTURE. The dominant culture is itself transformed by its interaction with minority groups.

acculturation difficulty A problem in adapting to a different CULTURE or environment. The problem is not based on any coexisting MENTAL DISORDER.

acetylcholine A NEUROTRANSMITTER in the BRAIN, where it helps to regulate MEMORY, and in the peripheral nervous system, where it controls the actions of skeletal and smooth muscle.

acetylcholinesterase inhibitors A class of medications used in the treatment of ALZHEIMER'S DISEASE (the most common dementing illness in the elderly), other dementias (e.g., LEWY BODY DEMENTIA), myasthenia gravis, glaucoma, and ANTICHOLINERGIC poisoning. Acetylcholinesterase inhibitors retard the breakdown of the NEUROTRANSMITTER ACETYLCHOLINE, which may improve COGNITION. They are also believed to have an effect on peptide processing, neurotransmitter RECEPTORS, and ion channels. See "Medications Used in Psychiatry."

achluophobia The FEAR of darkness.

acoustic agnosia See AUDITORY AGNOSIA.

acquired immunodeficiency syndrome (AIDS) A SECONDARY immunodeficiency SYNDROME resulting from HUMAN IMMUNODEFICIENCY VIRUS (HIV) infection and characterized by opportunistic infections, malignancies, neurological dysfunction (especially subcortical DEMENTIA), and a variety of other SYMPTOMS. Of the patients dying of AIDS, 90% show histological evidence of subacute ENCEPHALITIS, which produces a subcortical dementia, with slowed mental processing, poor SHORT-TERM MEMORY, loss of initiative, and APATHY. DEPRESSION is present in 20%–35% of AIDS patients.

acrophobia The FEAR of heights.

ACT See ASSERTIVE COMMUNITY TREATMENT (ACT).

ACTH See ADRENOCORTICOTROPIC HORMONE (ACTH).

actigraphy A method of monitoring rest/activity cycles. A small actigraph is worn by a patient to measure motor activity. It is used to clinically evaluate INSOMNIA, CIRCADIAN RHYTHM SLEEP DISORDERS, excessive daytime sleepiness, and RESTLESS LEGS SYNDROME.

acting out Expressions of UNCONSCIOUS emotional CONFLICTS or feelings in actions rather than words. The person is not consciously aware of the meaning of such acts (see CONSCIOUS). Acting out may be harmful or, in controlled situations, therapeutic (e.g., children's PLAY THERAPY).

action See "Legal Terms."

activities of daily living (ADLs) Any daily activity performed for self-care, such as feeding oneself, bathing, grooming, and dressing. Health professionals routinely refer to the ability or inability to perform ADLs as a measurement of the functional status of a person. This measurement is useful for assessing the elderly, the mentally ill, and those with chronic diseases in order to evaluate what type of health care services an individual may need and whether the person may live independently.

actualization Realization of one's full potential.

actus reus See "Legal Terms."

acupuncture An ancient Chinese practice of piercing the body with needles with the intent of relieving pain or treating disease. An ADJUNCTIVE therapy used in the treatment of chronic pain and other disorders, as well as in OPIOID DETOXIFICATION.

acute confusional state 1) A form of DELIRIUM in which the most prominent SYMPTOMS are disorders of MEMORY and ORIENTATION, usually with SHORT-TERM MEMORY DEFICIT, AMNESIA, and clouding of consciousness (i.e., reduced clarity of awareness of environment with reduced capacity to shift, focus, and sustain ATTENTION to environmental stimuli). Also known as *acute confusional disorder.*

2) An acute STRESS REACTION to new surroundings or new demands; it generally subsides as the person adjusts to the situation. See also IDENTITY CRISIS.

acute dystonic reaction (ADR) An idiosyncratic drug reaction that involves acute involuntary muscle movements and spasms. Although any muscle group in the body can be involved, the most common SYMPTOMS are torticollis, facial grimacing, and body arching. Approximately 3%–10% of patients exposed to CONVENTIONAL ANTIPSYCHOTICS, especially high-potency agents such as HALOPERIDOL (HALDOL), will experience an acute dystonic reaction. The movements typically occur at a time when the BLOOD LEVEL of medication is dropping.

acute stress disorder A type of ANXIETY DISORDER characterized by the development of severe dissociative, intrusive, avoidant, and HYPERAROUSAL SYMPTOMS in response to actual or threatened injury or death or after someone witnesses the serious injury or killing of another person. These symptoms usually develop within 1 month of the event and are associated with an elevated risk of developing POSTTRAUMATIC STRESS DISORDER (PTSD).

Adam A street name for 3,4-METHYLENEDIOXYMETHAMPHETAMINE (MDMA). See ECSTASY.

ADAMHA See ALCOHOL, DRUG ABUSE, AND MENTAL HEALTH ADMINISTRATION (ADAMHA).

Adapin Brand name (now discontinued) for the TRICYCLIC ANTIDEPRESSANT drug DOXEPIN.

adaptation Fitting one's behavior to meet the needs of one's environment, which often involves a modification of IMPULSES, EMOTIONS, or attitudes.

ADC AIDS dementia complex. See HIV DEMENTIA.

Adderall Brand name for AMPHETAMINE MIXED SALTS.

addiction DEPENDENCE on a substance to the extent that a physiological and/or psychological need is established. This may be manifested by any combination of the following SYMPTOMS: TOLERANCE, preoccupation with obtaining and using the substance, use of the substance despite anticipation of probable adverse consequences, repeated efforts to cut down or control substance use, and WITHDRAWAL SYMPTOMS when the substance is unavailable or not used.

addiction psychiatry An AMERICAN BOARD OF PSYCHIATRY AND NEUROLOGY (ABPN) subspecialty that focuses on evaluation and treatment of individuals with alcohol, drug, or other substance-related disorders, and of individuals with dual diagnosis of substance-related and other psychiatric disorders. Addiction psychiatrists often use a combination of medicine and psychotherapy to help patients fight their specific ADDICTION. This can include the use of drugs to combat WITHDRAWAL SYMPTOMS consistent with denying the body or mind its drug of choice. They also conduct extensive studies on the process of ADDICTION and how it can be prevented.

ADH See ALCOHOL DEHYDROGENASE (ADH).

ADHD   See ATTENTION-DEFICIT/HYPERACTIVITY DISORDER (ADHD).

adherence   Used most commonly when referring to a person's taking medications in the amount and frequency recommended. Sometimes called COMPLIANCE.

adiadochokinesia   The inability to perform rapid alternating movements of one or more of the extremities.

adjudication   See "Legal Terms."

adjunctive   Term used to describe an agent or therapy added to or administered in conjunction with the primary treatment.

adjustment   Alteration or accommodation by which one can better adapt oneself to the immediate environment and to one's inner self. See also ADAPTATION.

adjustment disorder   A MENTAL DISORDER in which emotional or behavioral SYMPTOMS develop in response to an identifiable stressor. The symptoms, which may include ANXIETY, depressed MOOD, and disturbance of conduct (or a combination of these symptoms), are clinically significant in that the distress exceeds what would be expected under the circumstances, or significant impairment in social or occupational functioning is produced. Duration of symptoms tends to be self-limited, not persisting more than 6 months after termination of the stressor or its consequences. Sometimes the disorder is designated as "acute" if duration is less than 6 months and as "chronic" if symptoms last for 6 months or longer.

adjuvant   Term used to describe an agent or technique that enhances the effectiveness of the primary treatment.

ADLs   See ACTIVITIES OF DAILY LIVING (ADLs).

administrative psychiatry   The branch of PSYCHIATRY that deals with the organization of MENTAL HEALTH services in a program, a hospital, or another facility. Its focus is on management and leadership and concerns the interaction of administration, clinical care, and the attitudes, values, and belief systems of the organization.

adolescence   A chronological period of accelerated physical and emotional growth leading to sexual and psychological maturity. It often begins at about age 12 years and ends at a loosely defined time, when the individual achieves independence and social productivity (usually in the early 20s). See also PSYCHOSEXUAL DEVELOPMENT; PSYCHOSOCIAL DEVELOPMENT.

adolescent psychiatry   See CHILD AND ADOLESCENT PSYCHIATRY.

ADR   See ACUTE DYSTONIC REACTION (ADR).

adrenaline See EPINEPHRINE.

adrenergic Referring to neural activation by CATECHOLAMINES such as EPINEPHRINE (ADRENALINE) and NOREPINEPHRINE (noradrenaline) as well as drugs with ADRENALINE-like action that are capable of binding ADRENERGIC RECEPTORS. Contrast with CHOLINERGIC.

adrenergic receptors RECEPTORS in the BRAIN and other organ systems (including, for example, the heart and blood vessels) that are the binding sites for the CATECHOLAMINES EPINEPHRINE and NOREPINEPHRINE as well as for ADRENERGIC drugs. Epinephrine plays an important role in the body's response to emergency situations. The FIGHT-OR-FLIGHT RESPONSE is initiated through activation of the SYMPATHETIC NERVOUS SYSTEM with release of epinephrine. Norepinephrine acts as both a HORMONE and a NEUROTRANSMITTER. As a stress hormone, norepinephrine increases the availability of food-energy stores and stimulates alertness and AROUSAL in the brain. As a neurotransmitter, norepinephrine plays an important role in attentiveness, emotions, sleeping, dreaming, and learning. Adrenergic receptors are divided into two main groups, alpha and beta, each of which has several subtypes. See also ALPHA-ADRENERGIC AGONISTS; BETA-BLOCKERS.

adrenocorticotropic hormone (ACTH) A HORMONE produced by the anterior part of the pituitary gland that stimulates hormone production in the adrenal cortex. A synthetic derivative of ACTH known as cosyntropin (Cortrosyn) is used for diagnostic testing of adrenal insufficiency, or Addison's disease.

adrenoleukodystrophy Formerly known as *Schilder's disease*; a rare, X-linked recessive metabolic disorder occurring in boys, characterized by adrenal atrophy and widespread, diffuse cerebral demyelination. It produces DEMENTIA, corticospinal tract dysfunction, and cortical blindness.

advance directive See "Legal Terms."

advanced sleep phase disorder See *advanced sleep phase pattern* under CIRCADIAN RHYTHM SLEEP DISORDERS.

adverse effect See SIDE EFFECT.

affect Behavior that expresses a subjectively experienced EMOTION. Affect is responsive to changing emotional states, whereas MOOD refers to a pervasive and sustained EMOTION. Common affects are EUPHORIA, anger, and sadness. Some types of disturbance of affect are the following:

blunted Severe reduction in the intensity of affective expression.

flat Absence or near absence of any SIGNS of affective expression; flat affect often manifests as a monotonous voice and an immobile face.

inappropriate Affective expression that is discordant with the content of the person's speech or ideation.

labile Abnormal variability, with repeated, rapid, and abrupt shifts in affective expression.

restricted or constricted Reduction in the expressive range and intensity of affects.

affective disorder A disorder in which MOOD change or disturbance is the primary manifestation. Now referred to as MOOD DISORDER.

aftercare Posthospitalization program of REHABILITATION designed to reinforce the effects of therapy and to help the patient adjust to his or her environment and prevent RELAPSE.

age-associated memory impairment (AAMI) The mild disturbance in MEMORY function that occurs normally with AGING. It is also called *benign senescent forgetfulness.*

ageism Systematic stereotyping of and discrimination against elderly people. It is distinguished from GERONTOPHOBIA, a specific pathological FEAR of old people and AGING.

aggression Forceful physical, verbal, or symbolic action. May be appropriate and self-protective (as in healthy self-assertiveness) or inappropriate (as in hostile or destructive behavior). May also be directed toward the environment, toward another person, or toward the self.

aging Characteristic pattern of life changes that occur normally in humans, plants, and animals as they grow older. Some age changes begin at birth and continue until death; other changes begin at maturity and end at death.

agitated depression A severe MAJOR DEPRESSIVE DISORDER in which PSYCHOMOTOR AGITATION is prominent.

agitation Excessive motor activity, usually nonpurposeful and associated with internal tension. Examples include inability to sit still, fidgeting, pacing, wringing of hands, and pulling of clothes. See PSYCHOMOTOR AGITATION.

agnosia The inability to recognize or identify objects despite intact sensory function. It may be seen in DEMENTIA.

agonist In pharmacology, a substance that stimulates or mimics a RECEPTOR-mediated biological response by binding to the cell receptors. Contrast with ANTAGONIST.

agoraphobia The FEAR of open spaces.

Agouti-related protein (AgRP) A neuropeptide produced in the BRAIN (in the arcuate nucleus of the HYPOTHALAMUS) by the AgRP/neuropeptide Y (NPY) neuron that increases appetite and decreases metabolism and energy expenditure. It is one of the most potent and long-lasting of appetite stimulators. An understanding of the role AgRP plays in weight gain may assist in developing pharmaceutical models for treating OBESITY.

agranulocytosis A reduction in the absolute number of circulating granulocytes (a category of white blood cells) that often leads to an increased susceptibility to bacterial and fungal infections and even death. The ATYPICAL ANTIPSYCHOTIC CLOZAPINE and the MOOD STABILIZER CARBAMAZEPINE may produce this condition and require hematological monitoring.

agraphesthesia The inability to identify a number written on the palm of one's hand. It is seen in CORTICOBASAL GANGLIONIC DEGENERATION, a "PARKINSON'S PLUS" SYNDROME.

agraphia The loss of a previously possessed facility for writing.

AgRP See AGOUTI-RELATED PROTEIN (AgRP).

AI See ARTIFICIAL INTELLIGENCE (AI).

AIDS See ACQUIRED IMMUNODEFICIENCY SYNDROME (AIDS).

AIDS dementia complex (ADC) See HIV DEMENTIA.

AIDS-related complex (ARC) A group of SYMPTOMS that appear to represent premonitory SIGNS of full-blown ACQUIRED IMMUNODEFICIENCY SYNDROME (AIDS), such as generalized lymphadenopathy (disease involving the lymph nodes), night sweats, persistent fevers, persistent cough, infection of the throat, and prolonged diarrhea.

ailurophobia The FEAR of cats.

AIMS See ABNORMAL INVOLUNTARY MOVEMENT SCALE (AIMS).

akathisia A subjective sense of restlessness accompanied by fidgeting of the legs, rocking from foot to foot, pacing, or being unable to sit or stand. SYMPTOMS develop within a few weeks of starting or raising the dose of a CONVENTIONAL ANTIPSYCHOTIC medication or of reducing the dose of medication used to treat EXTRAPYRAMIDAL SYMPTOMS (EPS) (see also EXTRAPYRAMIDAL SYNDROME).

akinesia A state of motor inhibition or reduced voluntary motor movement in a person. The SYMPTOMS may occur in a patient taking a CONVENTIONAL ANTIPSYCHOTIC medication.

akinetic mutism A state of apparent alertness with following eye movements but no speech or voluntary motor responses.

Akineton   Brand name for the ANTICHOLINERGIC drug BIPERIDEN.

AKT1 gene   A recently studied susceptibility GENE in SCHIZOPHRENIA. Family-based analyses have revealed a significant association of *AKT1* with schizophrenia. This association has been replicated in Asian, European, and Iranian groups.

alanine aminotransferase (ALT)   An ENZYME (formerly called *serum glutamic-pyruvic transaminase [SGPT]*) that is elevated in patients with liver disease or may be increased by certain psychiatric medications. Because most psychiatric medications are metabolized in the liver, PSYCHIATRISTS may periodically check the levels of this enzyme, especially in patients who are taking medications reported to increase this and other liver enzymes.

Al-Anon   A TWELVE-STEP PROGRAM for relatives of alcoholic persons operating in many communities under the philosophical and organizational structure of ALCOHOLICS ANONYMOUS (AA). A goal is to facilitate discussion and resolution of common problems.

Alateen   A TWELVE-STEP PROGRAM for teenaged children of alcoholic parents operating in some communities under the philosophical and organizational structure of ALCOHOLICS ANONYMOUS (AA). Alateen provides a setting in which the children may receive group support to achieve an understanding of their parents' problems and to learn better methods of coping.

alcohol amnestic disorder (Korsakoff's syndrome)   A disease associated with chronic alcohol DEPENDENCE (ALCOHOLISM) and resulting from a deficiency of vitamin B_1. Patients sustain damage to part of the THALAMUS and CEREBELLUM and have ANTEROGRADE and RETROGRADE AMNESIA, with an inability to retain new information. Other SYMPTOMS include inflammation of nerves, muttering DELIRIUM, INSOMNIA, ILLUSIONS, and HALLUCINATIONS. In alcohol amnestic disorder, unlike DEMENTIA, other intellectual functions may be preserved. See also SUBSTANCE-INDUCED PSYCHOTIC DISORDER; WERNICKE-KORSAKOFF SYNDROME.

alcohol dehydrogenase (ADH)   A primary ENZYME in the metabolism of alcohol, which oxidizes it to acetaldehyde. Eighty-five percent of the Japanese population and other Asian populations have an atypical ADH enzyme, which is about five times faster than normal. Consumption of alcohol by such persons leads to accumulation of acetaldehyde, which results in facial flushing, extensive vasodilation, and a racing heart (tachycardia).

alcohol dependence   DEPENDENCE on alcohol; also called ALCOHOLISM. See DEPENDENCE (on psychoactive substances).

Alcohol, Drug Abuse, and Mental Health Administration (ADAMHA)   An agency in the U.S. Department of HEALTH AND HUMAN SERVICES that was replaced in 1992 by the SUBSTANCE ABUSE AND MENTAL HEALTH SERVICES ADMINISTRATION (SAMHSA). In reorganizing ADAMHA into SAMHSA, the three ADAMHA research institutes—the NATIONAL INSTITUTE ON ALCOHOL ABUSE AND ALCOHOLISM (NIAAA), the NATIONAL INSTITUTE ON DRUG ABUSE (NIDA), and the NATIONAL INSTITUTE OF MENTAL HEALTH (NIMH)—were moved to the NATIONAL INSTITUTES OF HEALTH (NIH). The substance abuse and mental health services programs remain in SAMHSA.

alcohol hallucinosis   See SUBSTANCE-INDUCED PSYCHOTIC DISORDER.

Alcoholics Anonymous (AA)   A TWELVE-STEP PROGRAM for alcoholic persons who collectively assist other alcoholic persons through a structured fellowship of personal and group support. See also AL-ANON; ALATEEN.

alcohol psychosis   See SUBSTANCE-INDUCED PSYCHOTIC DISORDER.

alcohol-related disorders   In DSM-IV-TR, a group of MENTAL DISORDERS that includes alcohol DEPENDENCE, alcohol ABUSE, alcohol INTOXICATION, alcohol WITHDRAWAL, alcohol intoxication DELIRIUM, alcohol withdrawal DELIRIUM, alcohol-induced persisting DEMENTIA, alcohol-induced persisting AMNESTIC DISORDER, alcohol-induced PSYCHOTIC DISORDER, alcohol-induced MOOD DISORDER, alcohol-induced ANXIETY DISORDER, alcohol-induced SLEEP DISORDER, and alcohol-induced SEXUAL DYSFUNCTION. See INTOXICATION; ABUSE; DEPENDENCE; SUBSTANCE-INDUCED PSYCHOTIC DISORDER; and *alcohol* under WITHDRAWAL SYMPTOMS.

alcohol withdrawal syndrome   See *alcohol* under WITHDRAWAL SYMPTOMS.

alcoholism   A SYNDROME of chronic substance DEPENDENCE characterized by either TOLERANCE to alcohol or development of WITHDRAWAL SYMPTOMS on cessation of, or reduction in, alcohol intake. Other aspects of the syndrome are psychological dependence and impairment in social and/or vocational functioning. Vulnerability to alcoholism may have a GENETIC basis.

alexia   Loss of a previously possessed ability to grasp the meaning of written or printed words and sentences that cannot be explained by defective visual acuity. See also DYSLEXIA.

alexithymia   A disturbance in affective and COGNITIVE function that may occur in several disorders; it is common in PSYCHOSOMATIC disorders, addictive disorders, and POSTTRAUMATIC STRESS DISORDER (PTSD). The chief manifestations are difficulty in describing or recognizing on self-evaluation, and, in females, amenorrhea (failure to menstru-ate). Weight is typically 15% or more below normal, and it may de-crease to life-threatening extremes. In the *restricting* subtype, the person does not engage regularly in BINGE EATING. In the *binge-eating/ purging,* or *bulimic,* subtype, the person engages in recurrent epi-sodes of binge eating or purging during the episode of anorexia ner-vosa. See also BULIMIA NERVOSA.

anorgasmia   The inability to achieve ORGASM. See ORGASMIC DISORDERS.

anosmia   The partial or complete absence of the sense of smell, which is either congenital or the result of a TRAUMATIC BRAIN INJURY (TBI). If present following TBI, it predicts a poorer PROGNOSIS.

anosodiaphoria   A condition in which the patient appears uncon-cerned with or minimizes the significance of neurological and neuropsychological DEFICITS.

anosognosia   From the Greek "loss of knowledge," it usually occurs among people who have had a STROKE in the right hemisphere of the BRAIN, which has made them unable to use the left arm or leg (hemi-plegic). A small proportion of these hemiplegic patients cannot per-ceive that they are paralyzed.

ANS   See AUTONOMIC NERVOUS SYSTEM (ANS).

Antabuse   Brand name for DISULFIRAM.

antagonist   In pharmacology, a substance that opposes, blocks, or neutralizes a RECEPTOR-mediated biological response. For example, the MORPHINE antagonist NALOXONE competes with morphine for re-ceptor sites in the BRAIN and other tissues. By occupying these sites, naloxone prevents the NARCOTIC agent from binding to the receptors and exerting its effect. Contrast with AGONIST.

anterograde amnesia   See under AMNESIA.

antiandrogens   Drugs that reduce the production or block the action (RECEPTOR ANTAGONIST) of testosterone. In PSYCHIATRY, antiandrogens are used to control repetitive, deviant sexual behaviors such as PARAPHILIAS and paraphilia-related disorders. These drugs also are commonly used in the treatment of prostate cancer.

antianxiety medications   See ANXIOLYTICS and "Medications Used in Psychiatry."

anticholinergic effects or properties   Interference with the action of ACETYLCHOLINE in the BRAIN and peripheral nervous system by any drug. In PSYCHIATRY, the term generally refers to the SIDE EFFECTS of ANTIPSY-CHOTIC medications, TRICYCLIC ANTIDEPRESSANTS, and ANTIPARKINSONIAN

MEDICATIONS. Common SYMPTOMS of anticholinergic effects include dry mouth, blurred vision, constipation, and decreased ability to urinate.

anticholinergics   Medications that retard or block the activity of ACETYLCHOLINE within the CENTRAL NERVOUS SYSTEM (CNS) and the peripheral nervous system. Anticholinergics are classified as ANTIMUSCARINICS or ANTINICOTINICS, depending on the RECEPTORS affected. See "Medications Used in Psychiatry."

anticonvulsants   Drugs most commonly used for the treatment of SEIZURES. Anticonvulsants also may be effective in preventing or treating MANIA and DEPRESSION in patients with BIPOLAR DISORDER, hence their other name, MOOD STABILIZERS. They are used to treat REFRACTORY DEPRESSION as well. See "Medications Used in Psychiatry."

antidepressants   Medications used for the treatment of DEPRESSION. The mechanism of action of antidepressant medications appears to be due to various effects on pre- and postsynaptic RECEPTORS affecting the release and reuptake of BRAIN NEUROTRANSMITTERS such as DOPAMINE, NOREPINEPHRINE, and SEROTONIN. The main classes of antidepressant medications are TRICYCLIC ANTIDEPRESSANTS and TETRACYCLIC ANTIDEPRESSANTS, MONOAMINE OXIDASE INHIBITORS (MAOIs), and SELECTIVE SEROTONIN REUPTAKE INHIBITORS (SSRIs). Besides their use in the treatment of DEPRESSION, antidepressants are used to treat GENERALIZED ANXIETY DISORDER, PANIC DISORDER, OBSESSIVE-COMPULSIVE DISORDER, SOCIAL PHOBIA, POSTTRAUMATIC STRESS DISORDER (PTSD), PREMENSTRUAL DYSPHORIC DISORDER, ATTENTION-DEFICIT/HYPERACTIVITY DISORDER (ADHD), chronic pain, and other conditions. See "Medications Used in Psychiatry."

antihistamines   A class of medications that can attenuate or block the inflammatory response–triggering action of ENDOGENOUS HISTAMINE. Antihistamines are also useful as SEDATIVES or HYPNOTICS and may be used to reduce ANXIETY SYMPTOMS in patients with mild symptoms. See "Medications Used in Psychiatry."

antimanic medications   See MOOD STABILIZERS.

antimuscarinics   ANTICHOLINERGIC medications that selectively block MUSCARINIC RECEPTORS.

antinicotinics   ANTICHOLINERGIC medications that selectively block NICOTINIC RECEPTORS.

antioxidants   Compounds synthesized in the body or obtained from the diet, such as vitamins E and C, that are believed to decrease the production and effects of free radicals and, as a result, to improve COGNITIVE performance and slow the progression of ALZHEIMER'S DISEASE. *Free radicals* are extremely reactive and potentially toxic chem-

apolipoprotein E (*APOE*) gene   The gene that encodes apolipo-protein E (ApoE), a protein that plays an important role in the break-down of triglycerides, cholesterol, and other fats in the bloodstream. Of the gene's three alleles (called ε2, ε3, and ε4), the *APOE* ε4 variant represents the largest known risk factor for late-onset ALZHEIMER'S DIS-EASE in a variety of ethnic groups.

apomorphine   A DOPAMINE AGONIST medication (indicated for subcu-taneous use only) used as ADJUNCTIVE therapy in advanced PARKIN-SON'S DISEASE. Marketed under the brand name APOKYN.

apoplexy   See STROKE.

APP   See AMYLOID PRECURSOR PROTEIN (APP).

apperception   PERCEPTION as modified and enhanced by one's own EMOTIONS, MEMORIES, and biases.

apraxia   Loss of a previously possessed ability to carry out motor ac-tivities despite intact comprehension and motor function; may be seen in DEMENTIA. See also CONSTRUCTIONAL APRAXIA.

aprosodia   See AMELODIA.

arachnophobia   The FEAR of spiders.

ARC   See AIDS-RELATED COMPLEX.

Aricept   Brand name for the ACETYLCHOLINESTERASE INHIBITOR drug DONEPEZIL.

aripiprazole   An ATYPICAL ANTIPSYCHOTIC medication indicated for the treatment of SCHIZOPHRENIA, acute manic and mixed episodes of BIPOLAR DISORDER, irritability associated with AUTISTIC DISORDER, and AGITATION associated with schizophrenia or bipolar MANIA. Aripiprazole is also used as an ADJUNCTIVE treatment in MAJOR DEPRESSIVE DISORDER. Marketed under the brand name ABILIFY. See "Medications Used in Psychiatry."

arithmetic disorder   See MATHEMATICS DISORDER.

armodafinil   An atypical STIMULANT (the *R*-enantiomer [a stereo-isomer] of MODAFINIL) indicated for promoting wakefulness in pa-tients with excessive daytime sleepiness associated with OBSTRUCTIVE SLEEP APNEA; NARCOLEPSY; and CIRCADIAN RHYTHM SLEEP DISORDER, shift work type. Marketed under the brand name NUVIGIL. See "Medica-tions Used in Psychiatry."

arousal   A physiological and psychological state of being awake, alert, or reactive to stimuli. See also HYPERAROUSAL.

arousal disorders   A category of SLEEP DISORDERS (also known as PARA-SOMNIAS) that includes sleepwalking and sleep terrors. Most of the

SYMPTOMS are due to CENTRAL NERVOUS SYSTEM (CNS) activation, specifically motor and autonomic discharge. Arousal disorders have several features in common: mental confusion and DISORIENTATION, automatic behaviors, nonresponse to external stimuli, difficulty in being fully awakened, and AMNESIA the following morning. They usually occur in the first third of the sleep period, at the point of transition from Stage IV NREM SLEEP to REM SLEEP.

Artane   Brand name (now discontinued) for the ANTICHOLINERGIC drug TRIHEXYPHENIDYL.

arteriosclerosis   See CEREBRAL ARTERIOSCLEROSIS.

arteriosclerotic dementia   A form of DEMENTIA that is caused by thromboembolic cerebral vascular disease. It is usually associated with microinfarcts and vascular changes in areas of the BRAIN where no overt motor SIGNS, such as arm and leg weakness, are noted.

articulation disorder   See LOGICAL DISORDER.

artificial intelligence (AI)   A computer using ideas and methods of computation. Investigators use AI to understand and re-create the principles that make INTELLIGENCE possible.

asenapine   An ATYPICAL ANTIPSYCHOTIC medication approved for the treatment of SCHIZOPHRENIA and acute mania associated with BIPOLAR I DISORDER. Marketed under the brand name SAPHRIS (a sublingual tablet). See "Medications Used in Psychiatry."

Asendin   Brand name for the TETRACYCLIC ANTIDEPRESSANT drug AMOXAPINE.

Asperger's disorder   A PERVASIVE DEVELOPMENTAL DISORDER characterized by gross and sustained impairment in social interaction and restricted, repetitive, and stereotyped patterns of behavior, interests, and activities occurring in the context of preserved COGNITIVE and language development.

assault   See "Legal Terms."

assertive community treatment (ACT)   A team treatment approach designed to provide comprehensive, community-based psychiatric treatment, rehabilitation, and support to persons with serious and persistent mental illness (e.g., SCHIZOPHRENIA). Among the services ACT teams provide are case management, initial and ongoing assessments, psychiatric services, employment and housing assistance, family support and education, and substance abuse treatment services to allow individuals to live successfully in the community.

assertiveness training   A procedure in which individuals are taught appropriate interpersonal responses involving frank, honest, and direct expression of their feelings, both positive and negative.

assessment   The evaluation of a patient that leads to DIAGNOSIS and treatment.

assimilation   A term coined by the French developmental PSYCHOLOGIST Jean Piaget (1896–1980); it describes a person's ability to comprehend and integrate new experiences. The term is also used to describe the process that occurs when a minority person adopts the majority CULTURE.

association   Relationship between ideas and EMOTIONS by contiguity, continuity, or similarity. See also FREE ASSOCIATION; MENTAL STATUS.

astereognosis   From the Greek "without knowledge of solids," the inability to recognize objects by touching them even though the sense of touch is intact. This condition is caused by damage to the PARIETAL LOBE of the BRAIN. If the damage is in the right PARIETAL LOBE, a person with astereognosis cannot identify objects with his or her left hand, and vice versa. This condition is also known as *tactile* AGNOSIA, *stereognosis,* or *stereoanesthesia.*

asterixis   A TREMOR of the wrist when the wrist is extended (dorsiflexion), sometimes said to resemble a bird flapping its wings. Asterixis is seen most often in drowsy or stuporous patients with metabolic ENCEPHALOPATHIES, especially in decompensated cirrhosis or acute hepatic failure. It can also be a feature of WILSON'S DISEASE.

ataque de nervios   A CULTURE-SPECIFIC SYNDROME characterized by screaming uncontrollably, crying, trembling, and verbal or physical AGGRESSION. Dissociative experiences, seizure-like or fainting episodes, and suicidal gestures are also prominent in some *ataques.* It is principally reported among Latinos from the Caribbean but is also recognized among many Latin American and Latin Mediterranean groups.

Atarax   Brand name (now discontinued) for the ANTIHISTAMINE drug HYDROXYZINE.

ataraxia   A lucid state characterized by freedom from worry.

ataxia   Loss of muscle coordination; irregularity of muscle action.

athetosis   A muscular disorder characterized by irregular, twisting, slow movements of the toes and fingers. It results from a lesion in the extrapyramidal pathways (see EXTRAPYRAMIDAL SYSTEM). See also EXTRAPYRAMIDAL SYMPTOMS (EPS); EXTRAPYRAMIDAL SYNDROME.

Ativan   Brand name for the BENZODIAZEPINE ANXIOLYTIC drug LORAZEPAM.

atomoxetine   A nonstimulant selective NOREPINEPHRINE REUPTAKE INHIB-ITOR medication indicated for the treatment of ATTENTION-DEFICIT/HYPERACTIVITY DISORDER (ADHD). Marketed under the brand name STRATTERA. See "Medications Used in Psychiatry."

attachment   The behavior of an organism that relates in an affilia-tive or dependent manner to another object. This attachment devel-ops during critical periods of life and can be extinguished by lack of opportunity to relate. The quality of the attachment bond appears to have powerful implications for the quality of psychic structure and the subsequent relationships a person develops. If this separation occurs before maturation, it can provide for adaptive ADJUSTMENT, and PERSONALITY deviation can occur. See BONDING.

attachment disorder   See REACTIVE ATTACHMENT DISORDER.

attachment learning   The theory that the presence of someone to whom one is emotionally attached has a special effect on how one learns, especially in infancy.

attachment theory   A type of theory that is meant to describe and explain people's enduring patterns of relationships from birth to death. In attachment theory, ATTACHMENT is a bond between the child and the caregiver that guarantees safety and survival of the child. Variations of or failures in early attachment are thought to pre-dispose to, or be consistent with, later DEVELOPMENTAL DISORDERS or to particular modes of OBJECT RELATIONS.

attention   The ability to sustain focus on one activity. A disturbance in attention may appear as having difficulty in finishing tasks that have been started, being easily distracted, or having difficulty in concentrating.

attention-deficit/hyperactivity disorder (ADHD)   A person whose inattention and HYPERACTIVITY-impulsivity cause problems may have this disorder. SYMPTOMS appear before age 7 years and are inconsistent with the person's developmental level and severe enough to impair social or academic functioning.

predominantly inattentive type   Characteristic SYMPTOMS include DISTRACTIBILITY, difficulty in sustaining ATTENTION or following through on instructions in the absence of close supervision. Other symptoms include avoidance of tasks that require sustained men-tal effort, failure to pay close attention to details in schoolwork or other activities, difficulty in organizing activities, not listening to what is being said to him or her, loss of things that are necessary for assignments, and forgetfulness in daily activities.

predominantly hyperactive-impulsive type   Characteristic SYMP-TOMS include inappropriately leaving one's seat in the classroom or running about, fidgeting or squirming, difficulty engaging in leisure activities quietly, difficulty awaiting one's turn in games, and blurting out answers to questions before they are completed.

atypical   An adjective used to describe unusual or uncharacteristic variations of a disorder.

atypical antidepressants   A group of newer ANTIDEPRESSANT medications unrelated to SELECTIVE SEROTONIN REUPTAKE INHIBITORS (SSRIs), TRI-CYCLIC ANTIDEPRESSANTS, or MONOAMINE OXIDASE INHIBITORS (MAOIs). Examples of atypical antidepressants include SEROTONIN-NOREPINEPH-RINE REUPTAKE INHIBITORS (SNRIs; e.g., (DULOXETINE), NORADRENERGIC AND SPECIFIC SEROTONERGIC ANTIDEPRESSANTS (NaSSAs); e.g., MIRTAZAPINE), and SEROTONIN ANTAGONIST AND REUPTAKE INHIBITORS (SARIs; e.g., TRAZODONE). These agents are used to treat DEPRESSION, INSOMNIA, ANXIETY DISORDERS, chronic pain conditions, and other disorders. See "Medications Used in Psychiatry."

atypical antipsychotics   The newer generation of ANTIPSYCHOTIC medications (also called *second-generation antipsychotics [SGAs]*), known as SEROTONIN-DOPAMINE ANTAGONISTS (SDAs) because they have an effect on SEROTONIN RECEPTORS (in particular, 5-HT$_{2A}$ receptors) as well as DOPAMINE RECEPTORS (in particular, D$_2$ receptors). Currently available atypical antipsychotics include ARIPIPRAZOLE, ASENAPINE, CLO-ZAPINE, ILOPERIDONE, OLANZAPINE, PALIPERIDONE, QUETIAPINE, RISPERIDONE, and ZIPRASIDONE.

atypical depression   In DSM-IV-TR, depressive SYMPTOMS that do not meet the criteria for a specific DEPRESSIVE DISORDER. See also DEPRESSION.

atypical psychosis   In DSM-IV-TR, a psychotic disorder not otherwise specified; a residual category for psychotic SYMPTOMS that do not meet the criteria for a specific psychotic disorder. See also PSYCHOSIS.

audit (medical audit, patient care audit)   Periodic and systematic review of patterns of patient care to assess the quality of treatment.

auditory agnosia   The inability to recognize specific sounds in the context of intact hearing. There is a distinction in this SYNDROME between pure word deafness, which is considered an agnosia for auditory/verbal information, and auditory agnosia, which involves an agnosia for environmental, nonverbal sounds. *Cortical deafness* is also a term applied to patients who essentially do not respond to any auditory information even when hearing is intact. Also known as *acoustic agnosia*.

augmentation strategies   The addition of one or more medications to enhance or magnify the beneficial effects of a medication already being used, such as the addition of LITHIUM CARBONATE, LIOTHYRONINE, an ANTICONVULSANT, or a STIMULANT to augment ANTIDEPRESSANT response in a patient with REFRACTORY DEPRESSION. See also COACTIVE STRATEGY; COMBINATION TREATMENT.

aura   A premonitory, subjective brief sensation (e.g., a flash of light) that warns of an impending headache or convulsion. The nature of the sensation depends on the BRAIN area in which the attack begins. Seen in MIGRAINE and EPILEPSY.

authority figure   A person in a position of power (e.g., a parent or parent surrogate).

autism spectrum disorders   Another name for PERVASIVE DEVELOPMENTAL DISORDERS, which include AUTISTIC DISORDER, ASPERGER'S DISORDER, RETT'S DISORDER, and CHILDHOOD DISINTEGRATIVE DISORDER.

autistic disorder   A PERVASIVE DEVELOPMENTAL DISORDER consisting of gross and sustained impairment in social interaction and communication; restricted and stereotyped patterns of behavior, interest, and activities; and abnormal development prior to age 3 years manifested by delays or abnormal functioning in social development, language communication, or play. Specific SYMPTOMS may include impaired awareness of others, lack of social or emotional reciprocity, failure to develop peer relationships appropriate to developmental level, delay or absence of spoken language and abnormal nonverbal communication, stereotyped and repetitive language, idiosyncratic language, impaired imaginative play, insistence on sameness (e.g., nonfunctional routines or RITUALS), and stereotyped and repetitive motor mannerisms.

autistic fantasy   The substitution of excessive daydreaming for the pursuit of relationships with others, for solving problems, or for more direct and effective action.

autoerotic asphyxia   Asphyxia caused by intentionally strangling oneself while masturbating to intensify the ORGASM through reduced oxygen blood flow to the BRAIN. This practice carries a significant risk of death.

autoeroticism   Sensual self-gratification. Characteristic of, but not limited to, an early stage of emotional development. Includes satisfactions derived from genital play, masturbation, FANTASY, and oral, anal, and visual sources.

autogynephilia   One of the GENDER IDENTITY DISORDERS described by Ray Blanchard as a male propensity to "love oneself as a woman," or "a man's paraphilic tendency to be sexually aroused by the thought or image of himself as a woman."

automatism   Automatic and apparently undirected nonpurposeful behavior that is not consciously controlled. Seen in PSYCHOMOTOR EPILEPSY.

autonomic arousal disorder   A disorder characterized by persistent or recurrent SYMPTOMS other than pain that are mediated by the AUTONOMIC NERVOUS SYSTEM (ANS) and not a part of a GENERAL MEDICAL CONDITION. Symptoms may involve various systems or organs, including palpitations (cardiovascular), HYPERVENTILATION (respiratory), vomiting (gastrointestinal), urinary frequency (urogenital), or flushing (dermal). In earlier DSM classifications (DSM-I, DSM-II, and DSM-III), such symptoms were considered CONVERSION symptoms, PSYCHOSOMATIC symptoms, or PSYCHOPHYSIOLOGICAL DISORDERS.

autonomic dysfunction   Dysfunction of the AUTONOMIC NERVOUS SYSTEM (ANS); can be caused by various neurological disorders, such as PARKINSON'S DISEASE and multiple sclerosis.

autonomic nervous system (ANS)   The part of the nervous system that controls the cardiovascular, digestive, reproductive, and respiratory organs. It operates outside of consciousness and manages basic life-sustaining functions such as heart rate, digestion, and breathing. It includes the SYMPATHETIC NERVOUS SYSTEM and the PARASYMPATHETIC NERVOUS SYSTEM.

autonomous ego function   An aspect of the EGO that operates with little or no CONSCIOUS or UNCONSCIOUS CONFLICT.

autophobia   The FEAR of being alone or of solitude.

autoplastic   Referring to ADAPTATION by changing the self. A psychotherapeutic approach that has the goal of changing oneself to accommodate external circumstances. Contrast with ALLOPLASTIC.

autotopagnosia   Inability to localize and name the parts of one's own body.

Aventyl   Brand name for the TRICYCLIC ANTIDEPRESSANT drug NORTRIPTYLINE.

aversion therapy   A BEHAVIOR THERAPY procedure in which stimuli associated with undesirable behavior are paired with a painful or an unpleasant stimulus, resulting in the SUPPRESSION of the undesirable behavior.

avoidant disorder   SOCIAL PHOBIA occurring in childhood and adolescence.

avoidant personality disorder   See under PERSONALITY DISORDERS.

avolition   Lack of initiative or goals; one of the NEGATIVE SYMPTOMS of SCHIZOPHRENIA. The person may wish to do something, but the desire is without power or energy.

Axis I, II, III, IV, V   See MULTIAXIAL SYSTEM.

axon   The fiber-like extension of a NEURON through which the cell sends information to target cells.

azapirones   A class of psychoactive drugs derived from PIPERAZINE that are used as ANXIOLYTICS, ANTIDEPRESSANTS, and ANTIPSYCHOTICS. Medications in this class are also commonly used as augmentation to other antidepressants. An example is BUSPIRONE (BuSPAR). See "Medications Used in Psychiatry."

Azilect   Brand name for the ANTIPARKINSONIAN MEDICATION RASAGILINE.

B

baah-ji   A CULTURE-SPECIFIC SYNDROME. See *LATAH*.

bad object   One of the results of SPLITTING of the psychic representations of objects into their pleasurable, exciting, good, supportive, nurturing, and needs-meeting aspects (i.e., the good object) and their unpleasurable, frustrating, undesirable, painful, deprecatory, damaged, critical, hostile, incomplete, and disavowed aspects (i.e., the bad object). Splitting is a normal EGO mechanism during infantile development; in the adult, it is a manifestation of an inability to integrate positive and negative qualities of the object (or SELF) into a cohesive image.

bah-tschi   A CULTURE-SPECIFIC SYNDROME. See *LATAH*.

bah-tsi   A CULTURE-SPECIFIC SYNDROME. See *LATAH*.

Balint syndrome   Named after Rudolph Balint (1874–1929), a NEUROLOGIST and PSYCHIATRIST from Hungary, it is characterized by optic ATAXIA (the inability to move the hand to an object by using vision) and SIMULTANAGNOSIA (inability to comprehend more than one element of a visual scene at the same time or to integrate the parts into a whole). These visual difficulties are usually the result of damage to the superior part of the temporal-occipital lobes on both sides of the BRAIN.

barbiturates   An older class of medications, originally developed to treat SEIZURE disorders, ANXIETY, and INSOMNIA, that depress the activities of the CENTRAL NERVOUS SYSTEM (CNS). These medications are seldom used in clinical practice today because of their lethality in overdose and their high likelihood for ABUSE and DEPENDENCE.

basal forebrain   The basal forebrain is a group of structures that lie near the bottom of the front of the BRAIN. It includes the nucleus basalis, diagonal band, medial septum, and substantia innominata. It is considered to be the major CHOLINERGIC output of the CENTRAL NERVOUS SYSTEM (CNS). These structures are important in the production of ACETYLCHOLINE, which is then distributed widely throughout the brain. Basal forebrain damage can result in memory impairments such as AMNESIA and CONFABULATION.

basal ganglia   Clusters of NEURONS located deep in the BRAIN; they include the CAUDATE NUCLEUS and the PUTAMEN (CORPUS STRIATUM), the GLOBUS PALLIDUS, the subthalamic nucleus, and the SUBSTANTIA NIGRA. The basal ganglia appear to be involved in higher-order aspects of motor control, such as planning and execution of complex motor activity and the speed of movements.

Lesions of the basal ganglia produce various types of involuntary movements, such as ATHETOSIS, CHOREA, DYSTONIA, and TREMOR. The basal ganglia also are involved in the pathophysiology of PARKINSON'S DISEASE, HUNTINGTON'S DISEASE, and TARDIVE DYSKINESIA.

The internal capsule, containing all the fibers that ascend to or descend from the CEREBRAL CORTEX, runs through the basal ganglia and separates them from the THALAMUS.

basal nucleus of Meynert   A group of nerve cells in the substantia innominata of the BASAL FOREBRAIN that has wide projections to the NEOCORTEX and is rich in ACETYLCHOLINE and choline acetyltransferase. In PARKINSON'S DISEASE and ALZHEIMER'S DISEASE, the nucleus undergoes degeneration. A decrease in acetylcholine production is seen in ALZHEIMER'S DISEASE, LEWY BODY DEMENTIA, and some PARKINSON'S DISEASE patients showing abnormal BRAIN function, leading to a general decrease of mental capacity and learning. Most pharmacological treatments of DEMENTIA focus on compensating for a faltering basal nucleus function through artificially increasing ACETYLCHOLINE levels.

basic benefits   In insurance policies, the minimum set of benefits that must be made available to the insured.

basic trust   The infant's sense of security in his or her relationship with the mother (parents, caregiver) that makes it possible for the infant to begin to recognize the parent as other and separate from the self. It is the basis of REALITY TESTING, the ability to relate to others, and the feeling of self-worth and self-esteem.

bathophobia   The FEAR of depths.

battered child   See ABUSED CHILD.

battered woman syndrome   A collection of psychological SYMPTOMS, often considered a subcategory of POSTTRAUMATIC STRESS DISORDER (PTSD), which may occur in women who are exposed to repeated trauma, such as family violence.

battery   See "Legal Terms."

battle fatigue   A series of physical and mental SIGNS and SYMPTOMS experienced in combat and other dangerous, stressful missions. See also COMBAT FATIGUE.

BDD   See BODY DYSMORPHIC DISORDER (BDD).

BDNF   See BRAIN-DERIVED NEUROTROPHIC FACTOR (BDNF).

BEAM   See BRAIN ELECTRICAL ACTIVITY MAPPING (BEAM).

bebainan   A CULTURE-SPECIFIC DISSOCIATIVE DISORDER found in Bali, believed to be caused by sorcery. The most common symptoms are sudden feelings of confusion, crying, screaming and shouting, followed by inability of the sufferer to control his or her actions. Most sufferers are aware of their behavior during an attack, and remember the occurrence afterwards. *Bebainan* attacks provide sufferers with an opportunity to release feelings of frustration and anger without risk of widespread disapproval or stigmatization.

behavioral neurology   The branch of NEUROLOGY that concerns itself with functioning, such as language, MEMORY, and purposeful or motivated activity or AFFECT.

behavioral sciences   The study of human development, values, and interpersonal relationships. The behavioral sciences encompass fields such as PSYCHIATRY, PSYCHOLOGY, CULTURAL ANTHROPOLOGY, SOCIOLOGY, and political science.

behavior disorders of childhood   See ATTENTION-DEFICIT/HYPERACTIVITY DISORDER (ADHD); DISRUPTIVE BEHAVIOR DISORDERS.

behaviorism   An approach to PSYCHOLOGY first developed by John B. Watson (1878–1958) that rejected the notion of mental states and reduced all psychological phenomena to neural, muscular, and glandular responses. Contemporary behaviorism emphasizes the study of observable responses but is directed toward general behavior rather than discrete acts. It includes private events such as feelings and FANTASIES to the extent that these can be directly observed and measured.

behavior modification   A technique used in BEHAVIOR THERAPY that focuses on negative habits or behaviors and aims to reduce or eliminate them by the use of REINFORCEMENT (e.g., rewarding a desired behavior or punishing an unwanted one).

behavior therapy   A mode of treatment that focuses on substituting healthier ways of behaving for maladaptive patterns used in the past. Most likely to benefit are individuals who want to change habits, those with ANXIETY DISORDERS such as PHOBIAS or PANIC ATTACKS, and those with SUBSTANCE USE DISORDERS or EATING DISORDERS. The basic techniques include BEHAVIOR MODIFICATION, OPERANT CONDITIONING, SHAPING, TOKEN ECONOMY, SYSTEMATIC DESENSITIZATION, RELAXATION TRAINING, AVERSION THERAPY, EXPOSURE THERAPY, FLOODING, MODELING, social skills training, and PARADOXICAL INTENTION.

Behçet's disease   A multisystem disease that may involve all organs and affect the CENTRAL NERVOUS SYSTEM (CNS), causing MEMORY loss and impaired speech, balance, and movement. It is a rare, chronic, lifelong disorder that involves inflammation of blood vessels throughout the body. SYMPTOMS include recurrent oral ulcers and genital ulcers, eye inflammation, various types of skin lesions, arthritis, bowel inflammation, and meningitis. The effects of the disease may include blindness, STROKE, swelling of the SPINAL CORD, and intestinal complications.

Benadryl   Brand name for the ANTIHISTAMINE drug DIPHENHYDRAMINE.

benzodiazepine receptors   RECEPTORS located on NEURONS within the CENTRAL NERVOUS SYSTEM (CNS) to which BENZODIAZEPINES bind. Benzodiazepine receptors are linked to GABA (GAMMA-AMINOBUTYRIC ACID) RECEPTORS. Benzodiazepines enhance the affinity of GABA receptors for GABA, the principal inhibitory NEUROTRANSMITTER in the CNS, thereby increasing its inhibitory effects, which results in decreased ANXIETY and AROUSAL.

benzodiazepines   A class of medications with a similar chemical ring structure and similar therapeutic properties, including potent

HYPNOTIC, SEDATIVE, and ANXIOLYTIC effects. Benzodiazepines are also called ANXIOLYTICS or *antianxiety medications.* See "Medications Used in Psychiatry."

benztropine An ANTICHOLINERGIC medication used to treat muscle stiffness and other motor SIDE EFFECTS either from PARKINSON'S DISEASE or as a result of treatment with CONVENTIONAL ANTIPSYCHOTIC medications such as HALOPERIDOL (HALDOL). Marketed under the brand name COGENTIN. See "Medications Used in Psychiatry."

bereavement Feelings of deprivation, desolation, and GRIEF at the loss of a loved one. The grieving person does not need to seek professional help unless these feelings last for a long time or SYMPTOMS such as DEPRESSION or INSOMNIA become problematic.

bestiality ZOOPHILIA; sexual relations between a human being and an animal. See also PARAPHILIA.

best interests of the child See "Legal Terms."

best practice In PSYCHIATRY, a term used to describe the optimal clinical approach to the treatment of a particular MENTAL DISORDER. The practice is usually determined by expert consensus among a group of clinicians with special expertise in treating the disorder.

beta-adrenergic antagonists See BETA-BLOCKERS.

beta-amyloid Often abbreviated as *A-beta,* this is a protein that builds up in the BRAIN of persons with ALZHEIMER'S DISEASE, collecting in clumps called senile PLAQUES. Some researchers question whether beta-amyloid is the cause of the DEMENTIA, but most agree that it is involved in the disruption of thinking that is a hallmark of the disease.

beta-blockers A class of drugs that inhibits the action of beta-ADRENERGIC RECEPTORS, which modulate cardiac functions, respiratory functions, and the dilation and constriction of blood vessels. Beta-blockers are of value in the treatment of hypertension, cardiac arrhythmias, and MIGRAINE. In PSYCHIATRY, they have been used in the treatment of AGGRESSION and violence, ANXIETY-related TREMORS and LITHIUM-induced tremors, medication-induced AKATHISIA, SOCIAL PHOBIA, performance anxiety, PANIC states, and alcohol WITHDRAWAL. The medication PROPRANOLOL (INDERAL) is an example of a beta-blocker.

beyond a reasonable doubt See "Legal Terms."

bilis A CULTURE-SPECIFIC SYNDROME. See *MUINA.*

binge drinking A pattern of heavy alcoholic intake that occurs in bouts of a day or more that are set aside for drinking. During periods between bouts, the subject may abstain from alcohol.

binge eating   A period of overeating during which a larger amount of food is ingested than most people would eat during that time. The person feels that he or she cannot stop eating or has no control over what or how much is consumed. During the episode, the person may eat more rapidly than usual, eat until feeling uncomfortably full, eat large amounts of food although not feeling hungry, and eat alone because of embarrassment over how much is being eaten. After a bout of overeating, DEPRESSION, GUILT feelings, and feelings of disgust with oneself are common. When binge eating is accompanied by compensatory behavior such as purging or food restriction to control weight, it is termed BULIMIA NERVOSA.

binge-eating disorder   A proposed disorder (listed in DSM-IV-TR Appendix B, "Criteria Sets and Axes Provided for Further Study") characterized by recurrent episodes of BINGE EATING associated with subjective and behavioral indicators of impaired control over, and significant distress about, the binge eating and the absence of regular use of inappropriate compensatory behaviors (e.g., self-induced vomiting, misuse of laxatives, fasting, excessive exercise) that are characteristic of BULIMIA NERVOSA.

Binswanger's disease   A type of VASCULAR DEMENTIA, also known as *subcortical arteriosclerotic* ENCEPHALOPATHY. The damage is the result of the thickening and narrowing (atherosclerosis) of arteries that feed the subcortical areas of the brain. Patients have a history of hypertension, gait disturbance, urinary incontinence, and progressive COGNITIVE decline.

biochemistry   The chemistry of living organisms and of the changes occurring therein.

bioenergetic psychotherapy   See EXPERIENTIAL THERAPY.

biofeedback   The use of instrumentation to provide information (i.e., feedback) about variations in one or more of the subject's own physiological processes not ordinarily perceived (e.g., brain wave activity, muscle tension, blood pressure). Such feedback over a period of time can help the subject learn to control certain physiological processes even though he or she is unable to articulate how the learning was achieved.

biogenic amine hypothesis   The theory that abnormalities in the physiology and metabolism of BIOGENIC AMINES—particularly the CATECHOLAMINES DOPAMINE and NOREPINEPHRINE and the INDOLEAMINE SEROTONIN—are involved in the causes and courses of certain psychiatric illnesses. This hypothesis was derived originally from a serendipitous discovery that MONOAMINE OXIDASE INHIBITORS (MAOIs) and certain TRICYCLIC drugs had MOOD-elevating properties and that these agents exerted dramatic effects on BRAIN MONOAMINE functions. The finding that PHENOTHIAZINES and other CONVENTIONAL ANTIPSYCHOTICS inhibit DOPAMINE activity in the brain further supports this theory and suggests that a disorder of DOPAMINE metabolism may be implicated in the ETIOLOGY of PSYCHOSIS or MANIA. Also, disorders in norepinephrine and serotonin activity have been implicated in the etiology of DEPRESSION and MANIA.

biogenic amines   Organic substances of interest because of their possible role in BRAIN functioning; subdivided into CATECHOLAMINES (e.g., tyrosine, phenylalanine, DOPAMINE, EPINEPHRINE, NOREPINEPHRINE) and INDOLEAMINES (e.g., tryptophan, SEROTONIN).

The biosynthetic pathway for the CATECHOLAMINES is tyrosine → dihydroxyphenylalanine → DOPAMINE → NOREPINEPHRINE → EPINEPHRINE.

The biosynthetic pathway for the INDOLEAMINES is tryptophan → SEROTONIN (5-hydroxytryptamine) → 5-HIAA (5-HYDROXYINDOLEACETIC ACID).

biological psychiatry   A school of psychiatric thought that emphasizes physical, chemical, and neurological causes of psychiatric illness and treatment approaches.

biological rhythms   Cyclical variations in physiological and biochemical function, level of activity, and emotional state. *Circadian* rhythms have a cycle of about 24 hours, *ultradian* rhythms have a cycle that is shorter than 1 day, and *infradian* rhythms have a cycle that may last weeks or months.

biopsychosocial formulation   A creative synthesis of a clinical case, drawing on elements from the levels of biology, psychology, and sociology and expressed chronologically. It allows the clinician to get a comprehensive picture of the physical, mental, and environmental influences on a patient's health.

biperiden   An ANTICHOLINERGIC medication used as an ADJUVANT in the therapy of all forms of PARKINSONISM and to control medication-induced EXTRAPYRAMIDAL SYMPTOMS (EPS). Marketed under the brand name AKINETON. See "Medications Used in Psychiatry."

bipolar disorders   In DSM-IV-TR, a group of MOOD DISORDERS that includes bipolar disorder, single episode; bipolar disorder, recurrent; and CYCLOTHYMIC DISORDER.

In DSM-IV-TR, BIPOLAR I DISORDER includes a MANIC EPISODE at some time during its course. In any particular patient, the bipolar disorder may take the form of a single manic episode (rare), or it may consist of recurrent episodes that are either manic or depressive in nature (but at least one must have been predominantly manic).

In DSM-IV-TR, BIPOLAR II DISORDER denotes a mood disorder characterized by episodes of MAJOR DEPRESSIVE DISORDER and HYPOMANIA (rather than full MANIA). See HYPOMANIC EPISODE.

bipolar self In the SELF PSYCHOLOGY of Heinz Kohut (1913–1981), the final psychic structure that emerges following successful development and transformations of infantile constellations (equivalent to the mature human PSYCHE of ID, EGO, and SUPEREGO). The structure begins as the nuclear self made up of the GRANDIOSE SELF and the IDEALIZED PARENTAL IMAGO. In successful development, the grandiose self is transformed into self-assertive ambitions at one pole of the bipolar self. At the other pole are the internalized values and ideals that have grown out of the idealized parental imago. Between the two poles are the person's innate talents and skills.

birth trauma Term used by Otto Rank (1884–1939) to relate his theories of ANXIETY and NEUROSIS to what he believed to be the inevitable psychic shock of being born.

bisexuality Originally a concept of Sigmund Freud (1856–1939), indicating a belief that components of both sexes could be found in each person. Today, the term is often used to refer to persons who are capable of achieving ORGASM with a partner of either sex. See also GENDER ROLE; HOMOSEXUALITY.

blind spot Visual scotoma, a circumscribed area of blindness or impaired vision in the visual field; by extension, an area of the PERSONALITY of which the subject is unaware, typically because recognition of this area would cause painful EMOTIONS.

blocking A sudden obstruction or interruption in spontaneous flow of thinking or speaking, perceived as an absence or a deprivation of thought.

blood-brain barrier The protective barrier (boundary) surrounding the CENTRAL NERVOUS SYSTEM (CNS) (BRAIN and SPINAL CORD) that excludes many molecules and substances from freely diffusing or being transported into the brain tissues from the bloodstream.

blood levels The concentration of a drug in the plasma, serum, or blood. In PSYCHIATRY, the term is most often applied to levels of LITHIUM CARBONATE, TRICYCLIC ANTIDEPRESSANTS, and ANTICONVULSANTS. Maximum clinical responses to these agents have been correlated with specific ranges of blood levels. See also THERAPEUTIC WINDOW.

blood toxicology screening　A component of a substance ABUSE evaluation that seeks to determine whether detectable amounts of a substance or its metabolites are present in the blood.

blunted affect　See AFFECT.

board-certified psychiatrist　A PSYCHIATRIST who has passed examinations administered by the AMERICAN BOARD OF PSYCHIATRY AND NEUROLOGY (ABPN), and thus becomes certified as a medical specialist in PSYCHIATRY.

body dysmorphic disorder (BDD)　One of the SOMATOFORM DISORDERS, characterized by preoccupation with some imagined or slight defect in appearance that causes clinically significant distress or impairs social or occupational functioning.

body image　One's sense of the self and one's body; a multidimensional construct that encompasses PERCEPTIONS, thoughts, and feelings about the body.

body language　The expression of feelings or thoughts transmitted by one's motions, posture, or facial expressions that have meaning within the context in which they appear. See also KINESICS.

bondage　See SEXUAL MASOCHISM.

bonding　The unity of two people whose identities are significantly affected by their mutual interactions. Bonding often refers to the ATTACHMENT between a mother and her child.

borderline　See BORDERLINE PERSONALITY DISORDER under PERSONALITY DISORDERS.

borderline intellectual functioning　In DSM-IV-TR, an additional condition that may be a focus of clinical ATTENTION, especially when it coexists with a disorder such as SCHIZOPHRENIA. The INTELLIGENCE QUOTIENT (IQ) is in the 71–84 range.

borderline personality disorder　See under PERSONALITY DISORDERS.

borderline personality organization　As conceptualized by Otto Kernberg (1928–), a primitive CHARACTER structure represented by a fluid and labile sense of IDENTITY; desperate fear of isolation and aloneness, along with chaotic intimate relationships in which the other is both intensely needed and experienced as toxic and rejecting; and the use of archaic defenses of SPLITTING and PROJECTIVE IDENTIFICATION. Individuals with this personality organization often manifest eruptive anger in chaotic relationships, yet in nonintimate situations, they often function well.

boufée délirante　A CULTURE-SPECIFIC SYNDROME observed in West Africa and Haiti. This French term refers to a sudden outburst of agitated and aggressive behavior, marked confusion, and psychomotor excitement. It may sometimes be accompanied by visual and auditory HALLUCINATIONS or PARANOID IDEATION. These episodes may resemble an episode of BRIEF PSYCHOTIC DISORDER.

Brachmann de Lange syndrome   A relatively common birth defect syndrome with multiple malformations and INTELLECTUAL DISABILITY of unknown origin. Symptoms exhibited by affected individuals also include hyperactivity, SELF-INJURIOUS BEHAVIOR, aggression, sleep disturbance, and "autistic-like" behaviors (e.g., diminished social relatedness, repetitive and stereotyped behaviors).

bradykinesia   A neurological condition characterized by a generalized slowness of motor activity. It is seen especially in PARKINSON'S DISEASE and in LEWY BODY DEMENTIA.

bradyphrenia   The slowing of thought processes. Bradyphrenia can occur in PARKINSON'S DISEASE and is one of the extrapyramidal side effects of ANTIPSYCHOTIC medications (see EXTRAPYRAMIDAL SYMPTOMS [EPS]).

brain   The part of the nervous system contained in the skull; it includes the CEREBRUM, MIDBRAIN, CEREBELLUM, PONS, and MEDULLA OBLONGATA.

brain-derived neurotrophic factor (BDNF)   A protein that in humans is encoded by the *BDNF* gene. In the BRAIN, BNDF is active in the HIPPOCAMPUS, CEREBRAL CORTEX, and BASAL FOREBRAIN—areas vital to learning, memory, and higher thinking. Various studies have shown possible links between BDNF and conditions such as DEPRESSION, SCHIZOPHRENIA, OBSESSIVE-COMPULSIVE DISORDER, ALZHEIMER'S DISEASE, HUNTINGTON'S DISEASE, RETT'S DISORDER, and DEMENTIA, as well as ANOREXIA NERVOSA and BULIMIA NERVOSA.

brain electrical activity mapping (BEAM)   Computer-enhanced analysis and display of electroencephalographic and evoked response studies. In evoked response studies, a stimulus (e.g., flashing light) is presented to the individual, and the responses are recorded electrically from scalp electrodes. Computers translate the information into a topographic, colored display of electrical activity over the surface of the BRAIN. It is useful in diagnosing SEIZURE disorders and may be helpful in assessing certain psychiatric disorders. See also BRAIN IMAGING.

brain fag   A CULTURE-SPECIFIC SYNDROME observed initially in West Africa. It refers to a condition experienced by high school or university students in response to the challenges of schooling. Symptoms include difficulties in concentrating, remembering, and thinking. "Brain tiredness" or fatigue from "too much thinking" are idioms of distress in many cultures, and resulting syndromes resemble certain anxiety, depressive, and somatoform disorders.

brain imaging   Any technique that permits the in vivo visualization of the substance of the CENTRAL NERVOUS SYSTEM (CNS). The best known of such techniques is COMPUTED TOMOGRAPHY (CT). Newer methods of BRAIN imaging such as POSITRON EMISSION TOMOGRAPHY (PET), SINGLE PHOTON EMISSION COMPUTED TOMOGRAPHY (SPECT), and MAGNETIC RESONANCE IMAGING (MRI) are based on different physical principles but also yield a series of two-dimensional images (or "slices") of brain regions of interest.

Several other related techniques, such as ultrasound, angiography in its various forms, REGIONAL CEREBRAL BLOOD FLOW (rCBF) measurements, BRAIN ELECTRICAL ACTIVITY MAPPING (BEAM) and its variants, and even the older pneumoencephalogram (PEG), also provide images of some aspect of the CNS. However, these techniques are generally more invasive or limited in the structures visualized, the degree of resolution, or some other parameter, than CT, PET, SPECT, and MRI.

brain metabolism   The process by which the BRAIN synthesizes, degrades, and alters chemical substrates for repair and function.

brain stem   This part of the BRAIN includes the PONS and the MEDULLA OBLONGATA. The brain stem is the major route by which the FOREBRAIN sends information to and receives information from the SPINAL CORD and peripheral nerves. The brain stem controls, among other things, respiration and heart rhythm.

brain waves   See ELECTROENCEPHALOGRAM (EEG).

breach of contract   See "Legal Terms."

breathing-related sleep disorder   A DYSSOMNIA characterized by SLEEP disruption due to abnormal respiratory events during sleep, resulting in excessive daytime sleepiness or INSOMNIA. Types of abnormal breathing include *apneas* (episodes of breathing cessation), *hypopneas* (abnormally slow or shallow respiration), and *hypoventilation* (abnormal blood oxygen and carbon dioxide levels). Three forms of breathing-related sleep disorder have been described: OBSTRUCTIVE SLEEP APNEA, CENTRAL SLEEP APNEA, and CENTRAL ALVEOLAR HYPOVENTILATION SYNDROME.

brief   See "Legal Terms."

brief psychiatric hospitalization   In today's MANAGED CARE era, brief psychiatric hospitalization has become more prevalent. Although usually 5–10 days in duration, anything less than 1 month is considered brief. The goals are to stabilize the patient, identify precipitating factors, adjust for relevant environmental factors, and offer emotional support as well as to discharge the patient to a less restrictive setting as soon as possible.

brief psychotherapy   Any form of PSYCHOTHERAPY whose end point is defined either in terms of the number of sessions (generally no more than 15 or 20) or in terms of specified objectives. It is usually goal-oriented, circumscribed, active, focused, and directed toward a specific problem or SYMPTOM.

brief psychotic disorder   A transient psychotic disorder with duration limited from a few hours to 1 month and an eventual return to full functioning. SYMPTOMS during the episode indicate impaired REALITY TESTING that is not culturally sanctioned, DELUSIONS, HALLUCINATIONS, disorganized speech, or disorganized or CATATONIC BEHAVIOR.

Briquet's syndrome   See SOMATIZATION DISORDER.

Broca's aphasia   Loss of the ability to comprehend language coupled with the inability to produce words. See also APHASIA.

Broca's area   The area of the brain responsible for speech production, language processing, and language comprehension. Located in the left frontal operculum, Broca's area is named after Pierre Paul Broca, who in 1861 identified lesions in this region at autopsy in patients who had lost the ability to speak.

Brodmann areas   Regions of the CEREBRAL CORTEX defined on the basis of cytoarchitecture, or the organization of the cortex as observed when tissue is stained for nerve cells. Brodmann areas were originally defined and numbered by Korbinian Brodmann (1868–1918) and were referred to by numbers from 1 to 52. Brodmann published his maps of cortical areas in humans, monkeys, and other species in 1909. Many of the areas Brodmann defined based solely on their neuronal organization have since been correlated closely to diverse cortical functions, such as the *primary somatosensory cortex,* the *primary motor cortex,* the *primary visual cortex,* and the *primary auditory cortex.*

bromocriptine   A mixed DOPAMINE AGONIST-ANTAGONIST medication used to treat PARKINSON'S DISEASE and HYPERPROLACTINEMIA. Bromocriptine may also have utility in the treatment of NEUROLEPTIC MALIGNANT SYNDROME, COCAINE WITHDRAWAL, and DEPRESSION. Marketed under the brand names CYCLOSET and PARLODEL.

brujeria   A CULTURE-SPECIFIC SYNDROME. See ROOTWORK.

bruxism   Grinding of the teeth that occurs unconsciously while awake or during Stage 2 SLEEP. It may be SECONDARY to ANXIETY, tension, or dental problems.

bulimia nervosa   An EATING DISORDER characterized by recurrent episodes of BINGE EATING followed by compensatory behavior such as purging (i.e., self-induced vomiting or the use of diuretics and laxatives) or other methods of weight control (e.g., strict dieting, fasting, or vigorous exercise).

Buprenex   Brand name for the OPIOID AGONIST-ANTAGONIST ANALGESIC drug BUPRENORPHINE.

buprenorphine   An OPIOID AGONIST-ANTAGONIST ANALGESIC medication approved for the treatment of OPIATE ABUSE. In the United States, a special federal waiver (granted to physicians who meet specified training requirements) is required to prescribe buprenorphine in the outpatient setting for the treatment of opioid ADDICTION. Marketed under the brand name BUPRENEX. See "Medications Used in Psychiatry."

bupropion   An ATYPICAL ANTIDEPRESSANT of the aminoketone class that is believed to increase NOREPINEPHRINE and possibly DOPAMINE neurotransmission in the BRAIN. Bupropion is approved for the treatment of DEPRESSION (as brand name WELLBUTRIN) and nicotine ADDICTION (as brand name ZYBAN) and is also used off-label to treat ATTENTION-DEFICIT/HYPERACTIVITY DISORDER (ADHD). See "Medications Used in Psychiatry."

burden of proof   See "Legal Terms."

burnout   A STRESS REACTION that develops in persons working in an area of unrelenting occupational demands. SYMPTOMS include impaired work performance, fatigue, INSOMNIA, DEPRESSION, increased susceptibility to physical illness, and reliance on alcohol or other drugs of ABUSE for temporary relief.

BuSpar   Brand name for the nonbenzodiazepine ANXIOLYTIC drug BUSPIRONE.

buspirone   A nonbenzodiazepine ANXIOLYTIC medication of the AZAPIRONE class. Buspirone is believed to exert its anxiolytic effects through partial agonism of 5-HT$_{1A}$ SEROTONIN RECEPTORS in the brain. Marketed under the brand name BUSPAR. See "Medications Used in Psychiatry."

butorphanol tartrate   An OPIOID AGONIST-ANTAGONIST ANALGESIC medication used to treat MIGRAINE headaches and pain REFRACTORY to other standard treatments. Butorphanol may be habit forming. Marketed under the brand name STADOL NS; generic formulations are also available.

butyrophenones   A subgroup of CONVENTIONAL ANTIPSYCHOTIC drugs with a similar chemical structure (a piperidine ring with a three-carbon chain to which is attached a carbonyl-fluorobenzene ring). HALOPERIDOL (HALDOL) is the best-known member of this class and perhaps the most widely used CONVENTIONAL ANTIPSYCHOTIC medication.

C

Caenorhabditis elegans   Free-living, transparent nematode, about 1 mm in length, which lives in temperate soil environments. Research into the molecular and developmental biology of *C. elegans* was begun in 1974 by Sydney Brenner, and *C. elegans* has since been used extensively as a model organism. *C. elegans* is one of the simplest organisms with a nervous system. The organism has also been used as a model for nicotine dependence, as it has been found to experience the same symptoms humans experience when they quit smoking.

caffeine-induced disorders   In DSM-IV-TR, a group of MENTAL DISORDERS that includes caffeine INTOXICATION, caffeine-induced ANXIETY DISORDER, and caffeine-induced SLEEP DISORDER.

calcium channel blockers   A class of drugs (also known as *calcium antagonists*) that disrupt the flow of calcium (Ca^{2+}) through calcium channels. These drugs are of value in the treatment of hypertension and other cardiovascular disorders. In PSYCHIATRY, they have been found effective in the treatment of BIPOLAR DISORDER that has been REFRACTORY to LITHIUM CARBONATE or ANTICONVULSANT pharmacotherapy.

Campral   Brand name for the alcoholism treatment drug ACAMPROSATE.

candidate gene   A gene, located in a specific chromosome region, thought likely to cause a disease. Once a candidate gene can be linked to a specific disease, researchers can explore variations in the gene.

candidate gene studies   A research approach that focuses on testing the effects of genetic variants of a potentially contributing gene in an association study. Candidate gene studies have been conducted for MOOD DISORDERS, ALCOHOLISM, and other psychiatric illnesses.

cannabinoid receptors *Cannabinoids* are organic compounds that are present in *Cannabis sativa*. Two subtypes of cannabinoid RECEPTORS—CB_1 and CB_2—have been cloned from animal or human sources. The CB_1 receptor is expressed mainly in the BRAIN. Several studies have concluded that certain cannabinoids might have the ability to prevent ALZHEIMER'S DISEASE.

cannabis-related disorders In DSM-IV-TR, a group of MENTAL DISORDERS that includes cannabis DEPENDENCE, cannabis ABUSE, cannabis INTOXICATION, cannabis intoxication DELIRIUM, cannabis-induced PSYCHOTIC DISORDER with DELUSIONS or HALLUCINATIONS, and cannabis-induced ANXIETY DISORDER.

Cannabis sativa An India hemp plant from which MARIJUANA is derived. The main psychoactive component of cannabis is delta-9-tetrahydrocannabinol (THC). Marijuana may contain 0.1%–10% THC.

capacity See "Legal Terms."

Capgras' syndrome The DELUSION that impostors have replaced others or the self. The SYNDROME typically follows the development of negative feelings toward the other person that the subject cannot accept and attributes, instead, to the impostor.

capitation A uniform payment based on the number of people in the population being served. The health or MENTAL HEALTH care provider, or group of providers, accepts responsibility to deliver the health or mental health services needed by all members of a specified group, and an agreed-on payment is made at regular intervals to the provider. The payment is made even if no services have been given, but the payment is no greater than the agreed-on amount even if more extensive services have been provided.

carbamazepine An ANTICONVULSANT and ANALGESIC medication used in PSYCHIATRY as a MOOD STABILIZER to treat BIPOLAR DISORDERS. Marketed under the brand name TEGRETOL; may also be known by the discontinued brand name EQUETRO. See "Medications Used in Psychiatry."

carbidopa An agent used (usually in combination with LEVODOPA) to treat IDIOPATHIC PARKINSON'S DISEASE. Carbidopa blocks the peripheral conversion of levodopa to DOPAMINE, allowing greater amounts of levodopa to penetrate the brain. Because carbidopa does not itself cross the BLOOD-BRAIN BARRIER to any significant extent, it does not inhibit the conversion of levodopa to dopamine within the brain. Marketed under the brand name LODOSYN.

carbidopa-levodopa   A combined medication (of which LEVODOPA is the agent that primarily targets the brain) used to treat IDIOPATHIC PARKINSON'S DISEASE. The combination allows greater amounts of levodopa to reach the brain, where it is converted to DOPAMINE, resulting in increased dopamine levels, specifically in the DOPAMINERGIC neurons of the nigrostriatal pathway. Marketed under the brand name SINEMET.

caregiver   Any person involved in the treatment or REHABILITATION of a patient; includes the PSYCHIATRIST and other members of the traditional treatment team as well as community workers and other non-professionals.

case law   See "Legal Terms."

case management   In general, the process of following up a patient through various types of treatment and helping with care. It also refers to a type of health care delivery with emphasis on the development of alternative treatment plans for patients who have been identified (by preadmission certification, DIAGNOSIS, etc.) as potentially high-cost cases. Once such a case has been identified, the case manager confers with the patient's physician to develop a less expensive treatment plan and AFTERCARE.

castration   Removal of the sex organs. In psychological terms, the fantasized loss of the genitals. Also used metaphorically to denote a state of IMPOTENCE, powerlessness, HELPLESSNESS, or defeat.

castration anxiety   ANXIETY due to fantasized danger or injuries to the genitals and/or body. This fear is most intense in children ages 4–6 years but continues unconsciously through life and may be precipitated by everyday events that have symbolic significance and appear to be threatening, such as loss of a job, or an experience of ridicule or HUMILIATION.

CAT   Computerized axial tomography. See COMPUTED TOMOGRAPHY (CT).

catalepsy   A generalized condition of diminished responsiveness shown by trancelike states, posturing, or maintenance of physical attitudes for a prolonged period. May occur in either ORGANIC DISEASES or psychological disorders, as well as under HYPNOSIS. See also CATATONIC BEHAVIOR.

cataplexy   Sudden loss of postural tone without loss of consciousness, typically triggered by some emotional stimulus such as laughter, anger, or EXCITEMENT. It is a characteristic of NARCOLEPSY.

Catapres Brand name for the alpha$_2$-ADRENERGIC RECEPTOR AGONIST drug CLONIDINE.

catatonia Immobility with muscular RIGIDITY or inflexibility and, at times, excitability. See also SCHIZOPHRENIA.

catatonic behavior Marked motor abnormalities, generally limited to those occurring as part of a psychotic disorder. This term includes catatonic EXCITEMENT (apparently purposeless AGITATION not influenced by external stimuli), STUPOR (decreased reactivity and fewer spontaneous movements, often with apparent unawareness of the surroundings), NEGATIVISM (apparent motiveless resistance to instructions or attempts to be moved), posturing (the person's assuming and maintaining an inappropriate or a bizarre stance), RIGIDITY (the person's maintaining a stance or posture against all efforts to be moved), and WAXY FLEXIBILITY or *CEREA FLEXIBILITAS* (the person's limbs can be put into positions that are maintained).

catatonic disorder due to a general medical condition SECONDARY or symptomatic CATATONIA caused by a medical disorder or medication. Catatonic SYMPTOMS such as motoric immobility (e.g., CATALEPSY, *CEREA FLEXIBILITAS*), extreme AGITATION, extreme NEGATIVISM (e.g., RIGIDITY of posture), and peculiarities of voluntary movement (e.g., inappropriate or bizarre posturing, stereotyped movements, prominent mannerisms) occur because of a GENERAL MEDICAL CONDITION. This DIAGNOSIS emphasizes that catatonic symptoms are not confined to schizophrenic disorders. See also SECONDARY DISORDER.

catchment area A geographic area for which a MENTAL HEALTH program or facility has responsibility for its residents.

catecholamines A group of BIOGENIC AMINES derived from the amino acid tyrosine that includes the NEUROTRANSMITTERS DOPAMINE, EPINEPHRINE, and NOREPINEPHRINE, which exert an important influence on peripheral nervous system and CENTRAL NERVOUS SYSTEM (CNS) activity. See also BIOGENIC AMINE HYPOTHESIS.

catechol-O-methyltransferase (COMT) An enzyme that degrades and inactivates CATECHOLAMINES such as DOPAMINE, EPINEPHRINE, and NOREPINEPHRINE. COMT is also important in the metabolism of LEVODOPA (L-DOPA), a precursor of dopamine used in the treatment of PARKINSON's DISEASE. COMT inhibitors such as ENTACAPONE (COMTAN) inhibit degradation of levodopa, permitting greater and more sustained levels of levodopa to penetrate the brain, where it can be converted to DOPAMINE. Whether variations in COMT contribute to susceptibility to SCHIZOPHRENIA is currently a matter of considerable controversy.

categorical attitude   See ABSTRACT ATTITUDE.

catharsis   The healthful (therapeutic) release of ideas through "talking out" CONSCIOUS material accompanied by an appropriate emotional reaction. Also, the release into awareness of repressed ("forgotten") material from the UNCONSCIOUS. See also REPRESSION.

cathexis   ATTACHMENT, CONSCIOUS or UNCONSCIOUS, of emotional feeling and significance to an idea, an object, or, most commonly, a person. In TRANSFERENCE, patients withdraw their cathexis (or investment) from past figures and reinvest it in the clinician as a new figure.

CATIE   (Clinical   Antipsychotic   Trials   of   Intervention Effectiveness)   A nationwide public health–focused clinical trial that compared the effectiveness of "first generation" (introduced in the 1950s) and "second generation" (available since the 1990s) ANTIPSYCHOTIC medications. Phase I of CATIE analyzed the economic implications of ANTIPSYCHOTIC treatment and concluded that the older CONVENTIONAL ANTIPSYCHOTIC PERPHENAZINE was less expensive and no less effective than the newer ATYPICAL ANTIPSYCHOTICS OLANZAPINE, QUETIAPINE, RISPERIDONE, and ZIPRASIDONE during initial treatment, suggesting that older antipsychotics still have a role in treating SCHIZOPHRENIA. The study was funded by the NATIONAL INSTITUTE OF MENTAL HEALTH (NIMH).

caudate nucleus   An elongated, curved mass located within the BASAL GANGLIA, the caudate nucleus is an important component of the brain's learning and memory system, particularly during feedback processing. There is a caudate nucleus within each hemisphere of the BRAIN.

causalgia   A sensation of intense pain of either ORGANIC or psychological origin. See SOMATOFORM DISORDERS.

cause in fact   See "Legal Terms."

cause of action   See "Legal Terms."

CBGD   See CORTICOBASAL GANGLIONIC DEGENERATION (CBGD).

CBT   See COGNITIVE-BEHAVIORAL (PSYCHO)THERAPY (CBT).

CDC   See CENTERS FOR DISEASE CONTROL AND PREVENTION (CDC).

C. elegans   See *CAENORHABDITIS ELEGANS*.

Celexa   Brand name for the SELECTIVE SEROTONIN REUPTAKE INHIBITOR (SSRI) ANTIDEPRESSANT drug CITALOPRAM.

Centers for Disease Control and Prevention (CDC) A U.S. federal agency under the U.S. DEPARTMENT OF HEALTH AND HUMAN SERVICES (DHHS) and based in Atlanta, Georgia, the CDC works to protect public health and safety by providing information to enhance health decisions. It focuses national attention on developing and applying disease prevention and control (especially infectious diseases), environmental health, occupational safety and health, health promotion, prevention, and education activities designed to improve the health of the people of the United States.

Centers for Medicare and Medicaid Services (CMS) Formerly called the Health Care Financing Administration (HCFA); a federal agency within the U.S. DEPARTMENT OF HEALTH AND HUMAN SERVICES (DHHS) that administers MEDICARE, MEDICAID, the State Children's Health Insurance Program (SCHIP), and the Clinical Laboratory Improvement Amendments (CLIA).

central alveolar hypoventilation syndrome A BREATHING-RELATED SLEEP DISORDER characterized by an impairment in ventilatory control that results in abnormally low arterial oxygen levels, leading to frequent arousals from sleep. See also CENTRAL SLEEP APNEA; OBSTRUCTIVE SLEEP APNEA.

central nervous system (CNS) The BRAIN and the SPINAL CORD.

central sleep apnea A BREATHING-RELATED SLEEP DISORDER that occurs when the BRAIN does not send the signal to the muscles to take a breath, resulting in no muscular effort to take a breath. See also CENTRAL ALVEOLAR HYPOVENTILATION SYNDROME, OBSTRUCTIVE SLEEP APNEA.

cephalalgia Headache or head pain.

cerea flexibilitas The "WAXY FLEXIBILITY" often present in catatonic SCHIZOPHRENIA in which the patient's arm or leg remains in the position in which it is placed.

cerebellum A large part of the BRAIN situated anterior to and above the MEDULLA OBLONGATA concerned with the coordination of muscles and the maintenance of bodily equilibrium.

cerebral amyloid angiopathy A neurological condition in which AMYLOID protein builds up on the walls of the arteries in the brain and increases the risk of hemorrhagic STROKE. Because cerebral amyloid angiopathy can be caused by the same amyloid protein (AMYLOID PRECURSOR PROTEIN [APP]) that is associated with ALZHEIMER'S DISEASE, such brain hemorrhages are more common in people with ALZHEIMER'S DISEASE; however, they can also occur in people with no history of DEMENTIA.

cerebral angiography   A test most frequently used to confirm cases of STROKE, tumor, aneurysm (bulging of the artery walls), a clot, and a narrowing of the arteries and to evaluate the arteries of the head and neck before corrective surgery. It is used to obtain more exact information after an abnormality has been detected by a MAGNETIC RESONANCE IMAGING (MRI) or COMPUTED TOMOGRAPHY (CT) scan of the head, such as bleeding within the BRAIN. Under a local anesthetic, a needle is inserted into an artery, usually in the groin area. A catheter is inserted through the needle and then threaded through the main vessels of the abdomen and chest until it is properly placed in the arteries of the neck. The contrast medium is then injected into the neck area through the catheter, and X-ray pictures are taken.

cerebral arteriosclerosis   See VASCULAR DEMENTIA.

cerebral cortex   The external layer of GRAY MATTER that covers the human BRAIN hemispheres. This gray surface has a thickness varying from 1 to 4 mm. Its largest part is composed of NEURONS, which receive and transmit electrical IMPULSES from and to other brain regions and bony parts. The cerebral cortex is the part of the brain in which thought processes take place. In ALZHEIMER'S DISEASE, nerve cells in the cerebral cortex die.

cerebrospinal fluid (CSF)   Clear fluid occupying the space around and inside the BRAIN and SPINAL CORD.

cerebrovascular accident (CVA)   See STROKE.

cerebrovascular disease   See STROKE.

cerebrum   The expanded anterior portion of the BRAIN, which is considered the seat of CONSCIOUS mental processes.

chandelier cells   Specialized NEURONS found in all regions of the hippocampal formation, these cells form symmetrical SYNAPSES and have been shown to function as GABAergic (GABA (GAMMA-AMINOBUTYRIC ACID)–producing) inhibitory neurons, possibly preventing excessive excitatory activity in neuronal networks. In SCHIZOPHRENIA, scientists have observed changes in chandelier cell form and functionality, which may reflect altered information processing within the prefrontal cortex and its output connections to other brain regions. Nonspecific loss and/or reorganization of chandelier cells may also be involved in the development of EPILEPSY.

Chantix   Brand name for the smoking cessation drug VARENICLINE.

character   The sum of a person's relatively fixed PERSONALITY traits and habitual modes of response. Character develops over time, is related to infantile solutions to particular CONFLICTS, and is slow to change, even with psychoanalytic interventions.

character analysis Psychoanalytic treatment (see PSYCHOANALYSIS) aimed at the CHARACTER DEFENSES.

character defense Any PERSONALITY trait that serves an UNCONSCIOUS defensive purpose. See DEFENSE MECHANISM.

character disorder (character neurosis) An older term referring to PERSONALITY DISORDER manifested by a chronic, habitual, maladaptive pattern of reaction that is relatively inflexible, limits the optimal use of a person's potential, and often provokes responses from the environment that the person wants to avoid. In contrast to SYMPTOMS of NEUROSIS, symptoms of a character disorder are typically EGO-SYNTONIC. See also PERSONALITY.

Charles Bonnet syndrome Named after the eighteenth-century Swiss naturalist Charles Bonnet (1720–1793), the term is used to describe a situation in which people with sight problems start to see things that they know are not real (visual HALLUCINATIONS). People often do not report their visual hallucinations for FEAR that others will think that they are losing their minds.

chemical dependence A generic term for DEPENDENCE on (ADDICTION to) alcohol or other drugs. See DEPENDENCE (on psychoactive substances).

chibih A CULTURE-SPECIFIC SYNDROME. See *SUSTO*.

child abuse See ABUSED CHILD.

child analysis Application of modified psychoanalytic methods (see PSYCHOANALYSIS) and goals to problems of children to remove impediments to normal PERSONALITY development.

child and adolescent psychiatry The subspecialty of PSYCHIATRY that is involved in the DIAGNOSIS, PREVENTION, and treatment of MENTAL DISORDERS in persons younger than 18 years.

childhood disintegrative disorder A DEVELOPMENTAL DISORDER of childhood characterized by normal development for at least the first 2 years of life followed by loss of previously acquired skills in two or more of the following: EXPRESSIVE or RECEPTIVE language, social skills or adaptive behavior, bowel or bladder control, play, and motor skills. In addition, there is gross impairment in social interaction and communication, and restricted patterns of behavior, interest, and activities, all similar to manifestations described in AUTISTIC DISORDER.

childhood schizophrenia See SCHIZOPHRENIA.

chlordiazepoxide A long-acting BENZODIAZEPINE ANXIOLYTIC medication used commonly to treat alcohol WITHDRAWAL and used less frequently in PSYCHIATRY to treat ANXIETY DISORDERS. Marketed under the brand name LIBRIUM. See "Medications Used in Psychiatry."

chlorpromazine An older CONVENTIONAL ANTIPSYCHOTIC medication (a PHENOTHIAZINE of the aliphatic class) used in the treatment of SCHIZOPHRENIA AND OTHER PSYCHOTIC DISORDERS. Chlorpromazine is infrequently prescribed today. Although available only as generic, it may still be known by the discontinued brand name THORAZINE. See "Medications Used in Psychiatry."

cholinergic Referring to activation or transmission by the NEUROTRANSMITTER ACETYLCHOLINE. Contrast with ADRENERGIC.

cholinergic hypothesis The theory that the basic defect in ALZHEIMER'S DISEASE is an inadequacy of ACETYLCHOLINE for neurotransmission.

cholinergic receptors RECEPTORS in the BRAIN and AUTONOMIC NERVOUS SYSTEM (ANS) to which ACETYLCHOLINE binds. Acetylcholine plays an important role in COGNITION and MEMORY as well as in a host of other physical functions (e.g., heart, lung, gastrointestinal tract). Cholinergic receptors are classified as either *nicotinic* or *muscarinic,* depending on their differential sensitivities to the extrinsic molecules nicotine and muscarine. See also ANTICHOLINERGICS; ANTIMUSCARINICS; ANTINICOTINICS.

cholinesterase inhibitors See ACETYLCHOLINESTERASE INHIBITORS.

chorea Involuntary motor movement, usually of the arms and upper torso (and sometimes trunk and legs), that may be caused by rheumatic fever (SYDENHAM'S CHOREA) or HUNTINGTON'S DISEASE.

chromosome 21 The chromosome involved in DOWN SYNDROME (TRISOMY 21), which is most frequently due to nondisjunction of chromosome 21, resulting in 3, rather than 2, chromosomes (and making the total 47 chromosomes rather than the normal total of 46). The GENETIC defect in familial ALZHEIMER'S DISEASE is located on chromosome 21, the same chromosome that has an extra copy in DOWN SYNDROME. This finding supports the idea that at least one form of ALZHEIMER'S DISEASE is inherited and that a similar genetic defect may occur in both DOWN SYNDROME and familial ALZHEIMER'S DISEASE.

chromosomes Microscopic, intranuclear structures that carry the GENES. The normal human cell contains 46 chromosomes, consisting of 23 pairs of chromosomes—22 pairs of autosomes and 1 pair of sex chromosomes.

chronic Continuing over a long time or recurring frequently.

chronic fatigue syndrome   An illness of unknown ETIOLOGY characterized by fatigue, mild COGNITIVE dysfunction, and in some cases mild fever. Many patients with this SYNDROME may have DEPRESSION.

chronobiology   The science or study of temporal factors in life stages and disorders, such as the sleep-wake cycle and biological clocks and rhythms. See BIOLOGICAL RHYTHMS.

cingulate cortex   A part of the BRAIN situated in the medial aspect of the CEREBRAL CORTEX.

cingulate gyrus   A ridge in the medial part of the BRAIN. The cortical part of the cingulate gyrus is referred to as the CINGULATE CORTEX. The cingulate gyrus functions as an integral part of the LIMBIC SYSTEM, which is involved with EMOTION formation and processing, learning, and MEMORY.

circadian rhythms   See BIOLOGICAL RHYTHMS.

circadian rhythm sleep disorders   A family of SLEEP DISORDERS that affects the timing of sleep (among other things). Circadian rhythm sleep disorders may be characterized as either *extrinsic* or *intrinsic*.

extrinsic   Includes the following:

jet lag type   affects people who travel across several time zones.

shift work type   affects people who work nights or rotating shifts.

intrinsic   Includes the following:

advanced sleep phase pattern   characterized by difficulty staying awake in the evening and staying asleep in the morning.

delayed sleep phase pattern   characterized by a much later than normal timing of sleep onset and offset and a period of peak alertness in the middle of the night.

non-24-hour sleep-wake pattern   in which sleep occurs later and later each day, with the period of peak alertness also continuously moving around the clock from day to day.

irregular sleep-wake pattern   in which a person sleeps at very irregular times, and usually more than once per day, but with total time asleep typical for the person's age.

circumstantiality   A pattern of speech that is indirect and delayed in reaching its goal because of excessive or irrelevant detail or parenthetical remarks. The speaker does not lose the point, as is characteristic of LOOSENING OF ASSOCIATIONS, and clauses remain logically connected, but to the listener it seems that the end will never be reached. Compare with TANGENTIALITY.

cisternography   A radiological study used to evaluate the flow pattern of CEREBROSPINAL FLUID (CSF) by the introduction of a nondiffusible radiopharmaceutical agent into the subarachnoid space. Cisternography is used in the DIAGNOSIS of communicating HYDROCEPHALUS and CSF leaks and the postoperative evaluation of ventricular shunts.

citalopram   A SELECTIVE SEROTONIN REUPTAKE INHIBITOR (SSRI) ANTIDEPRESSANT medication approved to treat DEPRESSION and also used by clinicians to treat certain ANXIETY DISORDERS. Marketed under the brand name CELEXA. See "Medications Used in Psychiatry."

citicoline   A naturally occurring ENDOGENOUS nucleoside widely used in the treatment of loss of consciousness due to head trauma and BRAIN surgery. Citicoline also has been used in the treatment of patients recovering from ischemic STROKE, showing improvement in their COGNITIVE function.

civil action   See "Legal Terms."

civil commitment   See "Legal Terms."

civil law   See "Legal Terms."

clanging   A type of thinking in which the sound of a word, rather than its meaning, gives the direction to subsequent ASSOCIATIONS. Punning and rhyming may substitute for logic, and language may become increasingly a senseless COMPULSION to associate and decreasingly a vehicle for communication. For example, in response to the statement "That will probably remain a mystery," a patient said, "History is one of my strong points."

classical conditioning   See RESPONDENT CONDITIONING.

claustrophobia   The FEAR of closed spaces.

clear and convincing evidence   See "Legal Terms."

climacteric   Menopausal period in women. Sometimes used to refer to the corresponding age period in men. Also called *involutional period*.

Clinical Antipsychotic Trials of Intervention Effectiveness   See CATIE (CLINICAL ANTIPSYCHOTIC TRIALS OF INTERVENTION EFFECTIVENESS).

clinical psychologist   See PSYCHOLOGIST.

clinical social worker   A social worker who applies the theory and methods of SOCIAL WORK to the treatment and PREVENTION of psychosocial dysfunction, DISABILITY, or impairment with individuals, families, and small groups. Many states require a license to practice clinical social work. Usually, certification requires a master's degree in social work, at least 2 years' work experience, and the passing of an examination. See SOCIAL WORK.

clock drawing test   A simple test that can be used as a part of a neurological examination or as a screening tool for Alzheimer's disease and other types of dementia. The person undergoing testing is asked to draw a clock, put in all the numbers, and set the hands at ten past eleven. The clock drawing test can provide information about general cognitive and adaptive functioning, such as memory and the ability to process information and vision.

clomipramine   A tricyclic antidepressant medication approved for the treatment of obsessive-compulsive disorder. Marketed under the brand name Anafranil. See "Medications Used in Psychiatry."

clonazepam   A benzodiazepine anxiolytic medication used to treat various anxiety disorders, such as panic disorder and adjustment disorder with anxiety, as well as insomnia. Clonazepam is also used to treat seizure disorders. Marketed under the brand name Klonopin. See "Medications Used in Psychiatry."

clonidine   An alpha$_2$-adrenergic receptor agonist originally developed to treat hypertension but also effective in treating various other conditions, such as attention-deficit/hyperactivity disorder (ADHD) (for insomnia secondary to stimulant medications), tic disorders (including Tourette's disorder), alcohol withdrawal, opiate (narcotic) detoxification, and restless legs syndrome. Marketed under the brand name Catapres. See "Medications Used in Psychiatry."

clorazepate   A benzodiazepine anxiolytic medication used to treat anxiety disorders, insomnia, and acute alcohol withdrawal. Marketed under the brand name Tranxene. See "Medications Used in Psychiatry."

clouding of consciousness   See acute confusional state.

clozapine   An atypical antipsychotic medication used to treat refractory schizophrenia. Marketed under the brand names Clozaril and FazaClo. See "Medications Used in Psychiatry."

Clozaril   Brand name for the atypical antipsychotic drug clozapine.

cluster suicides   Multiple suicides, usually among adolescents, in a circumscribed time and area.

CME   See continuing medical education (CME).

CMHC   See community mental health center (CMHC).

CMS   See Centers for Medicare and Medicaid Services (CMS).

CNS   See central nervous system (CNS).

coactive strategy   The use of more than one medication to achieve a desired response. *Combination* is the use of two or more medications with different mechanisms of action but within the same overall class, such as the use of two ANTIDEPRESSANTS to treat REFRACTORY DEPRESSION. *Augmentation* is the addition of one or more medications to enhance the effects of a primary medication already being used, such as the addition of LITHIUM to an ANTIDEPRESSANT to treat REFRACTORY DEPRESSION.

cocaine   A naturally occurring STIMULANT drug found in the leaves of the coca plant, *Erythroxylon coca.* Its systemic effects include nervous system stimulation, manifested by garrulousness, restlessness, EXCITEMENT, delusional ideas, a false feeling of increased strength and mental capacity, and epileptic SEIZURES.

cocaine-related disorders   In DSM-IV-TR, a group of MENTAL DISORDERS that includes cocaine DEPENDENCE; cocaine ABUSE; cocaine INTOXICATION; cocaine WITHDRAWAL; cocaine intoxication DELIRIUM; cocaine-induced PSYCHOTIC DISORDER, with DELUSIONS or HALLUCINATIONS; cocaine-induced MOOD DISORDER; cocaine-induced ANXIETY DISORDER; cocaine-induced SEXUAL DYSFUNCTION; and cocaine-induced SLEEP DISORDER.

codependency   A term referring to the effects that people who are dependent on alcohol or other substances have on those around them, including the attempts of those people to manage the chemically dependent person. The term implies that the family's actions tend to perpetuate (enable) the person's DEPENDENCE.

Cogentin   Brand name for the ANTICHOLINERGIC drug BENZTROPINE.

Cognex   Brand name for the ACETYLCHOLINESTERASE INHIBITOR drug TACRINE.

cognition   A general term encompassing all the various modes of knowing and reasoning.

cognitive   Refers to the mental process of comprehension, JUDGMENT, MEMORY, and reasoning, in contrast to emotional and volitional processes. Contrast with CONATIVE.

cognitive-behavioral therapy (CBT)   A form of PSYCHOTHERAPY focused on changing thoughts and behaviors that are related to specific target SYMPTOMS. Treatment is aimed at symptom reduction and improved functioning. The patient is taught to recognize the negative and unrealistic thought patterns that contribute significantly to the development or maintenance of symptoms and to evaluate and modify such thinking patterns. Problematic behaviors are also focused on and changed with the use of behavioral strategies (e.g., response PREVENTION, scheduling pleasant activities).

cognitive deficits   Impairment of JUDGMENT, MEMORY, reasoning, and comprehension due to a variety of causes.

cognitive development   Beginning in infancy, the acquisition of INTELLIGENCE, CONSCIOUS thought, and problem-solving abilities. An orderly sequence in the increase in knowledge derived from sensorimotor activity has been empirically shown by Jean Piaget (1896–1980), who described four stages in the cognitive development of the child:

sensorimotor stage   The senses receive a stimulus, and the body reacts to it in a stereotyped way. It occurs from birth to 16–24 months. Object permanence develops during this time.

preoperational thought   Prelogical thought that occurs between ages 2 and 6 years. During this time, symbolic function and language develop and change the child's ability to interact. Egocentric thinking predominates, and the child believes that everything revolves around him or her. MAGICAL THINKING arises, and reality and FANTASY are interwoven.

concrete operations   Rational and logical thought process. It occurs between ages 7 and 11 and includes the development of the ability to understand another's viewpoint and the concept of conservation.

formal operations   Cognitive stage that includes abstract thinking, conceptual thinking, and deductive reasoning. Formal operational thinking is generally achieved by age 12, although some adults may never achieve this stage of cognitive development. See also PSYCHOSEXUAL DEVELOPMENT; PSYCHOSOCIAL DEVELOPMENT.

cognitive disorders   In DSM-IV-TR, this group includes DELIRIUM, DEMENTIA, and AMNESTIC DISORDER.

cognitive-emotional therapies   See EXPERIENTIAL THERAPY.

cognitive enhancers   Medications or supplements (also known as *memory enhancers* or *nootropics*) purported to improve mental functions such as COGNITION, MEMORY, intelligence, motivation, ATTENTION, and concentration. This category includes drugs used to treat people with cognitive difficulties, such as those with ALZHEIMER'S DISEASE, PARKINSON'S DISEASE, or ATTENTION-DEFICIT/HYPERACTIVITY DISORDER (ADHD).

cognitive errors   In COGNITIVE-BEHAVIORAL THERAPY, people with DEPRESSIVE DISORDERS or PERSONALITY DISORDERS are believed to have faulty assumptions or misconceptions that may be caused by past experiences and are not adapted to the actual situation of the person. These types of errors include magnification, overgeneralization, personalization, polarized thinking, and selective abstraction.

cognitive function   An intellectual process by which one becomes aware of, perceives, or comprehends ideas. It involves all aspects of perception, thinking, reasoning, and remembering.

cognitive processsing therapy (CPT)   A combination therapy often used with RAPE survivors who have POSTTRAUMATIC STRESS DISORDER (PTSD). CPT includes education and discussion of the assault with the group via writing and COGNITIVE RESTRUCTURING.

cognitive rehabilitation   Modification of COGNITIVE and ROLE functioning in seriously and persistently mentally ill patients, directed at improving visual and verbal MEMORY and social and emotional PERCEPTION.

cognitive restructuring   A technique of COGNITIVE THERAPY that enables one to identify negative, irrational beliefs and replace them with truthful, rational statements.

cognitive therapy   A type of PSYCHOTHERAPY, usually focused and problem oriented, directed primarily at identifying and modifying distorted thinking patterns and behavioral dysfunction. This technique is based on the assumption that certain thought patterns, called COGNITIVE structures or schemas, shape the way people react to the situations in their lives. Individuals with major DEPRESSION, ANXIETY DISORDERS, EATING DISORDERS, and SUBSTANCE USE DISORDERS are more likely to benefit.

cogwheel rigidity   Rigidity in which the muscles respond with cogwheel-like jerks to the use of force in bending the limb, as occurs in PARKINSON'S DISEASE.

Cohen syndrome   An inherited disorder affecting many parts of the body and characterized by DEVELOPMENTAL DELAY, INTELLECTUAL DISABILITY, and weak muscle tone (HYPOTONIA). Other features of the syndrome include progressive nearsightedness.

cohesive self   The stable sense of one's IDENTITY or core SELF, which develops through progressive consolidation of the GRANDIOSE SELF, the IDEALIZED PARENTAL IMAGO, and the person's talents and skills. A HOLDING ENVIRONMENT in which the child develops basic trust promotes optimal development.

colera   A CULTURE-SPECIFIC SYNDROME. See *MUINA*.

collective unconscious In Jungian theory (Carl Gustav Jung, 1875–1961), a portion of the UNCONSCIOUS common to all people. See also ANALYTIC PSYCHOLOGY.

coma A severe disturbance of consciousness with absence of voluntary activity (either motor or COGNITIVE) and diminished or absent responsiveness to tactile, thermal, proprioceptive, visual, auditory, olfactory, or verbal stimuli. Coma is indicative of widespread cerebral dysfunction and is often part of DELIRIUM.

combat fatigue An outmoded term for POSTTRAUMATIC STRESS DISORDER (PTSD). Disabling physical and emotional reaction incident to military combat. Paradoxically, the reaction may not necessarily include fatigue. See also SHELL SHOCK.

combination treatment Refers to the use of more than one treatment modality to achieve a desired effect, such as the pairing of COGNITIVE-BEHAVIORAL THERAPY (CBT) with ANTIDEPRESSANT pharmacotherapy to treat PANIC DISORDER. It also may refer to the use of two or more medications with different mechanisms of action but within the same overall class, such as the use of two different ANTIDEPRESSANTS to treat REFRACTORY DEPRESSION. See also AUGMENTATION STRATEGIES; COACTIVE STRATEGY.

commitment See "Legal Terms."

common law See "Legal Terms."

communication disorders In DSM-IV-TR, this group includes EXPRESSIVE LANGUAGE DISORDER, MIXED RECEPTIVE-EXPRESSIVE LANGUAGE DISORDER, PHONOLOGICAL DISORDER, and STUTTERING.

> **expressive language disorder** Characterized by scores on tests measuring EXPRESSIVE language development that are below those on tests of nonverbal INTELLIGENCE and RECEPTIVE language. SYMPTOMS may include limited vocabulary, speaking only in the present tense, errors in recalling words, and developmentally inappropriate sentence length.

> **mixed receptive-expressive language disorder** Characterized by testing performance on both RECEPTIVE and EXPRESSIVE language development batteries that is substantially below performance on nonverbal intellectual batteries. The typical manifestation is an inability to understand words or sentences.

> **phonological disorder** Characterized by failure to use developmentally expected speech sounds that are appropriate for age and dialect. Speech sounds may be omitted, substituted, or distorted, as in saying "w" for "r" or "f" for "th."

stuttering   Characterized by disturbance of the fluency and time patterning of speech. SYMPTOMS may include repetitions of sounds or syllables, sound prolongations, interjections, or circumlocutions to avoid difficult words.

community mental health center (CMHC)   A MENTAL HEALTH service delivery system first authorized by the federal Community Mental Health Centers Act of 1963 to provide a comprehensive program of mental health care to CATCHMENT AREA residents. The CMHC is typically a community facility or a network of affiliated agencies that serves as a locus for the delivery of the various services included in the concept of COMMUNITY PSYCHIATRY.

community psychiatry   That branch of PSYCHIATRY concerned with the provision and delivery of a coordinated program of MENTAL HEALTH care to residents of a geographic area. These efforts include working with patients, their families, and agencies within the community. Goals are the PREVENTION of mental illness as well as care and treatment for persons with MENTAL DISORDERS.

comorbidity   The simultaneous appearance of two or more illnesses, such as the co-occurrence of SCHIZOPHRENIA and substance ABUSE or of alcohol DEPENDENCE and DEPRESSION. The association may reflect a causal relation between one disorder and another or an underlying vulnerability to both disorders; however, the co-occurrence of the illnesses may be unrelated to any common ETIOLOGY or vulnerability.

compensation   A DEFENSE MECHANISM, operating unconsciously (see UNCONSCIOUS), by which one attempts to make up or compensate for real or perceived deficiencies. Also a CONSCIOUS process in which one strives to compensate for real or perceived defects of physique, performance skills, or psychological attributes. The two types frequently merge. See also INDIVIDUAL PSYCHOLOGY; OVERCOMPENSATION.

compensatory damages   See "Legal Terms."

competence   Having the capacity to function effectively as an individual and an organization within the context of the cultural beliefs, behaviors, and needs presented by individuals and their communities.

competency   See "Legal Terms."

competency to stand trial   See "Legal Terms."

complex   A group of associated ideas having a common, strong emotional tone. These ideas are largely UNCONSCIOUS and significantly influence attitudes and ASSOCIATIONS. See also OEDIPUS COMPLEX.

compliance   See ADHERENCE.

Comprehensive Crime Control Act of 1984 standard   See under INSANITY DEFENSE in "Legal Terms."

compulsion   Repetitive ritualistic behavior or thoughts, such as frequent hand washing, arranging objects according to a rigid formula, counting, or repeating words silently. The purpose of these behaviors or thoughts is to prevent or reduce distress or to prevent some dreaded event or situation. The person feels driven to perform such actions in response to an OBSESSION (a recurrent thought, IMPULSE, or image that is intrusive and distressing) or according to rules that must be applied rigidly, even though the behaviors or thoughts are recognized to be excessive or unreasonable. Failure to perform these actions often generates ANXIETY.

compulsive   Refers to intensity or repetitiveness of behavior rather than to compulsive behavior strictly defined. Thus, "compulsive drinking" and "compulsive gambling" refer to cravings that may be intense and often repeated, but they are not viewed as COMPULSIONS.

computed tomography (CT)   A technique for imaging anatomical structures with X ray. Objects are exposed to a series of X-ray beams on a single plane but with an origin at different points around a 180-degree arc. A computer algorithm reconstructs the beam absorption data so as to display an image of absorption values at each point in the plane. The process is repeated for each plane to be imaged. Used for detecting anatomical abnormalities such as STROKES, tumor, and atrophy of the BRAIN. See also BRAIN IMAGING.

computerized axial tomography (CAT) scanning   See COMPUTED TOMOGRAPHY (CT).

COMT   See CATECHOL-O-METHYLTRANSFERASE (COMT).

Comtan   Brand name for the ANTIPARKINSONIAN MEDICATION ENTACAPONE.

conative   Pertaining to one's basic strivings as expressed in behavior and actions.

Concerta   Brand name for the CENTRAL NERVOUS SYSTEM (CNS) STIMULANT drug METHYLPHENIDATE.

concrete operations   See COGNITIVE DEVELOPMENT.

concrete thinking   Thinking characterized by a focus on present objects and immediate experience with an inability to use concepts or make and understand generalizations.

concussion   An impairment of BRAIN function caused by injury to the head. The speed and degree of recovery depend on the severity of the brain injury. SYMPTOMS may include headache, DISORIENTATION, paralysis, and unconsciousness.

condensation   A psychological process, often present in dreams, in which two or more concepts are fused so that a single symbol represents the multiple components.

conditioning   Establishing new behavior as a result of psychological modifications of responses to stimuli.

conduct disorder   A DISRUPTIVE BEHAVIOR DISORDER of childhood characterized by repetitive and persistent violation of the rights of others or of age-appropriate social norms or rules. SYMPTOMS may include bullying others, truancy or work absences, staying out at night despite parental prohibition before age 13 years, using alcohol or other substances before age 13, breaking into another's house or car, fire setting with the intent of causing serious damage, physical cruelty to people or animals, stealing, or use more than once of a weapon that could cause harm to others (e.g., brick, broken bottle, or gun).

confabulation   The fabrication of false memories, perceptions, or beliefs about the self or the environment as a result of neurological or psychological dysfunction. It is difficult to distinguish confabulation from lies or delusions.

confidentiality   The ethical principle that a physician may not reveal any information disclosed in the course of medical attendance. See also CONFIDENTIALITY and PRIVILEGE in "Legal Terms."

conflict   A mental struggle that arises from the simultaneous operation of opposing IMPULSES, DRIVES, and external (environmental) or internal demands. Termed INTRAPSYCHIC when the conflict is between forces within the PERSONALITY and extrapsychic when it is between the self and the environment.

confrontation   A communication that deliberately pressures or invites another to self-examine some aspect of his or her behavior in which a discrepancy exists between self-reported and observed behavior. This technique is frequently used in the treatment of ALCOHOLISM and SUBSTANCE USE DISORDERS.

confusion   Disturbed ORIENTATION with respect to time, place, person, or situation. See DELIRIUM; DEMENTIA; MENTAL STATUS.

congenital   Literally, present at birth. Congenital conditions may include those that arise during fetal development or with the birth process as well as hereditary or genetically determined conditions. The term is not used to refer to conditions that appear after birth.

conjoint therapy A form of MARITAL THERAPY in which a therapist sees the partners together in joint sessions.

conscience The morally self-critical part of one's standards of behavior, performance, and value JUDGMENTS. Commonly equated with the SUPEREGO.

conscious The content of mind or mental functioning of which one is aware. In NEUROLOGY, awake, alert. See also UNCONSCIOUS.

consent decree See "Legal Terms."

conservatorship See "Legal Terms."

consortium See "Legal Terms."

constitution A person's intrinsic physical and psychological endowment; sometimes used more narrowly to indicate physical inheritance or intellectual potential.

constitutional types Constellations of morphological, physiological, and psychological traits as earlier proposed by various scholars, such as the Greek physician and philosopher Galen (129–210 A.D.): sanguine, melancholic, choleric, and phlegmatic types; German PSYCHIATRIST Ernst Kretschmer (1888–1961): pyknic (stocky), asthenic (slender), athletic, and dysplastic (disproportional) types; and American PSYCHOLOGIST William Sheldon (1898–1977): ectomorphic (thin), mesomorphic (muscular), and endomorphic (fat) types, based on the relative preponderance of outer, middle, or inner layers of embryonic cellular tissue.

constricted affect See AFFECT.

construct validity Term referring to how well a test or experiment measures up to its claim. Construct validity is a device used almost exclusively in social sciences, psychology, and education.

constructional apraxia An acquired difficulty in drawing two-dimensional objects or forms or in producing or copying three-dimensional arrangements of forms or shapes.

consultation-liaison psychiatry An area of special interest in general PSYCHIATRY that addresses the psychiatric and psychosocial aspects of medical care, particularly in a general hospital setting. This area is now called PSYCHOSOMATIC MEDICINE and has achieved subspecialty status. The consultation-liaison PSYCHIATRIST works closely with medical-surgical physicians and nonphysician staff to enhance the DIAGNOSIS, treatment, and management of patients with primary medical-surgical illness and concurrent psychiatric disorders or SYMPTOMS. Consultation-liaison psychiatry may occasionally lead to a recommendation for more specific AFTERCARE referral but more typically consists of short-term intervention by a "consultation team" with a BIOPSYCHOSOCIAL approach to illness.

consumer Someone who uses the services provided or whom the clinician is treating.

contingency reinforcement In operant or instrumental CONDITIONING, ensuring that desired behavior is followed by positive consequences and that undesired behavior is not rewarded.

continuing medical education (CME) Postgraduate educational activities aimed at maintaining, updating, and extending professional knowledge and skills. Many professional organizations and state licensing boards require participation in CME activities.

contract Explicit commitment between patient and therapist to a well-defined course of action to achieve the treatment goal. See also "Legal Terms."

conventional antipsychotics A group of older ANTIPSYCHOTIC drugs—also referred to as "traditional" or "first-generation" antipsychotics (FGAs) and sometimes called NEUROLEPTICS—that work principally by blocking DOPAMINE RECEPTORS in the BRAIN. Examples include CHLORPROMAZINE and HALOPERIDOL. These medications have the potential to cause adverse SIDE EFFECTS such as parkinsonian SYMPTOMS (muscle stiffness, RIGIDITY, slowed gait, and TREMOR) and TARDIVE DYSKINESIA (involuntary lip smacking, tongue movements, and upper-extremity movements). See "Medications Used in Psychiatry."

conversion A DEFENSE MECHANISM, operating unconsciously (see UNCONSCIOUS), by which INTRAPSYCHIC CONFLICTS that would otherwise give rise to ANXIETY are instead given symbolic external expression. The repressed ideas or IMPULSES, and the psychological defenses against them, are converted into a variety of somatic SYMPTOMS such as paralysis, pain, or loss of sensory function.

conversion disorder One of the SOMATOFORM DISORDERS (but in some classifications called a DISSOCIATIVE DISORDER), characterized by a SYMPTOM suggestive of a neurological disorder that affects sensation or voluntary motor function. The symptom is not consciously or intentionally produced, cannot be explained fully by any known GENERAL MEDICAL CONDITION, and is severe enough to impair functioning or require medical attention. Commonly seen conversion symptoms are blindness, double vision, deafness, impaired coordination, paralysis, and SEIZURES.

convulsive disorders   Include generalized SEIZURES, such as grand mal and petit mal, and the focal SEIZURES of Jacksonian and PSYCHOMOTOR EPILEPSY. These BRAIN disorders, with their characteristic electroencephalographic patterns (see ELECTROENCEPHALOGRAM [EEG]), are to be differentiated from a variety of other pathophysiological conditions in which a convulsive SEIZURE may occur. The latter may follow WITHDRAWAL from alcohol, BARBITURATES, and a wide variety of other drugs. Seizures also may occur in cerebral vascular disease, brain tumor, brain abscess, HYPOGLYCEMIA, HYPONATREMIA, and many other metabolic and intracranial disorders.

coping mechanisms   Ways of adjusting to environmental stress without altering one's goals or purposes. Includes both CONSCIOUS and UNCONSCIOUS mechanisms.

coprolalia   The involuntary use of profane words seen in patients with TOURETTE'S DISORDER.

coprophagia   Eating of filth or feces.

coprophilia   One of the PARAPHILIAS, characterized by marked distress over, or acting on, sexual urges involving feces.

copropraxia   Obscene gesturing seen in patients with TOURETTE'S DISORDER.

core conflictual relationship theme   In psychoanalytic therapy (see PSYCHOANALYSIS), any reference by the patient to earlier failures in interpersonal transactions. The patient typically expresses thoughts and feelings about earlier experiences (and especially about parent and child transactions) in a variety of ways, often indirect and veiled. It is the therapist's task to grasp the meaning of the patient's subjective experiences and to understand that the patient's wishes during earlier periods reflected phase-appropriate self-developmental needs and were not simply pleasures to be denied.

core gender identity   See GENDER IDENTITY.

corpus callosum   A structure of the BRAIN in the longitudinal fissure that connects the left and right cerebral hemispheres and facilitates communication between them. It is the largest WHITE MATTER structure in the brain, consisting of millions of nerve fibers. In REFRACTORY EPILEPSY, symptoms can be reduced by cutting the corpus callosum in an operation known as *corpus callosotomy*.

corpus striatum   A compound structure consisting of the CAUDATE NUCLEUS and the LENTIFORM NUCLEUS, which consists of the PUTAMEN and the GLOBUS PALLIDUS.

cortex   See CEREBRAL CORTEX.

corticobasal degeneration   See CORTICOBASAL GANGLIONIC DEGENERATION (CBGD).

corticobasal ganglionic degeneration (CBGD)   A   progressive neurological disorder characterized by nerve cell loss and atrophy of multiple areas of the BRAIN, including the CEREBRAL CORTEX and the BASAL GANGLIA. Symptoms are similar to those found in PARKINSON'S DISEASE, such as poor coordination, AKINESIA, rigidity, disequilibrium, and limb DYSTONIA. Other symptoms such as COGNITIVE and visual-spatial impairments, APRAXIA, hesitant and halting speech, MYOCLONUS (muscular jerks), and DYSPHAGIA may also occur. An individual with CBGD eventually becomes unable to walk. Also known as *corticobasal degeneration.*

corticotropin-releasing factor (CRF)   Synthesized in the HYPOTHALAMUS, CRF regulates the secretion of ADRENOCORTICOTROPIC HORMONE (ACTH) from the posterior pituitary. CRF has a variety of effects, including activation of the SYMPATHETIC NERVOUS SYSTEM and regulation of behavioral responses to stress.

cortisol   A steroid HORMONE produced in the adrenal glands. Increased levels of plasma cortisol have been reported in patients with MAJOR DEPRESSIVE DISORDER, whereas decreased levels have been reported in patients with POSTTRAUMATIC STRESS DISORDER (PTSD).

Cotard's syndrome   A NIHILISTIC DELUSION in which one believes that one's body, or parts of it, is disintegrating; that one is bereft of all resources; or that one's family has been exterminated. Neurologically, Cotard's syndrome is thought to be related to CAPGRAS' SYNDROME, and both are thought to result from a disconnect between the brain areas that recognize faces and the areas that associate emotions with that recognition (the AMYGDALA and other limbic structures). This disconnection creates a sense that the observed face is not the person's it purports to be; thus, if sufferers see their own face, they may feel no association between it and their sense of self, resulting in a sense that they themselves do not exist. Cotard's syndrome has been reported in DEPRESSIVE DISORDERS, SCHIZOPHRENIA, and brain lesions of the nondominant hemisphere. The syndrome is named after the French NEUROLOGIST Jules Cotard (1840–1887).

counseling   A form of SUPPORTIVE PSYCHOTHERAPY in which a person, adviser, or counselor offers guidance or advice to another based on discussion of the other's personal problems. PSYCHIATRISTS, PSYCHOLOGISTS, CLINICAL SOCIAL WORKER, and the clergy commonly use this method.

counterphobia   Deliberately seeking out and exposing oneself to, rather than avoiding, the object or situation that is consciously or unconsciously feared.

countertransference   The therapist's emotional reactions to the patient that are based on the therapist's UNCONSCIOUS needs and CONFLICTS, as distinguished from his or her CONSCIOUS responses to the patient's behavior. Countertransference may interfere with the therapist's ability to understand the patient and may adversely affect the therapeutic technique. However, countertransference also may have positive aspects and may be used by the therapist as a guide to a more empathic and accurate understanding of the patient.

couples therapy   See MARITAL THERAPY.

CPT   See COGNITIVE PROCESSING THERAPY (CPT).

crack   Slang for freebase or alkaloidal COCAINE. The name derives from the cracking sound cocaine makes when heated. Also known as "rock" because of its crystallized appearance, alkaloidal cocaine is ingested by inhalation of vapors produced from heating. The drug induces a sense of exhilaration in the user, primarily by blocking the reuptake of the NEUROTRANSMITTER DOPAMINE in the MIDBRAIN.

crank   Slang for an illicitly produced low-purity crystallized form of METHAMPHETAMINE, a STIMULANT that acts on the CENTRAL NERVOUS SYSTEM (CNS) to increase heart rate and alertness. Highs on this drug last between 8 and 24 hours and often conclude with a violent "crash" period during which the user tends to be prone to aggression. The drug received the nickname "crank" because it was often smuggled in the crank cases of vehicles.

cretinism   A type of INTELLECTUAL DISABILITY and bodily malformation caused by severe, uncorrected thyroid deficiency in infancy and early childhood.

Creutzfeldt-Jakob disease   A rare, fatal BRAIN disorder that causes a rapid, progressive DEMENTIA and associated neuromuscular disturbances. The disease is often referred to as SUBACUTE SPONGIFORM ENCEPHALOPATHY because it usually produces microscopic cavities in NEURONS that appear sponge-like. The illness is believed to be caused by PRIONS, proteinaceous infectious particles, which are abnormal forms of a human GENE.

CRF   See CORTICOTROPIN-RELEASING FACTOR (CRF).

cri du chat   A type of INTELLECTUAL DISABILITY that is caused by partial deletion of CHROMOSOME 5. The name is derived from a catlike cry emitted by children with this disorder.

criminal law   See "Legal Terms."

crisis   A state of sudden psychological disequilibrium; a turning point in a person's life.

crisis intervention   A form of BRIEF PSYCHOTHERAPY that emphasizes identification of a specific event precipitating the emotional trauma and uses methods to neutralize and cope with that trauma. Often used in hospital emergency departments.

critical incident stress debriefing   Psychological debriefing following a traumatic event, which was designed primarily for emergency response personnel, to allow traumatized individuals to discuss their thoughts, feelings, and behavior following the event.

cross-cultural psychiatry   The comparative study of mental illness and mental health among different societies, nations, and CULTURES. Often used synonymously with *transcultural psychiatry*.

cross-dependence   A drug's ability to suppress physical manifestations of substance DEPENDENCE produced by another drug and to maintain the physically dependent state. It provides the rationale for the treatment of DEPENDENCE on one substance (e.g., alcohol) by short-term substitution of a less dangerous and more controllable substance that is cross-dependent with that substance (e.g., the use of LIBRIUM [CHLORDIAZEPOXIDE] to treat alcohol WITHDRAWAL SYMPTOMS).

cross-dressing   See TRANSVESTISM.

cross-tolerance   TOLERANCE to a drug to which an individual has not been exposed because tolerance had developed to another substance over a period of long-term administration. A person who has developed tolerance to alcohol will have a diminished response to the usual dose of a BENZODIAZEPINE medication because tolerance to alcohol also has induced tolerance to the benzodiazepine's effect.

CSF   See CEREBROSPINAL FLUID (CSF).

CT   See COMPUTED TOMOGRAPHY (CT).

cult   A system of beliefs and rituals based on dogma or religious teachings that are usually contrary to those established within or accepted by the community.

cultural anthropology   The study of human society with emphasis on how values, customs, beliefs, language, and other patterns of behavior are transmitted by learning from past generations. See ETHNOLOGY; SOCIAL ANTHROPOLOGY.

cultural competence   A set of congruent behaviors, attitudes, and policies that come together in a system or agency or among professionals and that enable effective work in cross-cultural situations.

cultural diversity An understanding of the issues that arise between genders, ages, religions, lifestyles, beliefs, physical capabilities, and CULTURES.

cultural formulation A method of incorporating sociocultural issues into the clinical formulation. The cultural formulation begins with a review of the individual's CULTURAL IDENTITY, which involves not only ethnicity, acculturation/biculturality, and language but also age, gender, SOCIOECONOMIC STATUS, sexual orientation, religious and spiritual beliefs, disabilities, political orientation, and health literacy, among other factors.

cultural identity The CULTURE with which someone identifies and to which he or she looks for standards of behavior.

cultural psychiatry A branch of SOCIAL PSYCHIATRY concerned with mentally ill persons in relation to their cultural environment. SYMPTOMS of behavior regarded as psychopathological in one society may be regarded as acceptable and normal in another.

cultural sensitivity Acceptance that cultural differences and similarities exist, without assigning values to those cultural differences.

culture Integrated patterns of human behavior that include the language, thoughts, communications, actions, customs, beliefs, values, and institutions of racial, ethnic, religious, or social groups. Refers to the shared and largely learned attributes of a group of people. Anthropologists often describe culture as a system of shared meanings.

culture shock Feelings of isolation, rejection, and ALIENATION experienced by an individual or a group when transplanted from a familiar to an unfamiliar CULTURE (e.g., moving from one country to another).

culture-specific syndromes Forms of disturbed behavior and troubling experiences specific to certain cultural systems that do not conform to Western nosological entities (see NOSOLOGY) or diagnostic systems, such as DSM-IV-TR or ICD-10. See also DISSOCIATIVE TRANCE DISORDER.

curandero/curandera In Hispanic America, a traditional folk healer or shaman who is dedicated to curing physical or spiritual illnesses. *Curanderos* treat ailments like *ESPANTO*, *SUSTO*, and *MAL DE OJO* with religious rituals, ceremonial cleansing, and prayers. See CULTURE-SPECIFIC SYNDROMES.

Cushing's disease Clinical abnormalities due to chronic exposure to high level of CORTISOL. Caused by tumors of the anterior lobe of the pituitary gland. Patients with Cushing's disease often show COGNITIVE changes, particularly MEMORY impairment.

CVA   Cerebrovascular accident. See STROKE.

cybersex   A modern-day PARAPHILIA, characterized by DEPENDENCE on on-line sex-chat rooms.

Cycloset   Brand name for the mixed DOPAMINE AGONIST-ANTAGONIST drug BROMOCRIPTINE.

cyclothymic disorder   In DSM-IV-TR, one of the BIPOLAR DISORDERS characterized by HYPOMANIC EPISODES, which are less severe than mania, and periods of depressed MOOD or loss of interest or pleasure that do not meet criteria for MAJOR DEPRESSIVE DISORDER. See also DEPRESSIVE DISORDERS.

Cylert   Former brand name for the withdrawn STIMULANT drug PEMOLINE.

Cymbalta   Brand name for the SEROTONIN-NOREPINEPHRINE REUPTAKE IN-HIBITOR (SNRI) drug DULOXETINE.

cynophobia   The FEAR of dogs.

cyproheptadine   An antihistaminic and antiserotonergic agent used in the treatment of nightmares (including those related to POSTTRAU-MATIC STRESS DISORDER [PTSD]), SEXUAL DYSFUNCTION SECONDARY to ANTI-DEPRESSANT treatment, and psychogenic and nonpsychogenic anorexia as an appetite stimulant. Cyproheptadine has also been used in the management of moderate to severe cases of SEROTONIN SYNDROME. While not specifically used as a SEDATIVE, cyproheptadine causes drowsiness. Now available only as generic but may still be known by the discontinued brand name PERIACTIN.

cytochrome P450   ENZYME system in the liver that plays a key role in the metabolism of many medications. Many PSYCHOTROPIC medications are known to inhibit or stimulate the cytochrome P450 system, thus resulting in significant drug-DRUG INTERACTIONS that may result in clinically significant alterations of BLOOD LEVELS of medications.

Cytomel   Brand name for the synthetic thyroid HORMONE LIOTHYRONINE.

D

Da Costa's syndrome   Neurocirculatory asthenia (weakness); "soldier's heart"; a FUNCTIONAL DISORDER of the circulatory system that is usually a part of an ANXIETY state or SECONDARY to HYPERVENTILATION.

Dalmane Brand name for the BENZODIAZEPINE SEDATIVE-HYPNOTIC drug FLURAZEPAM.

damages See "Legal Terms."

day hospital See PARTIAL HOSPITALIZATION.

day residue Any element of a dream that is clearly derived from some event of the previous day. The event acquires significance from UNCONSCIOUS connection with repressed CONFLICTS and appears in the dream in a displaced and symbolic form.

Daytrana Brand name for METHYLPHENIDATE TRANSDERMAL SYSTEM.

DBS See DEEP BRAIN STIMULATION (DBS).

DBT See DIALECTICAL BEHAVIOR THERAPY (DBT).

DDAVP Brand name for DESMOPRESSIN ACETATE.

death instinct (Thanatos) In Freudian theory, the UNCONSCIOUS DRIVE toward death and self-destruction. It coexists with, and is in opposition to, the life instinct (Eros).

declarative memory Long-term or "declarative" MEMORY is characterized by active, conscious recall of all the facts, figures, and names we have ever learned. All of our experiences and CONSCIOUS memory fall into this category. Although no one knows exactly where this enormous database is stored, the HIPPOCAMPUS is believed to be necessary to store new memories as they occur. Declarative memory is often contrasted with PROCEDURAL MEMORY, which refers to implicit learned behaviors or rules for various functions.

decompensation The deterioration of existing defenses (see DEFENSE MECHANISM), leading to an exacerbation of pathological behavior.

deep brain stimulation (DBS) The use of an implanted electrode to deliver continuous high-frequency electrical stimulation to the THALAMUS to treat TREMOR in PARKINSON'S DISEASE.

de facto See "Legal Terms."

defendant See "Legal Terms."

defense mechanism UNCONSCIOUS INTRAPSYCHIC processes serving to provide relief from emotional CONFLICT and ANXIETY. CONSCIOUS efforts are frequently made for the same reasons, but true defense mechanisms are unconscious. Some of the common defense mechanisms defined in this glossary are COMPENSATION, CONVERSION, DENIAL, DISPLACEMENT, DISSOCIATION, IDEALIZATION, IDENTIFICATION, INCORPORATION, INTELLECTUALIZATION, INTROJECTION, PROJECTION, RATIONALIZATION, REAC-

TION FORMATION, REGRESSION, SUBLIMATION, SUBSTITUTION, SYMBOLIZATION, and UNDOING.

deficit   Insufficient quantity or inadequate supply. In NEUROLOGY, it refers to an inability to perform (e.g., a motor action or mental task) because of some interference in the chain of neurophysiological and neurochemical events that lies between stimulus and response.

deficit schizophrenia   See SCHIZOPHRENIA.

deinstitutionalization   Change in locus of MENTAL HEALTH care from traditional, institutional settings to community-based services. Sometimes called *transinstitutionalization* because it often merely shifts the patients from one institution (the hospital) to another (such as a prison).

déjà vu   A PARAMNESIA consisting of the sensation or ILLUSION that one is seeing what one has seen before.

de jure   See "Legal Terms."

delayed sleep phase disorder   See *delayed sleep phase pattern* under CIRCADIAN RHYTHM SLEEP DISORDERS.

delirium   A COGNITIVE DISORDER characterized by impairment in consciousness and ATTENTION and changes in COGNITION (e.g., MEMORY DEFICIT, DISORIENTATION, language or perceptual disturbance). The following types of delirium are recognized by DSM-IV-TR: delirium due to a GENERAL MEDICAL CONDITION, substance-induced delirium (in INTOXICATION and WITHDRAWAL states), delirium due to multiple ETIOLOGIES, and delirium not otherwise specified.

delirium tremens (DT)   Alcohol WITHDRAWAL DELIRIUM; alcohol delirium with onset during withdrawal. See *alcohol* under WITHDRAWAL SYMPTOMS; also see SUBSTANCE-INDUCED PSYCHOTIC DISORDER.

delusion   A false belief based on an incorrect inference about external reality, firmly sustained despite clear evidence to the contrary. The belief is not part of a cultural tradition such as an article of religious faith. Among the more frequently reported delusions are the following:

delusional jealousy   The false belief that one's sexual partner is unfaithful; also called the *Othello delusion*.

delusional parasitosis   A strong delusional belief that one is infested with parasites, whereas in reality no such parasites are present.

delusion of control The belief that one's feelings, IMPULSES, thoughts, or actions are not one's own but have been imposed by some external force.

delusion of poverty The conviction that one is, or will be, bereft of all material possessions.

delusion of reference The conviction that events, objects, or other people in the immediate environment have a particular and unusual significance (usually negative).

grandiose delusion An exaggerated belief of one's importance, power, knowledge, or IDENTITY.

nihilistic delusion A conviction of nonexistence of the self, part of the self, others, or the world. "I no longer have a brain" is an example.

persecutory delusion The conviction that one (or a group or institution close to one) is being harassed, attacked, persecuted, or conspired against.

somatic delusion A false belief involving the functioning of, or some other aspect of, one's body, such as the conviction of a postmenopausal woman that she is pregnant, or a person's conviction that he has snakes in his colon.

systematized delusion A single false belief with multiple ELABORATIONS or a group of false beliefs that the person relates to a single event or theme. This event is believed to have caused every problem in life that the person experiences.

delusional depression A severe form of DEPRESSIVE DISORDER characterized by psychotic thinking (e.g., DELUSIONS or HALLUCINATIONS) as well as neurovegetative SYMPTOMS. Listed in DSM-IV-TR as MAJOR DEPRESSIVE DISORDER, severe with psychotic features.

delusional disorder Although in clinical practice it is often difficult to differentiate from the PARANOID type of SCHIZOPHRENIA, the DELUSIONS in this disorder are characteristically systematized rather than bizarre. Also, other characteristics of the active phase of SCHIZOPHRENIA are absent or only fleetingly present, and PERSONALITY functioning remains relatively intact outside the area of the delusional theme. An example would be a man's belief that his wife is having an affair despite no evidence to support this conclusion. As indicated under DELUSION, subtypes are recognized on the basis of the predominant delusional theme.

dementia   A COGNITIVE DISORDER characterized by DEFICITS in MEMORY, APHASIA, APRAXIA, AGNOSIA, and deficits in executive functioning. Various forms of dementia are recognized in DSM-IV-TR: 1) dementia of the ALZHEIMER'S type; 2) VASCULAR DEMENTIA; 3) dementia due to other GENERAL MEDICAL CONDITIONS, including HUMAN IMMUNODEFICIENCY VIRUS (HIV) infection, head injury, PICK'S DISEASE, CREUTZFELDT-JAKOB DISEASE, HUNTINGTON'S DISEASE, and PARKINSON'S DISEASE; 4) substance-induced persisting dementia (seen with alcohol, inhalants, and SEDATIVES, HYPNOTICS, or ANXIOLYTICS); 5) dementia due to multiple ETIOLOGIES; and 6) dementia not otherwise specified. See also SENILE DEMENTIA.

dementia praecox   Obsolete descriptive term for SCHIZOPHRENIA. Introduced as *"démence précoce"* by Benedict Augustine Morel in 1857 and later popularized by Emil Kraepelin (1856–1926).

dementia with Lewy bodies   See LEWY BODY DEMENTIA.

demography   The study of a population and those variables that bring about change in that population. See also EPIDEMIOLOGY.

demophobia   The FEAR of crowds.

dendrite   A branch of the nerve cell that receives nerve IMPULSES from the AXON of a neighboring nerve; a treelike extension of the NEURON cell body. It receives information, along with the cell body, from other neurons.

denial   A DEFENSE MECHANISM, operating unconsciously, used to resolve emotional CONFLICT and allay ANXIETY by disavowing thoughts, feelings, wishes, needs, or external reality factors that are consciously intolerable.

deoxyribonucleic acid (DNA)   Chemical substance found in CHROMOSOMES within cell nuclei; its molecular structure contains the organism's GENETIC information.

Depacon   Brand name for the ANTICONVULSANT drug VALPROATE.

Depade   Brand name (now discontinued) for the OPIOID ANTAGONIST drug NALTREXONE.

Depakene   Brand name for the ANTICONVULSANT drug VALPROIC ACID.

Depakote   Brand name for the ANTICONVULSANT drug DIVALPROEX SODIUM.

Department of Health and Human Services (DHHS)   A federal department established in 1953 as the U.S. Department of Health, Education and Welfare (DHEW) to supervise and coordinate the following agencies: Agency for Healthcare Research and Quality (AHRQ); Agency for Toxic Substances and Disease Registry

(ATSDR); U.S. FOOD AND DRUG ADMINISTRATION (FDA); SUBSTANCE ABUSE AND MENTAL HEALTH SERVICES ADMINISTRATION (SAMHSA); NATIONAL INSTITUTES OF HEALTH (NIH); CENTERS FOR DISEASE CONTROL AND PREVENTION (CDC); CENTERS FOR MEDICARE AND MEDICAID SERVICES (CMS) (formerly the HEALTH CARE FINANCING ADMINISTRATION [HCFA]); Health Resources and Services Administration (HRSA); and Indian Health Service (IHS). In 1979, a separate Department of Education was established, and DHEW became the DEPARTMENT OF HEALTH AND HUMAN SERVICES (DHHS). In 1995, the Social Security Administration became an independent agency.

dependence   Reliance on someone or something else for support. In PSYCHIATRY, the term is used to refer to needs for protection, security, food, and so forth, as in the child's dependence on a caregiver (see DEPENDENT PERSONALITY DISORDER under PERSONALITY DISORDERS).

dependence (on psychoactive substances)   CHEMICAL DEPENDENCE; sometimes defined in terms of physiological dependence, as evidenced by TOLERANCE or WITHDRAWAL; at other times, defined in terms of impairment in social and occupational functioning resulting from the pathological and repeated use of a substance. In the latter definition, TOLERANCE and WITHDRAWAL SYMPTOMS may be present but are not essential.

The behaviors and effects associated with substance DEPENDENCE include taking of the substance to relieve or avoid WITHDRAWAL SYMPTOMS; taking larger amounts or using it over a longer period than intended; unsuccessful efforts to cut down or control intake; interference with meeting major ROLE obligations at work, school, or home; recurrent use in situations in which it poses a physical hazard (e.g., driving, operating machinery); or substance use taking precedence over important social, occupational, or recreational activities.

dependency needs   Vital needs for mothering, love, affection, shelter, protection, security, food, and warmth. May be a manifestation of REGRESSION when they reappear excessively in adults.

dependent personality disorder   See under PERSONALITY DISORDERS.

depersonalization   Feelings of unreality or strangeness concerning the environment, the self, or both. This state is characteristic of DEPERSONALIZATION DISORDER but also may occur in SCHIZOTYPAL PERSONALITY DISORDER, in SCHIZOPHRENIA, and in persons experiencing overwhelming ANXIETY, stress, or fatigue.

depersonalization disorder   One of the DISSOCIATIVE DISORDERS, characterized by persistent or recurrent feelings of being detached from one's body or mental processes. The affected person often describes a sense of being an automaton or an outside observer of him- or herself.

L-deprenyl   See SELEGILINE.

depression   When used to describe a MOOD, *depression* refers to feelings of sadness, despair, and discouragement. As such, depression may be a normal feeling state. The overt manifestations are highly variable and may be CULTURE specific. Depression may be a SYMPTOM seen in a variety of mental or physical disorders, a SYNDROME of associated symptoms SECONDARY to an underlying disorder, or a specific MENTAL DISORDER. Slowed thinking, anhedonia, decreased energy and concentration, decreased purposeful physical activity, GUILT, lack of appetite, weight loss, and sleep disturbance may be seen in the depressive syndrome. DSM-IV-TR classifies depression by severity, recurrence, and association with HYPOMANIA, MANIA, or PSYCHOSIS. Other categorizations, which are less often used today, divide depression into REACTIVE depression and ENDOGENOUS depression on the basis of precipitants or symptom clusters. Depression in children may be indicated by refusal to go to school, ANXIETY, excessive reaction to separation from parental figures, ANTISOCIAL BEHAVIOR, and somatic complaints.

depression with psychotic features   Major depressive episode with DELUSIONS or HALLUCINATIONS whose content may be consistent with the depressive themes of inadequacy, GUILT, disease, or death. Features such as persecutory DELUSIONS, thought insertion, thought broadcasting, and delusions of control may be present.

depressive disorders   In DSM-IV-TR, a group of MOOD DISORDERS that includes MAJOR DEPRESSIVE DISORDER (single episode or recurrent), DYSTHYMIC DISORDER, and DEPRESSIVE DISORDER NOT OTHERWISE SPECIFIED (NOS).

major depressive disorder   (in other classificatory systems called *major depression; depressed manic-depressive disorder*) occurs in a person who has never had an episode of MANIA and is characterized by significant lowering of the MOOD and loss of interest or pleasure in daily activities, plus a range of other SYMPTOMS that may include significant weight or appetite changes, INSOMNIA or HYPERSOMNIA, PSYCHOMOTOR AGITATION or retardation, fatigue or loss of energy, feelings of worthlessness or excessive and inappropriate GUILT, diminished ability to think or concentrate, indecisiveness, and recurrent thoughts of death or SUICIDE. Some patients have only a single episode of depression, whereas others have recurrent episodes.

dysthymic disorder   is characterized by a CHRONIC course of at least 2 years' duration (i.e., seldom without SYMPTOMS) with depressive MOOD and a range of other symptoms that may include feelings of inadequacy, loss of self-esteem, or self-deprecation; feelings of hopelessness or despair; feelings of GUILT, brooding about past events, or self-pity; low energy and chronic tiredness; being less active or talkative than usual; poor concentration and indecisiveness; and inability to enjoy pleasurable activities. The severity of the depression does not meet the criteria for MAJOR DEPRESSIVE DISORDER.

depressive disorder not otherwise specified (NOS) includes disorders with depressive features that do not meet criteria for MAJOR DEPRESSIVE DISORDER, DYSTHYMIC DISORDER, or ADJUSTMENT DISORDER with depressed mood (or with mixed ANXIETY and depressed mood) or depressive symptoms about which there is inadequate or contradictory information.

depressive personality disorder A proposed disorder (listed in DSM-IV-TR Appendix B, "Criteria Sets and Axes Provided for Further Study") consisting of a persistent, enduring characteristic MOOD tone that is gloomy, cheerless, unhappy, or dejected. The person's self-concepts include persistent beliefs of inadequacy, worthlessness, and low self-esteem. Attitudes toward others are negative, critical, and judgmental. The person is brooding, worrisome, pessimistic, and prone to feelings of GUILT. Depressive personality disorder has considerable overlap with DYSTHYMIC DISORDER.

depressive position A term applied by Melanie Klein (1882–1960) and her followers to the stage of development that peaks about the sixth month of life. The infant begins to FEAR destroying and losing the beloved object and wants to appease it and preserve it.

depth psychology An inexact term referring to the PSYCHOLOGY of UNCONSCIOUS mental processes. Also a system of psychology in which the study of such processes plays a major role, as in PSYCHOANALYSIS.

derealization A feeling of estrangement or DETACHMENT from one's environment. May be accompanied by DEPERSONALIZATION.

dereflection See EXISTENTIAL PSYCHOTHERAPY.

dereistic Referring to mental activity that is not in accordance with reality, logic, or experience. See also AUTISTIC DISORDER.

dermatillomania A disorder (classified as an IMPULSE-CONTROL DISORDER not otherwise specified [NOS] in DSM-IV-TR) in which the patient inflicts excessive scratching, picking, and squeezing on healthy skin. May be a SYMPTOM of a variety of psychiatric disorders, including STEREOTYPIC MOVEMENT DISORDER, BODY DYSMORPHIC DISORDER (BDD), and Tourette's disorder. Many patients with dermatillomania have a comorbid mood, anxiety, or somatoform disorder. Also known as *psychogenic excoriation* or *compulsive skin picking.*

descriptive psychiatry   A system of psychiatry based on the study of readily observable external factors. Often used to refer to the systematized descriptions of mental illness formulated by Emil Kraepelin (1856–1926).

desensitization   See systematic desensitization.

designer drugs   Addictive drugs that are synthesized or manufactured to give the same subjective effects as well-known illicit drugs. Because the process is covert and illegal, tracing the manufacturer to check the drugs for adverse effects is difficult. Common examples are ecstasy and "Eve," both of which are similar to amphetamines.

desipramine   A tricyclic antidepressant medication used in the treatment of depression. Marketed under the brand name Norpramin. See "Medications Used in Psychiatry."

desmopressin acetate   A synthetic analogue of the natural hormone 8-arginine vasopressin (an antidiuretic hormone that reduces urine production by limiting the amount of water eliminated in the urine) that is used to treat primary nocturnal enuresis, a disorder believed to be caused by inadequate release of this hormone by the pituitary. Marketed under the brand name DDAVP.

Desoxyn   Brand name for the longer-acting, legally produced form of the psychostimulant drug methamphetamine.

desvenlafaxine   A synthetic form of an active metabolite of venlafaxine (an atypical antidepressant of the serotonin-norepinephrine reuptake inhibitor [SNRI] class) approved for the treatment of major depressive disorder. Marketed under the brand name Pristiq. See "Medications Used in Psychiatry."

Desyrel   Brand name (now discontinued) for the atypical antidepressant drug trazodone.

detachment   A behavior pattern characterized by general aloofness in interpersonal contact; may include intellectualization, denial, and superficiality.

determinism   The theory that one's emotional life does not result from chance alone but rather from specific causes or forces, known or unknown.

detoxification   The process of providing medical care during the removal of dependence-producing substances from the body so that

WITHDRAWAL SYMPTOMS are minimized and physiological function is safely restored. Treatment includes medication, rest, diet, fluids, and nursing care.

devaluation A mental mechanism in which one attributes exaggeratedly negative qualities to oneself or others.

developmental arrest An interruption, as a result of trauma, constitution, or both, in the expectable unfolding of psychological development of an individual. A developmental arrest may profoundly affect the quality of the adult personality of the individual.

developmental coordination disorder A MOTOR SKILLS DISORDER consisting of a level of motor coordination in daily activities that is significantly lower than expected, given the subject's age, INTELLIGENCE, and age-appropriate education. Manifestations include delayed motor milestones (e.g., crawling, walking), clumsiness, and poor handwriting. The term is applied only to presentations that are not due to a GENERAL MEDICAL CONDITION such as cerebral palsy or muscular dystrophy.

developmental delay Delay in the development of functions such as speaking, reading, arithmetic ability, motor skills, and social and communication skills.

developmental disorders A category of childhood disorders characterized by delay or ABNORMALITY in the development of functions such as speaking, reading, arithmetic ability, motor skills, and social and communication skills.

developmental lines The different stages through which an organism passes during its life span, often described separately for different organ systems or functions. Each stage usually shows characteristic features and presents its own challenges that must be met if development is to proceed normally.

Dexedrine Brand name for the psychostimulant drug DEXTROAMPHETAMINE.

dexmethylphenidate A mild STIMULANT of the CENTRAL NERVOUS SYSTEM (CNS) used to treat ATTENTION-DEFICIT/HYPERACTIVITY DISORDER. Marketed under the brand name FOCALIN. See "Medications Used in Psychiatry."

dextroamphetamine A form of AMPHETAMINE used to treat NARCOLEPSY and ATTENTION-DEFICIT/HYPERACTIVITY DISORDER (ADHD) in children and adults. In some cases, this drug has been used to treat DEPRESSION or as an ADJUNCTIVE therapy in the treatment of EXOGENOUS OBESITY. This medication is known as a CENTRAL NERVOUS SYSTEM (CNS)

STIMULANT. Marketed under the brand names DEXEDRINE (dextroamphetamine) and ADDERALL (DEXTROAMPHETAMINE and AMPHETAMINE MIXED SALTS); may also be known by the discontinued brand name DEXTROSTAT. See "Medications Used in Psychiatry."

DextroStat Brand name (now discontinued) for the psychostimulant drug DEXTROAMPHETAMINE.

dhat A folk diagnostic term used in India to refer to severe anxiety and hypochondriacal concerns associated with the discharge of semen, whitish discoloration of the urine, and feelings of weakness and exhaustion. Similar to *JIRYAN* (India), *SUKRA PRAMEHA* (Sri Lanka), and *SHEN-K'UEI* (China). See CULTURE-SPECIFIC SYNDROMES.

diagnosis The process of determining, through examination and analysis, the nature of a patient's illness.

diagnosis-related group (DRG) Medical-based classification, representing 23 major diagnostic categories, that aggregates patients into case types based on DIAGNOSIS. A DRG is a subset of a major diagnostic category.

Diagnostic and Statistical Manual of Mental Disorders **(DSM)** The AMERICAN PSYCHIATRIC ASSOCIATION's official classification of MENTAL DISORDERS. The DSM is an evolving text that is periodically revised to reflect the most recent knowledge regarding mental disorders.

DSM-I The first edition, published in 1952.

DSM-II The second edition, published in 1968.

DSM-III The third edition, published in 1980.

DSM-III-R The revised DSM-III, published in 1987.

DSM-IV The fourth edition, published in 1994.

DSM-IV-TR The evidence-based revision of the DSM-IV text, published in 2000.

DSM-5 The fifth edition, scheduled for publication in 2013.

dialectical behavior therapy (DBT) A form of PSYCHOTHERAPY that teaches behavioral and COGNITIVE coping skills, developed specifically for patients with BORDERLINE PERSONALITY DISORDER.

diazepam A long-acting BENZODIAZEPINE ANXIOLYTIC medication used to treat various ANXIETY DISORDERS as well as alcohol WITHDRAWAL SYMPTOMS. Marketed under the brand name VALIUM. See "Medications Used in Psychiatry."

dibenzoxazepines A subgroup of CONVENTIONAL ANTIPSYCHOTIC medications that includes LOXAPINE.

DID See DISSOCIATIVE IDENTITY DISORDER (DID).

diencephalon The part of the FOREBRAIN that contains such important structures as the THALAMUS, HYPOTHALAMUS, and posterior portion of the pituitary gland.

differential diagnosis The process whereby multiple possible disorders are considered by a clinician to formulate a final DIAGNOSIS.

differentiation The degree to which an individual identifies the SELF as separate or distinct from others. See SEPARATION-INDIVIDUATION.

diffuse axonal injury One of the most common and devastating types of TRAUMATIC BRAIN INJURY (TBI), where damage occurs over a more widespread area than in focal brain injury. Diffuse axonal injury, which refers to extensive lesions in WHITE MATTER tracts, is one of the major causes of unconsciousness and persistent vegetative state after head trauma. It occurs in about half of all cases of severe head trauma and also occurs in moderate and mild TBI.

diffusion tensor imaging (DTI) A MAGNETIC RESONANCE IMAGING (MRI) technique that enables measurement of the restricted diffusion of water in tissue in order to produce neural tract images instead of using these data solely for the purpose of assigning contrast or colors to pixels in a cross-sectional image. DTI is mainly used in imaging of the white matter of the brain. DTI data can also be used to track a fiber, or path, through which information travels in the brain. See also DIFFUSION-WEIGHTED IMAGING (DWI).

diffusion-weighted imaging (DWI) A MAGNETIC RESONANCE IMAGING (MRI) technique that produces in vivo magnetic resonance images of biological tissues weighted with the local characteristics of water diffusion. Areas of cerebral infarction have decreased apparent diffusion, which results in increased signal intensity on DWI scans. DWI has been demonstrated to be more sensitive for the early detection of STROKE than standard pulse sequences and is closely related to temperature mapping. See also DIFFUSION TENSOR IMAGING (DTI).

DiGeorge syndrome See VELOCARDIOFACIAL SYNDROME (VCFS).

dihydroindolones A subgroup of CONVENTIONAL ANTIPSYCHOTIC medications that includes the discontinued drug MOLINDONE.

Dilantin Brand name for the ANTICONVULSANT drug PHENYTOIN.

diminished capacity See "Legal Terms."

diphenhydramine An ANTIHISTAMINE medication used in general medical practice to treat cold or allergy SYMPTOMS and pruritus (itching) and used in PSYCHIATRY as an ANXIOLYTIC or to treat SLEEP disturbance. Marketed under the brand name BENADRYL. See "Medications Used in Psychiatry."

diphenylbutylpiperidines A subgroup of CONVENTIONAL ANTIPSYCHOTIC drugs that includes PIMOZIDE (ORAP).

diphenylhydantoin See PHENYTOIN.

diplopia Double vision due to paralysis of the ocular muscles; seen in inhalant INTOXICATION and other conditions affecting the oculomotor nerve.

disability (psychiatric) Lack of intellectual or emotional capacity or fitness. As defined by the federal government, "Inability to engage in any substantial gainful activity by reason of any medically determinable physical or mental impairment which can be expected to last or has lasted for a continuous period of not less than 12 full months."

DISC1 See DISRUPTED-IN-SCHIZOPHRENIA 1 (*DISC1*) GENE.

disconnection syndrome A term coined by the NEUROLOGIST Norman Geschwind (1926–1984) to describe the interruption of information transferred from one BRAIN region to another.

disinhibition 1) In psychological terms, refers to freedom to act according to one's inner DRIVES or feelings, with less regard for restraints imposed by cultural norms or one's SUPEREGO.

2) In NEUROLOGY, refers to removal of an inhibitory, constraining, or limiting influence, as in the failure of cortical control over emotions or behaviors regulated by more primitive BRAIN structures. An example is a person with frontal lobe injury from an automobile accident expressing violent rage over a child's playing with food during a family dinner.

3) In neurobiology, may refer to uncontrolled firing of impulses, as when a drug interferes with the usual limiting or inhibiting action of GABA (GAMMA-AMINOBUTYRIC ACID) within the CENTRAL NERVOUS SYSTEM (CNS).

disintegration anxiety See FRAGMENTATION.

disintegrative disorder See CHILDHOOD DISINTEGRATIVE DISORDER.

disorder of written expression A LEARNING DISORDER characterized by a substantially lower than expected level of writing skills given the subject's chronological age, measured INTELLIGENCE, and age-appropriate education.

disorientation Loss of awareness of the position of the SELF in relation to space, time, or other persons; confusion. See also DELIRIUM; DEMENTIA.

displacement A DEFENSE MECHANISM, operating unconsciously (see UNCONSCIOUS), in which EMOTIONS, ideas, or wishes are transferred from their original object to a more acceptable substitute; often used to allay ANXIETY. This mechanism is commonly observed in dreams and in the formation of PHOBIAS.

Disrupted-in-Schizophrenia 1 (*DISC1*) gene A GENE that controls the birth of new neurons in addition to integration of those neurons into existing BRAIN circuitry. This finding suggests that loss of the gene, as occurs in some cases of SCHIZOPHRENIA as well as BIPOLAR DISORDERS and MAJOR DEPRESSIVE DISORDER, may lead to an increased risk of compromised COGNITION and behavioral abnormalities.

disruptive behavior and attention-deficit disorders In DSM-IV-TR, a group of MENTAL DISORDERS that includes ATTENTION-DEFICIT/HYPERACTIVITY DISORDER (ADHD), CONDUCT DISORDER, and OPPOSITIONAL DEFIANT DISORDER.

disruptive behavior disorders In children and adolescents, the disruptive behavior disorders are characterized by willful disobedience and externally directed behavior, including blaming of others for problems. In DSM-IV-TR, this category includes CONDUCT DISORDER and OPPOSITIONAL DEFIANT DISORDER.

moderate conduct disturbance SYMPTOMS may include truancy or work absences, alcohol or other substance use before age 13 years, stealing without confrontation, destruction of others' property, fire setting with intent of causing serious damage, initiating fights outside of home, and being physically cruel to animals.

oppositional defiant disorder SYMPTOMS may include losing temper; arguing with adults and actively refusing their requests; deliberately annoying others; blaming others for one's mistakes; being easily annoyed, resentful, or spiteful; and physically fighting with other members of the household.

severe conduct disturbance SYMPTOMS may include running away from home overnight at least twice, breaking into another's property, being physically cruel to people, stealing with confrontation, repeatedly using a dangerous weapon, and forcing someone into sexual activity.

dissociation The splitting off of clusters of mental contents from CONSCIOUS awareness. Dissociation is a mechanism central to CONVERSION DISORDERS and DISSOCIATIVE DISORDERS. The term is also used to describe the separation of an idea from its emotional significance and AFFECT as seen in the INAPPROPRIATE AFFECT of schizophrenic patients.

Often a result of psychic trauma, dissociation may allow the individual to maintain allegiance to two contradictory truths while remaining unconscious of the contradiction. An extreme manifestation of dissociation is DISSOCIATIVE IDENTITY DISORDER (DID), in which a person may exhibit several independent personalities, each unaware of the others.

dissociative amnesia   Formerly known as *psychogenic amnesia*. A MEMORY impairment, characterized by sudden and brief loss of personal information, with no other COGNITIVE disturbance, often in response to traumatic or stressful events.

dissociative disorders   In DSM-IV-TR, this category includes DISSOCIATIVE AMNESIA, DISSOCIATIVE FUGUE, DISSOCIATIVE IDENTITY DISORDER (DID; MULTIPLE PERSONALITY DISORDER), DEPERSONALIZATION DISORDER, and dissociative disorder not otherwise specified.

dissociative fugue   A DISSOCIATIVE DISORDER marked by sudden, unexpected travel away from one's customary environment, with inability to RECALL one's past. The disturbance is accompanied by confusion about one's personal IDENTITY or even the assumption of a new identity.

dissociative identity disorder (DID)   Formerly known as *multiple personality disorder*. It consists of the existence within one person of two or more distinct personalities or PERSONALITY states (*alters* or *alter personalities*). Each personality state has its own relatively enduring pattern of perceiving, relating to, and thinking about the environment and the self, and at least two of them alternate in taking control of the person's behavior. Characteristically, there is an amnesic barrier between personalities, which may be absolute or, more commonly, unilateral, denying one personality access to the MEMORIES of the other but allowing the other personality full access to the memory systems of both.

dissociative symptoms   Any altered form of consciousness that changes the sense of self or the ability to integrate MEMORIES and PERCEPTIONS.

dissociative trance disorder   A proposed disorder (listed in DSM-IV-TR Appendix B, "Criteria Sets and Axes Provided for Further Study") characterized by a disturbance of the normally integrative functions of MEMORY, IDENTITY, or consciousness or by a conviction of having been taken over by a spirit, a deity, or another person (i.e., possession). In a TRANCE, consciousness is altered and responsivity is markedly diminished or selectively focused. Other dissociative phenomena may include amnestic episodes and the assumption of a different identity. The SYMPTOMS cause significant distress or impairment in functioning, and they fall outside the sanctioned religious practices of the community.

Many different CULTURE-SPECIFIC SYNDROMES, indigenous to particular locations and CULTURES and predominated by trance and possession phenomena, have been described.

distractibility   Inability to maintain ATTENTION. The person shifts from one area or topic to another with minimal provocation. Distractibility may be a manifestation of an underlying medical disease, medication SIDE EFFECT, or a MENTAL DISORDER such as an ANXIETY DISORDER, MANIA, or SCHIZOPHRENIA.

distributive analysis and synthesis   The therapy used by the psychobiological school of PSYCHIATRY developed by Adolf Meyer (1866–1950). It entails extensive guided and directed investigation and analysis of the patient's entire past experience, stressing assets and liabilities to make possible a constructive synthesis. See PSYCHOBIOLOGY.

disulfiram   A medication used to reinforce alcohol abstinence in patients with ALCOHOLISM because it produces severe nausea and vomiting when the person drinks. Disulfiram inhibits ALCOHOL DEHYDROGENASE, an ENZYME involved in alcohol metabolism in the liver, and the resultant buildup of acetaldehyde produces symptoms of nausea and vomiting, with severity depending on concentration. Patients must be counseled against using topical agents containing alcohol (e.g., perfume, aftershave) or consuming liquids or foods containing alcohol (e.g., mouthwashes, foods cooked in alcohol). Marketed under the brand name ANTABUSE. See "Medications Used in Psychiatry."

divalproex sodium   An ANTICONVULSANT medication used in PSYCHIATRY as a MOOD STABILIZER to treat BIPOLAR DISORDER. Marketed under the brand name DEPAKOTE. See "Medications Used in Psychiatry."

dizygotic twins   Twins who develop from two separately fertilized ova. Also called *fraternal* twins.

DNA   See DEOXYRIBONUCLEIC ACID (DNA).

doli incapax   See "Legal Terms."

dominance   In psychological terms, a predisposition to play a prominent or controlling ROLE when interacting with others. In NEUROLOGY, the (normal) tendency of one-half of the BRAIN to be more important than the other in mediating various functions (cerebral dominance). In GENETICS, the ability of one GENE (dominant gene) to express itself in the PHENOTYPE of an individual when paired with another (recessive) gene that would have expressed itself in a different way.

donepezil   An ACETYLCHOLINESTERASE INHIBITOR used in the treatment of DEMENTIA. Marketed under the brand name ARICEPT. See "Medications Used in Psychiatry."

L-dopa   See LEVODOPA.

dopamine (3,4-dihydroxyphenylethylamine)   A CATECHOLAMINE NEUROTRANSMITTER found in the BRAIN. Neuropathology involving DOPAMINERGIC systems in the brain is associated with some forms of PSYCHOSIS and MOVEMENT DISORDERS. Dopamine is the primary neurotransmitter involved in the reward pathways in the brain. Consequently, drugs that increase dopamine signaling (i.e., DOPAMINE AGONISTS) may produce euphoric effects. See also BIOGENIC AMINES.

dopamine agonists   Drugs that bind to DOPAMINE RECEPTORS in place of DOPAMINE and directly stimulate those receptors. Some dopamine AGONISTS are currently used to treat PARKINSON'S DISEASE.

dopamine antagonists   Drugs that block or reverse the actions of DOPAMINE by preventing dopamine from attaching to DOPAMINE RECEPTORS. In psychiatry, dopamine ANTAGONISTS (i.e., ANTIPSYCHOTICS) have traditionally been used to treat SCHIZOPHRENIA. It has been hypothesized that people with schizophrenia may have an overactive dopamine system. Dopamine antagonists can help regulate this system by "turning down" dopamine activity.

dopamine hypothesis   A theory postulating that the pathogenesis of SCHIZOPHRENIA and other psychotic states is due to excesses in DOPAMINE activity in various areas of the BRAIN. This theory is based in part on observations that the ANTIPSYCHOTIC properties of specific drugs may be related to their ability to block the action of dopamine (and hence treat the SYMPTOMS of PSYCHOSIS) and the opposite effects observed with PSYCHOTOMIMETIC drugs such as AMPHETAMINES that increase the action of dopamine (which may produce symptoms of psychosis).

dopamine receptors   Sites located on the surface membranes of NEURONS in the CENTRAL NERVOUS SYSTEM (CNS) and in cells outside the CNS (e.g., kidneys) to which the NEUROTRANSMITTER DOPAMINE binds, activating dopamine signaling and cellular response. Dopamine receptors (of which there are five known subtypes: D_1–D_5) are involved in many neurological processes, including motivation, pleasure, cognition, memory, learning, and fine motor control, as well as in modulation of neuroendocrine signaling. Dopamine receptors have been recognized as important components in the etiology of ATTENTION-DEFICIT/HYPERACTIVITY DISORDER (ADHD). Drugs used to treat ADHD (including METHYLPHENIDATE and AMPHETAMINE) have significant effects on dopamine signaling in the brain.

dopaminergic   Referring to the NEUROTRANSMITTER DOPAMINE (3,4-DIHYDROXYPHENYLETHYLAMINE).

Doral   Brand name for the BENZODIAZEPINE SEDATIVE-HYPNOTIC drug QUAZEPAM.

double bind   Interaction in which one person demands a response to a message containing mutually contradictory signals, while the other person is unable either to comment on the incongruity or to escape from the situation.

double-blind   Referring to a study design in which several treatments, usually one or more drugs and a PLACEBO, are compared in such a way that neither the patient nor the persons directly involved in the study know which treatment is being administered.

Down syndrome   Also known as TRISOMY 21, a common form of INTELLECTUAL DISABILITY caused by a chromosomal abnormality formerly called MONGOLISM. Two types are recognized, based on the nature of the chromosomal aberration: the translocation type and the nondisjunction type. Physical findings include widely spaced eyes with slanting openings, small head with flattened occiput, lax joints, flabby hands, small ears, and CONGENITAL anomalies of the heart. See also CHROMOSOME 21.

doxepin   A TRICYCLIC ANTIDEPRESSANT medication used in the treatment of DEPRESSION. Now available only as generic but may still be known by the discontinued brand names ADAPIN and SINEQUAN. See "Medications Used in Psychiatry."

dream anxiety disorder   NIGHTMARE DISORDER. See PARASOMNIAS.

DRG   See DIAGNOSIS-RELATED GROUP (DRG).

drive   Basic urge, INSTINCT, motivation; a term used to avoid confusion with the more purely biological concept of INSTINCT.

drug abuse   See ABUSE (of psychoactive substances).

drug court   A court given responsibility to handle cases involving substance-abusing offenders through comprehensive supervision, drug testing, treatment services, and immediate sanctions and incentives. Drug court offers individuals facing criminal charges for drug use and possession an opportunity to enter a substance abuse recovery program in lieu of serving straight jail time. The first drug court in the United

States took shape in Miami–Dade County, Florida, in 1989 as a response to the growing CRACK COCAINE problem plaguing the city.

drug dependence   Habituation to, ABUSE of, and/or ADDICTION to a chemical substance. Largely because of psychological craving, the life of the drug-dependent person revolves around the need for the specific effect of one or more chemical agents on MOOD or state of consciousness. The term thus includes not only the addiction (which emphasizes the physiological DEPENDENCE) but also drug ABUSE (in which the pathological craving for drugs seems unrelated to physical dependence). Substances capable of inducing dependence include alcohol, OPIATES, synthetic ANALGESICS with morphine-like effects, BARBITURATES, other HYPNOTICS, SEDATIVES, certain ANXIOLYTICS, COCAINE, psychostimulants, MARIJUANA, and PSYCHOTOMIMETIC drugs. See also DEPENDENCE (on psychoactive substances).

drug holiday   Discontinuance of a therapeutic drug for a limited time. Sometimes a drug holiday is used as a method of evaluating baseline behavior or as a means of controlling or reducing the dosage of psychoactive drugs and SIDE EFFECTS.

drug-induced parkinsonism (pseudoparkinsonism)   A SYNDROME resembling PARKINSON'S DISEASE, resulting from the DOPAMINE-blocking action of ANTIPSYCHOTICS, particularly the CONVENTIONAL ANTIPSYCHOTIC medications. The SYMPTOMS include AKINESIA (reduced voluntary motor movements), masklike FACIES, and a coarse, pill-rolling TREMOR. The tremor is less common in this syndrome than in the naturally occurring disorder.

drug interaction   The effects of two or more drugs taken concomitantly, producing an alteration in the usual effects of either drug taken alone. The interacting drugs may have a potentiating or additive effect and produce SIDE EFFECTS. An example of drug interaction is alcohol and SEDATIVE drugs taken together, leading to intensification of CENTRAL NERVOUS SYSTEM (CNS) depression.

drug levels   See BLOOD LEVELS.

drug tolerance   See TOLERANCE.

DSM   See *DIAGNOSTIC AND STATISTICAL MANUAL OF MENTAL DISORDERS* (DSM).

DT   See DELIRIUM TREMENS (DT).

DTI   See DIFFUSION TENSOR IMAGING (DTI).

dual addiction   Coexisting substance ABUSE and MENTAL ILLNESS.

dual diagnosis   The co-occurrence within one's lifetime of a psychiatric disorder and a SUBSTANCE USE DISORDER. COMORBIDITY is the preferred term.

due process of law   See "Legal Terms."

duloxetine   A SEROTONIN-NOREPINEPHRINE REUPTAKE INHIBITOR (SNRI) medication indicated for the treatment of MAJOR DEPRESSIVE DISORDER and GENERALIZED ANXIETY DISORDER. It is also approved for the treatment of pain in diabetic PERIPHERAL NEUROPATHY, FIBROMYALGIA, and chronic musculoskeletal conditions. Marketed under the brand name CYMBALTA. See "Medications Used in Psychiatry."

dummy   British term for PLACEBO.

durable power of attorney   See "Legal Terms."

dura mater   The outermost layer of the meninges that cover the BRAIN and SPINAL CORD. The subdural space lies below it and separates it from the arachnoid membrane.

duress   See "Legal Terms."

Durham **rule**   See under INSANITY DEFENSE in "Legal Terms."

duty   See "Legal Terms."

duty to warn   See "Legal Terms."

DWI   See DIFFUSION-WEIGHTED IMAGING (DWI).

dyad   A two-person relationship, such as the therapeutic relationship between doctor and patient in individual PSYCHOTHERAPY.

dynamic psychiatry   The study of PSYCHIATRY from the point of view of motivation, emphasizing both psychological meaning and biological INSTINCTS as forces relevant to understanding human behavior in health and illness.

dynamic psychotherapy   See PSYCHODYNAMIC PSYCHOTHERAPY.

dynamics   See PSYCHODYNAMICS.

dys–   Prefix typically used to indicate that a function has not developed normally (e.g., dyscalculia, DYSGRAPHIA, and DYSLEXIA) or to indicate a lack of normal function.

dysarthria   Difficulty in speech production caused by lack of coordination of the speech apparatus.

dyscalculia   See LEARNING DISABILITY.

dysgeusia   Impaired taste. Also known as *parageusia.*

tal and social prohibitions (the SUPEREGO), and of reality. The compromises between these forces achieved by the ego tend to resolve INTRAPSYCHIC CONFLICT and serve an adaptive and executive function. Psychiatric usage of the term should not be confused with common usage, which connotes self-love or selfishness.

ego-alien   See EGO-DYSTONIC.

ego analysis   Intensive psychoanalytic study and analysis of the ways in which the EGO resolves or attempts to deal with INTRAPSYCHIC CONFLICTS, especially in relation to the development of mental mechanisms and the maturation of capacity for rational thought and action. Modern PSYCHOANALYSIS gives more emphasis to considerations of the defensive operations of the ego than did earlier techniques, which emphasized instinctual forces to a greater degree.

ego boundaries   Hypothesized lines of demarcation between the EGO and 1) the external world (external ego boundary) and 2) the internal world, including the repressed UNCONSCIOUS, the ID, and much of the SUPEREGO (internal ego boundary).

egocentric   Self-centered.

ego-dystonic   Referring to aspects of a person's behavior, thoughts, and attitudes that are viewed by the SELF as repugnant or inconsistent with the total PERSONALITY and sense of self. Contrast with EGO-SYNTONIC.

ego functions   According to the theoretical system of Carl Gustav Jung (1875–1961), the EGO has four inseparable functions (i.e., four different fundamental ways of perceiving and interpreting reality): thinking, feeling, sensation, and intuition. Thinking is the opposite of feeling, and sensation is the opposite of intuition. Jung suggested that most people start life developing one of these four ego functions and at various stages throughout life may develop others. The undeveloped ego functions have less effect on the individual's COGNITION.

ego ideal   The part of the PERSONALITY that comprises the aims and goals for the SELF; usually refers to the CONSCIOUS or UNCONSCIOUS emulation of significant figures with which one has identified. The EGO ideal emphasizes what one should be or do in contrast to what one should not be or not do.

egomania   Pathological preoccupation with self. See –MANIA.

ego psychology   The study and elucidation of those slowly changing functions known as *psychic structures* that usually shape, channel, and organize mental activity into meaningful and tolerable patterns of experience. The usual structures referred to in this sense are MEM-

ORY, speech, locomotion, COGNITION, DRIVE, restraint, discharge, and the capacity to make JUDGMENTS and decisions.

ego strength   The ability of the EGO to execute its functions, to mediate between the external world, the ID, and the SUPEREGO effectively and efficiently, so that energy is left over for creativity and other integrative activities. Among specific functions that may be assessed in determining ego strength are JUDGMENT, REALITY TESTING, regulation of DRIVES, defensive functions, thought processes, and OBJECT RELATIONS.

ego-syntonic   Referring to aspects of a person's behavior, thoughts, and attitudes that are viewed by the SELF as acceptable and consistent with the total PERSONALITY and sense of self. Contrast with EGO-DYSTONIC.

eidetic image   Unusually vivid and apparently exact mental image; may be a MEMORY, FANTASY, or dream.

ejaculatio retardata   See ORGASMIC DISORDERS.

ejaculatory incompetence (impotence)   MALE ORGASMIC DISORDER (see under ORGASMIC DISORDERS).

elaboration   An UNCONSCIOUS process consisting of expansion and embellishment of detail, especially with reference to a symbol or representation in a dream.

Elavil   Brand name (now discontinued) for the TRICYCLIC ANTIDEPRESSANT drug AMITRIPTYLINE.

Eldepryl   Brand name for the MONOAMINE OXIDASE (MAO) B inhibitor drug SELEGILINE.

elective mutism   See SELECTIVE MUTISM.

Electra complex   The female OEDIPUS COMPLEX; an infrequently used term describing the pathological relationship between a woman and a man based on unresolved developmental CONFLICTS.

electroconvulsive therapy (ECT)   The use of electric current with anesthetics and muscle relaxants to induce convulsive SEIZURES. It is most effective in the treatment of DEPRESSION. It was introduced in 1938 by Italian PSYCHIATRISTS Ugo Cerletti (1877–1963) and Lucio Bini (1908–1964). The American Psychiatric Association Task Force on ECT (2000) found ECT useful for the treatment of major depression, MANIA or BIPOLAR DISORDER, SCHIZOPHRENIA with CATATONIA or prominent affective symptomatology, SCHIZOPHRENIFORM DISORDER, and SCHIZOAFFECTIVE DISORDER. Modifications are electronarcosis, which produces sleep-like states, and ELECTROSTIMULATION, which avoids convulsions.

electroencephalogram (EEG)   A graphic (voltage vs. time) depiction of the BRAIN's electrical potentials (BRAIN WAVES) recorded by scalp electrodes. It is used for the DIAGNOSIS of neurological and neuropsychiatric disorders (especially SEIZURE disorders) and in neurophysiological research. Sometimes used interchangeably with *electrocorticogram* and *depth record,* in which the electrodes are in direct contact with brain tissue.

electromyogram (EMG)   An electrophysiological recording of muscle potentials that measures the amount and nature of muscle activity at the site from which the recording is taken.

electroshock treatment   See ELECTROCONVULSIVE THERAPY (ECT).

electrostimulation   See ELECTROCONVULSIVE THERAPY (ECT).

elimination disorders   Included in this group are FUNCTIONAL ENCOPRESIS and functional ENURESIS.

elopement   A patient's unauthorized departure from a psychiatric facility.

emancipated minor   See "Legal Terms."

EMDR   See EYE MOVEMENT DESENSITIZATION AND REPROCESSING (EMDR).

emergence   See EPIGENESIS.

EMG   See ELECTROMYOGRAM (EMG).

emotion   A state of AROUSAL determined by a set of subjective feelings, often accompanied by physiological changes, that impels one toward action. Examples are FEAR, anger, love, and hate. See AFFECT.

emotional-control therapies   See EXPERIENTIAL THERAPY.

emotional deprivation   Lack of adequate and appropriate interpersonal and/or environmental experience, usually in the early developmental years.

emotional disturbance   See MENTAL DISORDER.

emotional illness   See MENTAL DISORDER.

emotional lability   A condition characterized by excessive emotional reactions and frequent MOOD changes. It is often seen in patients with ALZHEIMER'S DISEASE, STROKE, brain injury, ATTENTION-DEFICIT/HYPERACTIVITY DISORDER (ADHD), or BORDERLINE PERSONALITY DISORDER.

emotional-release therapies   See EXPERIENTIAL THERAPY.

empathic failure   As conceptualized by Heinz Kohut (1913–1981), lack of responsivity to a child's phase-appropriate needs. In a treatment setting, the term refers to a therapist's lack of responsivity to the patient. See HOLDING ENVIRONMENT; MIRRORING.

empathy   Insightful awareness of the meaning and significance of the feelings, EMOTIONS, and behavior of another person. Contrast with SYMPATHY.

employee assistance program (EAP) Confidential help provided by companies and other employers to their employees for personal problems that might influence their ability to work effectively. These programs were started in the early 1900s as employee counseling, became focused in the 1960s on helping employees who were having problems with alcohol, and expanded subsequently to include other personal problems.

EMSAM Brand name for SELEGILINE TRANSDERMAL SYSTEM.

encephalitis Acute or chronic inflammation of the BRAIN caused by viruses, bacteria, spirochetes, fungi, or protozoa. Neurological SIGNS and SYMPTOMS and various mental and behavioral changes occur during the illness and may persist. See also ENCEPHALOPATHY.

encephalopathy An imprecise term referring to any disorder of BRAIN function (metabolic, toxic, neoplastic) but often implying a chronic degenerative process.

encopresis A developmental problem, characterized by the repeated voluntary or involuntary defecation into clothing or in other inappropriate places, occurring in children ages 4 years and older.

encounter group therapy See EXPERIENTIAL THERAPY.

endemic See under EPIDEMIOLOGY.

Endep Brand name (now discontinued) for the TRICYCLIC ANTIDEPRESSANT drug AMITRIPTYLINE.

endocrine disorders Disturbances of the function of the ductless glands, which may be metabolic in origin and may be associated with, or aggravated by, emotional factors, producing mental and behavioral disturbances in addition to physical SIGNS.

Of particular significance in PSYCHIATRY is the HYPOTHALAMIC-PITUITARY-ADRENAL AXIS (HPA AXIS), consisting of a self-regulating cycle of NEUROHORMONES released from the HYPOTHALAMUS and stimulating the release of HORMONES from the anterior pituitary. These in turn stimulate hormone secretion in target organs (thyroid, adrenal glands, and gonads). The HPA axis is involved in the regulation of sexual activity, thirst, hunger, SLEEP, learning, MEMORY, and perhaps ANTIDEPRESSANT activity.

endogenous Originating or beginning within the organism. Contrast with EXOGENOUS.

endogenous depression See DEPRESSION.

endogenous psychoses The various forms of SCHIZOPHRENIA and MOOD DISORDERS and primary degenerative disorders of the CENTRAL

NERVOUS SYSTEM (CNS) that, so far as it is known, arise within the organism itself. This term is becoming increasingly obsolete as the neurobiological basis of many psychiatric disorders is being established. Hence, most psychiatric disorders will be found to be ENDOGENOUS. Contrast with EXOGENOUS PSYCHOSES.

endomorphic   See CONSTITUTIONAL TYPES.

endorphins   OPIOID peptides secreted in the BRAIN that have a pain-relieving effect similar to that of MORPHINE. These peptides may be released in response to prolonged exercise, such as the "runner's high" experienced by long-distance runners.

engram   A MEMORY trace; a neurophysiological process that accounts for persistence of memory.

enkephalin   ENDOGENOUS OPIOID peptide found in the BRAIN that may serve as a NEUROTRANSMITTER.

entacapone   An inhibitor of CATECHOL-O-METHYLTRANSFERASE (COMT) used as an ADJUNCT to CARBIDOPA-LEVODOPA therapy in the treatment of PARKINSON'S DISEASE for patients who experience the signs and symptoms of end-of-dose "wearing-off." Entacapone primarily inhibits the peripheral metabolism of levodopa by COMT, allowing greater and more sustained levels of levodopa to penetrate the brain, where it can be converted to DOPAMINE. Marketed under the brand name COMTAN.

entitlement   The right or claim to something. In health law, the term *entitlement programs* refers to legislatively defined rights to health care, such as MEDICARE and MEDICAID programs.

   In psychodynamic PSYCHIATRY, *entitlement* usually refers to an unreasonable expectation or unfounded claim. An example is a person with NARCISSISTIC PERSONALITY DISORDER who feels deserving of preferred status and special treatment in the absence of apparent justification for such treatment.

entomophobia   The FEAR of insects.

enuresis   The repeated voiding of urine into bed or clothes in children at least 5 years old, not due to any GENERAL MEDICAL CONDITION. May be associated with various psychosocial factors, such as early childhood hospitalization, the birth of a younger sibling, or serious trauma.

enzyme   An organic compound that interacts with a biological substrate to form a new chemical, either (and more commonly) through the process of synthesis or through degradation. For example, the enzyme MONOAMINE OXIDASE degrades BIOGENIC AMINES.

epidemic hysteria   Also called *mass psychogenic illness*; the development of SYMPTOMS in a group of persons in response to a stimulus in a closed environment, such as the development of breathing difficulties in students after exposure to nontoxic fumes at their school.

Epidemiologic Catchment Area (ECA) study   This study was initiated in response to the 1977 report of the President's Commission on Mental Health. The purpose was to collect data on the PREVALENCE and INCIDENCE of MENTAL DISORDERS and on the use of, and need for, services by the mentally ill. Research teams at five universities (Yale University, Johns Hopkins University, Washington University, Duke University, and the University of California at Los Angeles), in collaboration with the NATIONAL INSTITUTE OF MENTAL HEALTH (NIMH), conducted the studies with a core of common questions and sample characteristics. All data were collected between 1980 and 1985.

epidemiology   In PSYCHIATRY, the study of the INCIDENCE, distribution, PREVALENCE, and control of MENTAL DISORDERS in a given population. Common terms in epidemiology are

endemic   Native to or restricted to a particular area.

epidemic   The outbreak of a disorder that affects significant numbers of persons in a given population at any time.

pandemic   Occurring over a very wide area, in many countries, or universally.

epigenesis   Originally from the Greek *epi* (on, upon, on top of) and *genesis* (origin); the theory that the embryo develops progressively by stages, forming structures that were not originally present in the ovum or the sperm. The concept has been extended to other areas of medicine, with somewhat different meanings. Some of the other meanings are 1) any change in an organism that is due to outside influences rather than to genetically determined ones; 2) the occurrence of SECONDARY SYMPTOMS as a result of disease; 3) developmental factors, and specifically the GENE–environment interactions, that contribute to development; 4) the appearance of new functions that are not predictable on the basis of knowledge of the part-processes that have been combined; and 5) the appearance of specific features at each stage of development, such as the different goals and risks that Erik Erikson (1902–1994) described for the eight psychosocial stages of human life (e.g., trust vs. mistrust, autonomy vs. doubt). The life cycle theory adheres to the epigenetic principle in that each stage of development is characterized by crises or challenges that must be satisfactorily resolved if development is to proceed normally.

epigenetics   The study of the factors that cause development. See EPIGENESIS.

epilepsy   A neurological disorder characterized by periodic motor or sensory SEIZURES or their equivalents, sometimes accompanied by alterations of consciousness. The ELECTROENCEPHALOGRAM (EEG) may show an abnormal BRAIN WAVE pattern during or between seizures. IDIOPATHIC epilepsy has no known organic cause; epilepsy is termed *symptomatic* when it is SECONDARY to brain lesions.

Epilepsy is generally divided into partial and generalized seizures. In partial seizures, consciousness may not be impaired. In seizures with complex SYMPTOMS (TEMPORAL LOBE EPILEPSY, PSYCHOMOTOR SEIZURES), consciousness usually is impaired. Among the many forms of generalized seizures are absences (formerly called *petit mal epilepsy*) and tonic-clonic seizures (formerly called *grand mal* seizures). STATUS EPILEPTICUS refers to prolongation of a grand mal seizure and its failure to end spontaneously.

epileptic equivalent   Episodic, sensory, or motor phenomena that a person with EPILEPSY may experience instead of convulsive SEIZURES.

Jacksonian epilepsy   A type of grand mal EPILEPSY that typically begins with abnormal clonic movements of the thumb and forefinger, the angle of the mouth, or the big toe and spreads to include the rest of the limb and finally the other side of the body. At this point, consciousness is usually lost. Named after the NEUROLOGIST J. Hughlings Jackson (1835–1911).

major epilepsy (grand mal)   Convulsive SEIZURES with loss of consciousness and vegetative control.

minor epilepsy (petit mal)   Nonconvulsive epileptic SEIZURES or equivalents; may be limited to only momentary lapses of consciousness.

temporal lobe epilepsy   Also called *complex partial seizures*. Usually originating in the TEMPORAL LOBES, temporal lobe epilepsy involves recurrent periodic disturbances of behavior, during which the patient carries out movements that are often repetitive and highly organized but semiautomatic in character. See INTERICTAL BEHAVIOR SYNDROME.

epinephrine   One of the CATECHOLAMINES secreted by the adrenal gland and by NEURONS of the SYMPATHETIC NERVOUS SYSTEM. It is responsible for many of the physical manifestations of FEAR and ANXIETY. Also known as *adrenaline.*

epistemology The theory of knowledge; the study of the method and grounds of knowledge.

EPS See EXTRAPYRAMIDAL SYMPTOMS (EPS).

Equanil Brand name (now discontinued) for the nonbenzodiazepine SEDATIVE-HYPNOTIC drug MEPROBAMATE.

Equetro Brand name (now discontinued) for the ANTICONVULSANT/ MOOD STABILIZER drug CARBAMAZEPINE.

erectile dysfunction See MALE ERECTILE DISORDER under SEXUAL AROUSAL DISORDERS.

ergotamine An alkaloid (naturally occurring nitrogen-containing compounds) produced by ergot (a toxic fungus) that contains lysergic acid and is used in the PREVENTION of MIGRAINES.

erogenous zone An area of the body particularly susceptible to EROTIC AROUSAL when stimulated, especially the oral, anal, and genital areas. Sometimes called the *erotogenic zone.*

erotic Consciously or unconsciously invested with sexual feeling; sensually related.

erotomania An abnormally strong sexual desire. See –MANIA.

erotomanic delusion See DELUSIONAL DISORDER.

erythrophobia The FEAR of blushing.

escitalopram oxalate A newer SELECTIVE SEROTONIN REUPTAKE INHIBITOR (SSRI) medication (the isolated *S*-enantiomer of CITALOPRAM) approved for treatment of MAJOR DEPRESSIVE DISORDER in adults and adolescents and GENERALIZED ANXIETY DISORDER in adults. Marketed under the brand name LEXAPRO. See "Medications Used in Psychiatry."

Eskalith Brand name (now discontinued) for LITHIUM CARBONATE.

ESP See EXTRASENSORY PERCEPTION (ESP).

espanto A CULTURE-SPECIFIC SYNDROME. See *SUSTO.*

essential tremor A progressive neurological disorder most commonly manifested by TREMOR of the arms, which can also occur in the head, jaw, and voice. Also known as KINETIC TREMOR. Anxiety and depressive symptoms as well as cognitive difficulties have been linked to essential tremor. Recent studies have indicated that onset after age 65 years may be associated with an increased risk of DEMENTIA.

estazolam A short-acting BENZODIAZEPINE SEDATIVE-HYPNOTIC medication used to treat INSOMNIA. Now available only as generic but may still be known by the discontinued brand name PROSOM. See "Medications Used in Psychiatry."

eszopiclone　A short-acting nonbenzodiazepine SEDATIVE-HYPNOTIC medication used in the treatment of INSOMNIA. Marketed under the brand name LUNESTA. See "Medications Used in Psychiatry."

ethnicity　A common heritage shared by a particular group. Heritage includes similar history, language, rituals, and preferences for music and foods.

ethnology　A science that concerns itself with the division of human beings into races and their origin, distribution, relations, and characteristics. See CULTURAL ANTHROPOLOGY; SOCIAL ANTHROPOLOGY.

ethology　The scientific study of animal behavior; also the empirical study of human behavior.

etiology　Causation, particularly with reference to disease.

Etrafon　Brand name (now discontinued) for PERPHENAZINE–AMITRIPTYLINE COMBINATION.

euphoria　An exaggerated feeling of physical and emotional well-being, usually of psychological origin. Also seen in DELIRIUM and DEMENTIA and in toxic and drug-induced states. See also BIPOLAR DISORDERS.

evaluation　See ASSESSMENT.

event-related potential　Electrical activity produced by the BRAIN in response to a sensory stimulus or associated with the execution of a motor, COGNITIVE, or psychophysiological task. See also ELECTROENCEPHALOGRAM (EEG); EVOKED POTENTIAL.

evidence-based practice　A term used to describe a clinical practice based on studies published in the scientific literature. The publications must be peer reviewed by experts to ensure their quality. Quality depends on scientifically rigorous methods of data collection, analysis, and interpretation. No single study, regardless of the quality of its design, is sufficient by itself to serve as the basis for evidence. Findings must be replicated in several studies, and findings must be consistent. The strength or degree of evidence amassed for any intervention is referred to as the *level of evidence.*

evocative memory　The capacity to retrieve a memory by virtue of conscious will, in the absence of an externally perceived cue.

evoked potential　Electrical activity produced by the BRAIN in response to any sensory stimulus; a more specific term than EVENT-RELATED POTENTIAL, as the "event" is a sound. See also ELECTROENCEPHALOGRAM (EEG).

excitement　Agitation. See CATATONIC BEHAVIOR; PSYCHOMOTOR AGITATION.

excitotoxicity A cascade of neuronal injury that leads to neurodegeneration and DEMENTIA. Abnormal stimulation of the CENTRAL NERVOUS SYSTEM (CNS) following a traumatic stimulus, such as a STROKE, which triggers a cascade of cell death.

executive ego function A psychoanalytic term (see PSYCHOANALYSIS) for the EGO's management of the mental mechanisms in order to meet the needs of the organism.

executive functioning Higher-level COGNITIVE abilities such as planning or decision making. These functions are often impaired during the early stages of DEMENTIA.

Exelon Brand name for the ACETYLCHOLINESTERASE INHIBITOR drug RIVASTIGMINE.

exhibitionism Pleasure in attracting attention to oneself. One of the PARAPHILIAS, characterized by marked distress over, or acting on, urges to expose one's genitals to an unsuspecting stranger.

existential psychiatry (existentialism) A school of PSYCHIATRY that evolved from traditional psychoanalytic thought. It stresses the way in which a person experiences the phenomenological world and takes responsibility for existence. Philosophically, it is holistic and self-deterministic in contrast to biological or culturally deterministic points of view. See also PHENOMENOLOGY.

existential psychotherapy A type of PSYCHOTHERAPY that emphasizes the person's inherent capacities to become healthy and fully functioning. It concentrates on the present, on achieving consciousness of life as being partially under one's control, on accepting responsibility for decisions, and on learning to tolerate ANXIETY.

exogenous Originating or beginning outside the organism. Contrast with ENDOGENOUS.

exogenous psychoses Obsolete term referring to disorders that have as their cause factors outside the organism (e.g., disorders SECONDARY to infection, INTOXICATION, or trauma) or outside the neuropsychiatric "system" itself (e.g., hormonal, metabolic, or cardiovascular disorders). Contrast with ENDOGENOUS PSYCHOSES.

experiential group A group whose main purpose is concerned with sharing whatever happens in a spontaneous fashion.

experiential therapy A generic term for a group of therapies that use controlled or released EMOTION or "spiritual" experiences and power of CONSCIOUS COGNITION and responsibility as the primary vehicles for inner growth and self-actualization. Included are 1) emotional-release therapies that are usually short term and intense (encounter group therapy, gestalt therapy, primal scream therapy) and may emphasize body contact as the most direct vehicle for the release of emotional and muscular tensions (bioenergetic psychotherapy, ROLFING); 2) emotional-control therapies that focus on gaining greater control over the body through training (YOGA, transcendental meditation, tai chi, and chi kung); 3) religious and inspirational therapies (faith healing, Christian Science); and 4) cognitive-emotional therapies such as Albert Ellis's (1913–2007) rational-emotive psychotherapy and William Glasser's (1925–) reality therapy. Many of these therapies are not considered to constitute standard or accepted psychiatric treatment.

expert testimony   See "Legal Terms."

expert witness   See "Legal Terms."

exposure hierarchy   A master list of all the exposure exercises that an individual will perform to reduce his or her ANXIETY or PANIC symptoms. These exercises are ordered from most to least difficult to do. See EXPOSURE THERAPY.

exposure therapy   A COGNITIVE-BEHAVIORAL (PSYCHO)THERAPY (CBT) technique that involves gradually exposing an individual to situations that previously have been avoided because of ANXIETY or PANIC. See also EXPOSURE HIERARCHY. Most often used in treating PHOBIAS, such as FEAR of flying or heights and AGORAPHOBIA. Exposure therapy identifies the thoughts, emotions, and physiological AROUSAL that accompany a fear-inducing stimulus and attempts to break the pattern of escape that strengthens the fear response through measured exposure to progressively stronger stimuli until habituation is reached.

expressed emotions   The feelings that a family shows toward one of their members; specifically, overinvolvement with and HOSTILITY and criticism toward a family member with SCHIZOPHRENIA.

expressive aphasia   See BROCA'S APHASIA.

expressive (communication)   The process of producing and communicating a message. Contrast with RECEPTIVE (communication/language).

expressive language disorder   See under COMMUNICATION DISORDERS.

expressive psychoanalytic psychotherapy   A form of therapy that relies on the psychoanalytic concepts of TRANSFERENCE, COUNTERTRANSFERENCE, and unconscious motivation, even though it may not adhere to some conventions of formal PSYCHOANALYSIS, such as the use of a couch. It seeks to encourage the expression, understanding, and working-through of thoughts and feelings that may have been previously unavailable to conscious awareness.

expressive writing disorder   See DISORDER OF WRITTEN EXPRESSION.

externalization   A mental process in which the individual attributes internal phenomena to the external world.

extinction   The weakening of a reinforced operant response as a result of ceasing REINFORCEMENT. See also OPERANT CONDITIONING. Also, the elimination of a conditioned response by repeated presentations of a conditioned stimulus without the unconditioned stimulus. See also RESPONDENT CONDITIONING.

extrapyramidal symptoms (EPS)   A set of side effects commonly associated with ANTIPSYCHOTIC medications. Extrapyramidal symptoms are usually divided into DYSKINESIAS (MOVEMENT DISORDERS) and DYSTONIAS (muscle tension disorders). "Tardive" symptoms are those that appear during long-term treatment (often after several years). Unlike earlier symptoms, tardive symptoms are more likely to be permanent, remaining even after the medication is stopped.

extrapyramidal syndrome   A variety of SIGNS and SYMPTOMS—including muscular RIGIDITY, TREMORS, drooling, shuffling gait (PARKINSONISM), restlessness (AKATHISIA), unusual involuntary postures (DYSTONIA), motor inertia (AKINESIA), and many other neurological disturbances—resulting from dysfunction of the EXTRAPYRAMIDAL SYSTEM. This syndrome may occur as a reversible SIDE EFFECT of certain CONVENTIONAL ANTIPSYCHOTIC drugs, particularly PHENOTHIAZINES. See also TARDIVE DYSKINESIA.

extrapyramidal system   The portion of the CENTRAL NERVOUS SYSTEM (CNS) responsible for coordinating and integrating various aspects of motor behavior or body movements. This system is usually described in terms of cortical, BASAL GANGLIA, and MIDBRAIN levels of integration.

extrasensory perception (ESP)   PERCEPTION without recourse to the conventional use of any of the five physical senses. See also PARAPSYCHOLOGY; TELEPATHY.

extraversion   A state in which ATTENTION and energies are largely directed outward from the self as opposed to inward toward the self, as in INTROVERSION. Also known as *extroversion.*

extroversion   See EXTRAVERSION.

eye movement desensitization and reprocessing (EMDR)   A recent approach to the treatment of POSTTRAUMATIC STRESS DISORDER (PTSD). The technique involves the patient's imagining a scene from the trauma, focusing on the accompanying COGNITION and AROUSAL, and tracking the therapist's rapidly moving finger. This is repeated until ANXIETY decreases, at which point the patient is told to think about a positive thought and associate it with the scene while moving the eyes.

eye tracking   Various movements of the eyes (also called SMOOTH PURSUIT EYE MOVEMENTS [SPEM]) that enable the viewer to keep a moving target in focus. Eye-tracking abnormalities, such as jumpy extraneous eye movements that interfere with tracking, have been reported in 70%–80% of patients with SCHIZOPHRENIA and in 15%–50% of their first-degree relatives but in only 6% of nonschizophrenic subjects.

F

---

facies   Distinctive facial expressions associated with specific medical or psychiatric disorders (e.g., masklike facies in PARKINSON'S DISEASE).

facilitating environment   As conceptualized by D.W. Winnicott (1896–1971), a milieu that promotes the child's development of self-esteem and self-assertive ambitions. See HOLDING ENVIRONMENT; MIRRORING.

factitious disorders   A group of disorders characterized by intentional production or feigning of physical or psychological SYMPTOMS or SIGNS related to a need to assume the SICK ROLE. No obvious SECONDARY GAIN, such as economic support or obtaining better care, is usually noted. The symptoms produced may be predominantly psychological, predominantly physical, or a combination of both. An example is MUNCHAUSEN SYNDROME, a factitious disorder with physical symptoms, or GANSER SYNDROME, a factitious disorder with psychological symptoms.

factor analysis   A statistical technique that examines population clusters to extract patterns of commonality.

Fahr's disease   A rare degenerative neurological disorder characterized by abnormal calcium deposits and associated cell loss in certain areas of the BRAIN, such as the BASAL GANGLIA. SYMPTOMS include progressive deterioration of COGNITIVE abilities leading to DEMENTIA and loss of acquired motor skills.

failure to thrive   A common problem in pediatrics in which infants or young children show delayed physical growth, often with impaired social and motor development. Nonorganic failure to thrive is thought to be associated with lack of adequate emotional nurturing. See REACTIVE ATTACHMENT DISORDER.

faith healing See EXPERIENTIAL THERAPY.

falling out A SYNDROME (seen in southern United States or Caribbean groups) characterized by a sudden collapse, sometimes preceded by dizziness. The individual's eyes are open, but the person claims an inability to see. This syndrome may correspond to a diagnosis of CONVERSION DISORDER or a DISSOCIATIVE DISORDER. See CULTURE-SPECIFIC SYNDROMES.

false imprisonment See "Legal Terms."

family therapy Treatment of more than one member of a family in the same session. The treatment may be supportive, directive, or interpretive. The assumption is that a MENTAL DISORDER in one member of a family may be a manifestation of disorders or problems in other members and may affect interrelationships and functioning.

Fanapt Brand name for the ATYPICAL ANTIPSYCHOTIC drug ILOPERIDONE.

fantasy An imagined sequence of events or mental images (e.g., daydreams) that serves to express UNCONSCIOUS CONFLICTS, to gratify unconscious wishes, or to prepare for anticipated future events.

FazaClo Brand name for an orally disintegrating tablet formulation of the ATYPICAL ANTIPSYCHOTIC drug CLOZAPINE.

FDA See FOOD AND DRUG ADMINISTRATION (FDA).

fear Unpleasant emotional and physiological response to recognized sources of danger, to be distinguished from ANXIETY. See also PHOBIA.

feeding disorder of infancy or early childhood Persistent failure to eat adequately, with loss of weight or failure to gain weight, that is not due to an associated gastrointestinal or other GENERAL MEDICAL CONDITION. In DSM-IV-TR, feeding and EATING DISORDERS include PICA and RUMINATION DISORDER.

femaleness Anatomical and physiological features that relate to the female's procreative and nurturing capacities. See also FEMININE.

female orgasmic disorder See under ORGASMIC DISORDERS.

female sexual arousal disorder See under SEXUAL AROUSAL DISORDERS.

feminine Referring to a set of sex-specific social ROLE behaviors unrelated to procreative and nurturing biological functions. See also FEMALENESS; GENDER IDENTITY; GENDER ROLE.

fetal alcohol syndrome   A CONGENITAL disorder resulting from alcohol teratogenicity (i.e., the production, actual or potential, of pathological changes in the fetus, most frequently in the form of abnormal development of one or more organ systems; commonly referred to as *birth defects*), with the following possible dysmorphic categories: CENTRAL NERVOUS SYSTEM (CNS) dysfunction, birth deficiencies (such as low birth weight), facial abnormalities, and variable major and minor malformations. A safe level of alcohol use during pregnancy has not been established, and it is generally advisable for women to refrain from alcohol use during pregnancy.

fetishism   One of the PARAPHILIAS, characterized by marked distress over, or acting on, sexual urges involving the use of nonliving objects (fetishes), such as underclothing, stockings, or boots. See also TRANSVESTIC FETISHISM.

FGAs   First-generation ANTIPSYCHOTICS; see CONVENTIONAL ANTIPSYCHOTICS.

fibromyalgia   A chronic pain disorder characterized by widespread pain, multiple tender points, abnormal pain processing, sleep disturbances, fatigue, and psychological distress.

fiduciary   See "Legal Terms."

fight-or-flight response   The body's response to perceived threats or danger. During this reaction, certain HORMONES, such as adrenaline (EPINEPHRINE) and CORTISOL, are released, speeding the heart rate, slowing digestion, shunting blood flow to major muscle groups, and changing various other AUTONOMIC NERVOUS SYSTEM (ANS) functions, giving the body a burst of energy and strength. This response is often present in PANIC ATTACKS or ANXIETY.

finger agnosia   AUTOTOPAGNOSIA restricted to the fingers.

first-generation antipsychotics (FGAs)   See CONVENTIONAL ANTIPSYCHOTICS.

fixation   The arrest of PSYCHOSOCIAL DEVELOPMENT. This condition may be considered pathological, depending on the degree of intensity, and is often a consequence of early trauma.

flagellation   See SEXUAL MASOCHISM.

flashback   Reexperiencing, after ceasing the use of a HALLUCINOGEN, one or more of the perceptual SYMPTOMS that had been part of the hallucinatory experience while using the drug. It also commonly occurs as a symptom of ACUTE STRESS DISORDER or POSTTRAUMATIC STRESS DISORDER (PTSD).

flexibilitas cerea   See CEREA FLEXIBILITAS.

flight of ideas   A nearly continuous flow of accelerated speech with abrupt changes from one topic to another, usually based on understandable ASSOCIATIONS, distracting stimuli, or playing on words. When severe, however, this may lead to disorganized and incoherent speech. Flight of ideas is characteristic of MANIC EPISODES, but it also may occur in DEMENTIA, SCHIZOPHRENIA, other PSYCHOSES, and, rarely, acute reactions to stress.

flooding (implosion)   A BEHAVIOR THERAPY procedure for PHOBIAS and other problems involving maladaptive ANXIETY, in which the causes of the anxiety are presented in intense forms, either in imagination or in real life. The presentations, which act as desensitizers, are continued until the stimuli no longer produce disabling anxiety.

flunitrazepam   A short- to intermediate-acting BENZODIAZEPINE derivative available in some countries for the treatment of severe INSOMNIA under the brand name ROHYPNOL. In the United States, flunitrazepam is considered to be an illegal drug. Although its illicit use has been implicated in cases of "date rape," flunitrazepam is more often used recreationally (in street slang, it is commonly referred to as a "roofie").

fluoxetine   A SELECTIVE SEROTONIN REUPTAKE INHIBITOR (SSRI) ANTIDEPRESSANT medication used to treat DEPRESSION, OBSESSIVE-COMPULSIVE DISORDER, and EATING DISORDERS. Marketed under the brand name PROZAC. See "Medications Used in Psychiatry."

fluphenazine   A CONVENTIONAL ANTIPSYCHOTIC medication (a PHENOTHIAZINE of the piperazine class) used to treat SCHIZOPHRENIA AND OTHER PSYCHOTIC DISORDERS. Now available only as generic but may still be known by the discontinued brand name PROLIXIN. See "Medications Used in Psychiatry."

flurazepam   A long-acting BENZODIAZEPINE SEDATIVE-HYPNOTIC medication frequently used to treat INSOMNIA. Marketed under the brand name DALMANE. See "Medications Used in Psychiatry."

fluvoxamine   A SELECTIVE SEROTONIN REUPTAKE INHIBITOR (SSRI) medication approved for the treatment of OBSESSIVE-COMPULSIVE DISORDER but also used by clinicians to treat DEPRESSION, PANIC DISORDER, and EATING DISORDERS. Marketed under the brand name LUVOX. See "Medications Used in Psychiatry."

FMR1   See FRAGILE X MENTAL RETARDATION 1 (*FMR1*) GENE.

fMRI   See FUNCTIONAL MAGNETIC RESONANCE IMAGING (fMRI).

focal psychotherapy   BRIEF PSYCHOTHERAPY that concentrates on a central or core issue or a circumscribed area of CONFLICT as the only or major object of intervention efforts. *Focalization* refers to the ability of the therapist and patient to agree on a psychodynamic target for the treatment.

Focalin   Brand name for the CENTRAL NERVOUS SYSTEM (CNS) STIMULANT drug DEXMETHYLPHENIDATE.

folie à deux   See SHARED PSYCHOTIC DISORDER.

follow-up examination   Clinical ASSESSMENT, often repeated at specific intervals following discharge from inpatient or OUTPATIENT treatment. Its major purposes are to evaluate the need for adjustment of medication dosage, to detect SIGNS of RELAPSE, to measure improvement over time, and to identify (and, when possible, control) significant contributory factors to the maintenance or recurrence of SYMPTOMS.

Food and Drug Administration (FDA)   One of a number of health administrations under the assistant secretary of health (of the U.S. Department of HEALTH AND HUMAN SERVICES) that set standards for and license the sale of drugs and food substances and in general safeguard the public from the use of dangerous drugs and food substances.

forebrain   The largest part of the BRAIN that includes the CEREBRUM, the THALAMUS, and the HYPOTHALAMUS and that (especially in higher vertebrates) is the main control center for sensory and associative information processing, visceral functions, and voluntary motor functions.

forensic psychiatry   A branch of PSYCHIATRY that focuses on interrelationships with civil, criminal, and administrative law as well as evaluation and specialized treatment of individuals involved with the legal system or incarcerated in jails, prisons, and forensic psychiatry hospitals. See also "Legal Terms."

formal operations   See COGNITIVE DEVELOPMENT.

formal thought disorder   An inexact term referring to a disturbance in the form of thinking rather than to ABNORMALITY of content. See BLOCKING; INCOHERENCE; LOOSENING OF ASSOCIATIONS; POVERTY OF SPEECH.

formication   The tactile HALLUCINATION or ILLUSION that insects are crawling on the body or under the skin.

fragile X–associated tremor/ataxia syndrome (FXTAS)   A newly recognized GENETIC disorder that affects mostly men and causes tremor, loss of coordination, and DEMENTIA. FXTAS results from a premutation of the *FMR1* GENE on the X CHROMOSOME. A more extensive MUTATION in this gene causes FRAGILE X SYNDROME in children.

fragile X mental retardation 1 (*FMR1*) gene The GENE responsible for encoding fragile X mental retardation protein (FMRP), which is required for normal neural development. FRAGILE X SYNDROME occurs when *FMR1* cannot produce enough FMRP.

fragile X syndrome The most common form of inherited INTELLECTUAL DISABILITY, caused by an abnormality of the X CHROMOSOME. The connection between the tip of the long arm of the abnormal chromosome and the rest of the chromosome is very slender and is easily broken, hence the term *fragile X*.

Clinical manifestations of fragile X syndrome include moderate to severe INTELLECTUAL DISABILITY and a large head, long face, prominent ears, and, in affected males, large testicles. Some subjects with the abnormal GENE are of normal INTELLIGENCE but show one or more forms of LEARNING DISABILITY. Many also have ATTENTION-DEFICIT/HYPERACTIVITY DISORDER (ADHD).

fragmentation Separation into different parts or detachment of one or more parts from the rest. A FEAR of fragmentation of the PERSONALITY, also known as *disintegration* ANXIETY, is often observed in patients whenever they are exposed to repetitions of earlier experiences that interfered with development of the SELF. This fear may be expressed as feelings of falling apart, as a loss of IDENTITY, or as a fear of impending loss of one's vitality and of psychological depletion.

fraud See "Legal Terms."

free association In psychoanalytic therapy (see PSYCHOANALYSIS), spontaneous, uncensored verbalization by the patient of whatever comes to mind.

free-floating anxiety Severe, generalized, persistent ANXIETY not specifically ascribed to a particular object or event and often a precursor of PANIC. See GENERALIZED ANXIETY DISORDER (GAD).

Friedreich's ataxia An inherited disease characterized by gait disturbance, clumsiness, and weakness of the lower extremities.

frigophobia The FEAR of cold weather.

frontal convexity syndrome One of the principal FRONTAL LOBE SYNDROMES. It is characterized by APATHY, occasional brief outbursts of anger, PSYCHOMOTOR RETARDATION, discrepant motor and verbal behavior, and poor abstraction and categorization.

frontal lobe   The area of the BRAIN located at the front of each cerebral hemisphere and positioned anterior to the PARIETAL LOBES and
above and anterior to the TEMPORAL LOBES. It is separated from the PA-
RIETAL LOBE by the primary motor cortex, which controls voluntary
movements of specific body parts.
    The frontal lobe contains most of the DOPAMINE-sensitive neurons in
the CEREBRAL CORTEX. The dopamine system is associated with reward,
attention, long-term memory, planning, impulse control, and drive.
Dopamine reduction in the prefrontal cortex is related to poorer performance and inefficient functioning of that brain region during working
memory tasks, and to a slightly increased risk for schizophrenia.

frontal lobe syndrome   A pattern of emotional, behavioral, and PER-
SONALITY CHANGES that occur following an injury to the prefrontal
lobes. The three principal SYNDROMES are FRONTAL CONVEXITY SYNDROME,
MEDIAL FRONTAL SYNDROME, and ORBITOFRONTAL SYNDROME. Impairment
of frontal lobe functioning is also found in a range of psychiatric conditions, including SCHIZOPHRENIA, ATTENTION-DEFICIT/HYPERACTIVITY DIS-
ORDER (ADHD), and ANTISOCIAL PERSONALITY DISORDER.

frontotemporal dementia (FTD)   A group of related conditions resulting from the progressive shrinking and degeneration of the TEM-
PORAL LOBE and FRONTAL LOBE of the BRAIN. These areas of the brain
play a significant role in decision making, behavioral control, emotion, and language. Behavioral symptoms and PERSONALITY CHANGES
may include decreased concern for social norms or other people and
lack of insight into one's own behaviors. Language symptoms tend
to include difficulty naming familiar objects. FTD patients may also
show difficulty walking, rigidity, TREMOR, or muscle weakness. FTD
was originally known as PICK'S DISEASE.

frontotemporal lobar degeneration (FTLD)   A group of clinically,
pathologically, and genetically heterogeneous disorders associated
with atrophy in the FRONTAL LOBE and TEMPORAL LOBE of the brain, with
sparing of the PARIETAL LOBE and occipital lobe. FTLD is one of the
most common causes of dementia after ALZHEIMER'S DISEASE, LEWY
BODY DEMENTIA, and VASCULAR DEMENTIA. Three clinical subtypes of
FTLD are described: FRONTOTEMPORAL DEMENTIA, SEMANTIC DEMENTIA,
and PROGRESSIVE NONFLUENT APHASIA.

frotteurism   One of the PARAPHILIAS, consisting of recurrent, intense
sexual urges involving touching and rubbing against a nonconsenting person. Common sites in which such activities take place are
crowded trains, buses, and elevators. Fondling the victim may be
part of the condition and is called *toucherism*.

frozen watchfulness An alertness or even hypervigilance that is maintained despite an overall inhibition of motor activity that may include MUTISM.

FTD See FRONTOTEMPORAL DEMENTIA (FTD).

FTLD See FRONTOTEMPORAL LOBAR DEGENERATION (FTLD).

fugue See DISSOCIATIVE FUGUE.

functional In medicine, referring to changes in the way an organ system operates that are not attributable to known structural alterations. See also FUNCTIONAL DISORDER.

functional assessment and impairments Measuring both the ability of a person to perform tasks necessary to meet the demands of daily life and the impairments that prevent such activities.

functional disorder Abnormal performance or operation of an organ or organ system that is not a result of known changes in structure. Contrast with ORGANIC MENTAL DISORDER.

functional magnetic resonance imaging (fMRI) One of the most recently developed forms of NEUROIMAGING, fMRI is a type of specialized MAGNETIC RESONANCE IMAGING (MRI) scan. It measures the hemodynamic response in the brain that corresponds to mental operations. fMRI is based on the increase in blood flow to the local vasculature that accompanies neural activity in the brain. fMRI has come to dominate the field of brain mapping as a result of its reduced invasiveness, absence of radiation exposure, and relatively wide availability.

fusion The union and integration of the INSTINCTS and DRIVES so that they complement each other and help the organism to deal effectively with both internal needs and external demands.

FXTAS See FRAGILE X–ASSOCIATED TREMOR/ATAXIA SYNDROME (FXTAS).

G

GABA (gamma-aminobutyric acid) The major inhibitory NEUROTRANSMITTER in the BRAIN, implicated in several psychiatric and neurological conditions. See also DISINHIBITION.

gabapentin An ANTICONVULSANT/MOOD STABILIZER medication sometimes used to treat BIPOLAR II DISORDER and REFRACTORY PANIC DISORDER.

Marketed under the brand name NEURONTIN. See "Medications Used in Psychiatry."

GABA receptors   RECEPTORS to which GABA (GAMMA-AMINOBUTYRIC ACID), the major inhibitory NEUROTRANSMITTER in the CENTRAL NERVOUS SYSTEM (CNS), binds. Two subtypes of GABA receptors—GABA$_A$ and GABA$_B$—have been identified. GABA$_A$ receptors also contain binding sites within the receptor complex for BENZODIAZEPINES, BARBITURATES, ethanol, and other GABAergic drugs, which potentiate the inhibitory response to GABA in the presence of these drugs.

GAD   See GENERALIZED ANXIETY DISORDER (GAD).

GAF Scale   See GLOBAL ASSESSMENT OF FUNCTIONING (GAF) SCALE.

galactorrhea   The secretion of breast milk in men or in women who are not breast-feeding an infant. Patients with galactorrhea have a high level of PROLACTIN in the blood, which can be caused by a tumor in the pituitary gland or from taking certain medications, such as CONVENTIONAL ANTIPSYCHOTICS.

galantamine   An ACETYLCHOLINESTERASE INHIBITOR used to improve thinking and MEMORY in patients with early SIGNS of ALZHEIMER'S DISEASE. Marketed under the brand name RAZADYNE (formerly named REMINYL). See "Medications Used in Psychiatry."

galvanic skin response (GSR)   The change in the electrical resistance of the skin following stimulation; an easily measured variable widely used in experimental studies.

gambling   See PATHOLOGICAL GAMBLING.

gamma-aminobutyric acid   See GABA (GAMMA-AMINOBUTYRIC ACID).

Ganser syndrome   A form of FACTITIOUS DISORDER in which a patient feigns psychological SYMPTOMS, such as DEMENTIA or PSYCHOSIS, for no apparent gain, except to be a patient.

gatekeeper   In a MANAGED CARE system, the person who decides what medical services a patient may have access to. Often it is the PRIMARY CARE PHYSICIAN, but it also may be a nonphysician case manager. See also CASE MANAGEMENT.

gateway drugs   A term referring to tobacco, alcohol, marijuana, inhalants, and ANABOLIC STEROIDS that emphasizes that these drugs are often the stepping-stones to more severe ADDICTION.

Gault **decision**   See "Legal Terms."

gegenhalten   "Active" resistance to passive movement of the extremities that does not appear to be under voluntary control. This phenomenon may occur in disorders of the CEREBRAL CORTEX.

gender identity (core gender identity)   The inner sense of MALE-NESS or FEMALENESS that identifies the person as being male, female, or ambivalent. DIFFERENTIATION of gender identity usually takes place in infancy and early childhood and is reinforced by the hormonal changes of puberty. Gender identity is distinguished from sexual identity, which is biologically determined. See also GENDER IDENTITY DISORDER; GENDER ROLE.

gender identity disorder   A disorder characterized by a strong and persistent IDENTIFICATION with the opposite sex (cross-gender identification) and discomfort with one's assigned sex or a sense of inappropriateness in that GENDER ROLE. Although onset is usually in childhood or ADOLESCENCE, the disorder may not present clinically until adulthood. Manifestations include a repeated desire to be of the opposite sex, insistence that one has the typical feelings and reactions of the opposite sex, a belief that one was born the wrong sex, and preoccupation with one's primary and secondary sex characteristics in order to simulate the opposite sex.

gender role   The image a person presents to others and to the SELF that declares him or her to be boy or girl, man or woman. Gender role is the public declaration of GENDER IDENTITY, but the two do not necessarily coincide.

generalized anxiety disorder (GAD)   A disorder characterized by unrealistic or excessive anxiety, apprehensive expectations, and worry about many life circumstances (e.g., academic, athletic, or social performance). A mother may worry excessively about her child, who is in no danger. The worry is associated with SYMPTOMS such as trembling, muscle tension, restlessness, feelings of being smothered, light-headedness, INSOMNIA, exaggerated startle response, or difficulty in concentration. The worrying is difficult to control, and with associated symptoms, often social or occupational functioning is impaired.

When it occurs in children, GAD is termed OVERANXIOUS DISORDER. Symptoms include multiple unrealistic anxieties concerning the quality of one's performance in school, at work, or in sports, and of one's health or appearance, accompanied by the need to be reassured.

general medical condition   Any condition or disorder that is listed outside the MENTAL DISORDERS section of the *INTERNATIONAL CLASSIFICATION OF DISEASES* (ICD). The phrase is used in DSM-IV-TR as a term of convenience only. It does not imply that there is any fundamental distinction between mental disorders and general medical conditions or that mental disorders are unrelated to physical or biological factors or processes. See also SECONDARY DISORDER.

general paralysis (general paresis)　A form of tertiary neurosyphilis. It is a GENERAL MEDICAL CONDITION occasionally associated with other neurological SIGNS of syphilitic involvement of the nervous system and detectable with laboratory tests of the blood or spinal fluid.

genes　Located at various points along the CHROMOSOMES, genes are fragments of DEOXYRIBONUCLEIC ACID (DNA) that carry the hereditary code. It is estimated that the human has approximately 23,000 genes, known collectively as the *genome.*

genetic(s)　In biology, pertaining to GENES or to inherited characteristics. Also, in PSYCHIATRY, pertaining to the historical development of one's psychological attributes or disorders.

genetic counseling　Advice given to a prospective parental couple regarding the inheritance of a pathological condition related to the couple's GENETIC ENDOWMENT.

genetic endowment　Inherited traits, potentials, and capacities.

genetic marker　A DEOXYRIBONUCLEIC ACID (DNA) sequence that is associated with the presence of or vulnerability to a disease. More often than not, the abnormality is not the GENE actually responsible for the disorder but a DNA segment that remains physically close to the responsible gene and thus signals the presence of that gene.

genetic testing　The analysis of human DEOXYRIBONUCLEIC ACID (DNA), RIBONUCLEIC ACID (RNA), CHROMOSOMES, proteins, and certain metabolites in order to detect heritable disease-related GENOTYPES, MUTATIONS, or PHENOTYPES for clinical purposes. Such purposes include predicting risk of disease, identifying carriers, and establishing prenatal and clinical DIAGNOSIS or PROGNOSIS. Prenatal, newborn, and carrier screening, as well as testing in high-risk families, are included.

genetic viewpoint　A psychoanalytic metapsychological hypothesis that is concerned with the origin and development of psychic phenomena in terms of how the past is contained in the present and why an individual adopts certain CONFLICTS and ADAPTATIONS.

genital phase　The final phase of PSYCHOSEXUAL DEVELOPMENT, as conceived by Sigmund Freud (1856–1939), and the psychic characteristics of this phase. The genital phase begins at the onset of puberty. The integration of OBJECT love with genital sexuality is a primary developmental attainment of this phase.

genotype　The total set of GENES present at the time of conception, producing the GENETIC constitution. See PHENOTYPE.

Geodon　Brand name for the ATYPICAL ANTIPSYCHOTIC drug ZIPRASIDONE.

geriatric psychiatry Also called *geropsychiatry*; an AMERICAN BOARD OF PSYCHIATRY AND NEUROLOGY (ABPN) subspecialty of PSYCHIATRY that focuses on the prevention, evaluation, diagnosis, and treatment of mental and emotional disorders in the elderly, as well as improvement of psychiatric care for healthy and ill elderly people.

geriatrics A branch of medicine dealing with the AGING process and diseases of the aging human being.

gerontology The study of AGING.

gerontophobia The FEAR of old people and AGING.

geropsychiatry See GERIATRIC PSYCHIATRY.

Gerstmann's syndrome A neurological disorder characterized by four primary SYMPTOMS: ACALCULIA, AGRAPHIA, an inability to distinguish right from left, and FINGER AGNOSIA. Gerstmann's syndrome has been attributed to lesions in the angular gyrus of the dominant inferior PARIETAL LOBE. This disease is classified as a SPONGIFORM ENCEPHALOPATHY.

Gerstmann-Straussler-Scheinker syndrome A rare familial neurological disorder characterized by widespread degeneration of the nervous system, difficulty walking, progressive DEMENTIA, and absence of leg reflexes.

gestalt psychology A German school of PSYCHOLOGY that emphasizes a total perceptual configuration and the interrelationships of its component parts.

ghost sickness A preoccupation with death and the deceased (sometimes associated with witchcraft) frequently observed among Native American tribes. Symptoms attributed to it include bad dreams, weakness, feelings of danger, loss of appetite, fainting, dizziness, fear, anxiety, hallucinations, loss of consciousness, confusion, feelings of futility, and a sense of suffocation. See CULTURE-SPECIFIC SYNDROMES.

Gilles de la Tourette's syndrome A genetically determined SYNDROME usually beginning in early childhood characterized by repetitive TICS, other abnormal movements, uncontrolled grunts, unintelligible sounds, and occasionally verbal obscenities. Also known as TOURETTE'S DISORDER, from part of the last name of Georges Gilles de la Tourette (1857–1904).

ginkgo biloba An herbal medication sometimes used to treat mild DEMENTIA or MEMORY impairment. The active ingredient is the dry extract from the leaf of the ginkgo biloba tree. The extract is made up of several active compounds, including flavonoids, bioflavonoids, and terpenoids.

Global Assessment of Functioning (GAF) Scale   A numerical AS-SESSMENT, on a scale of 1 to 100, with 100 being the highest score, of the patient's overall symptomatology and psychological, social, and occupational functioning on a hypothetical continuum of MENTAL HEALTH–illness.

globus hystericus   The disturbing sensation of a lump in the throat.

globus pallidus   With the CAUDATE NUCLEUS, the PUTAMEN, the subthalamic nucleus, and the SUBSTANTIA NIGRA, a major element of the BASAL GANGLIA. The basal ganglia appear to be involved in motor control, such as planning and execution of complex motor activity.

glossolalia   Gibberish-like speech or "speaking in tongues."

glutamate   The major excitatory NEUROTRANSMITTER in the CENTRAL NERVOUS SYSTEM (CNS), which plays a key role in maintenance of NEURONAL PLASTICITY and is important in learning and memory. Excessive excitatory neurotransmission and glutamate concentration may lead to excitotoxic conditions and neurodegenerative processes, which, for example, may be involved in ALZHEIMER'S DISEASE. Among other functions, glutamate appears to play a role in protecting against the SYMPTOMS of PSYCHOSIS. This is borne out by the evidence that GLUTAMATERGIC ANTAGONISTS (NMDA RECEPTOR ANTAGONISTS) may produce psychotic symptoms similar to those of schizophrenia, and GLUTAMATERGIC AGONISTS may be useful in treating schizophrenia.

glutamate receptors   RECEPTORS in the CENTRAL NERVOUS SYSTEM (CNS) to which GLUTAMATE binds. Glutamate receptors play a vital role in the mediation of excitatory synaptic transmission and are important for neural communication, memory formation, and learning. The two primary glutamate receptors are named after the agonists that bind to them with high specificity: AMPA (ALPHA-AMINO-3-HYDROXY-5-METHYL-4-ISOXAZOLEPROPIONIC ACID) and NMDA (N-METHYL-D-ASPARTATE).

glutamatergic   Referring to the NEUROTRANSMITTER GLUTAMATE.

grand mal   See EPILEPSY.

grandiose delusion   See DELUSIONAL DISORDER.

grandiose self   As conceptualized in Heinz Kohut's (1913–1981) SELF PSYCHOLOGY, one part of the BIPOLAR SELF. The efforts of the child to elicit continuing praise from the parents by being perfect. The mother's generally positive responses to those efforts affirm the child's worth and promote the development of self-esteem and self-assertive ambitions, pursuit of goals, and enjoyment of physical and mental activities.

grandiosity Exaggerated belief or claims of one's importance or IDENTITY, often manifested by DELUSIONS of great wealth, power, or fame. See BIPOLAR DISORDERS; MANIA.

granular cortex The outer layer of the CEREBRAL CORTEX.

gray matter The CEREBRAL CORTEX of the BRAIN, which contains nerve cell bodies whose function is to route sensory or motor stimulus to the CENTRAL NERVOUS SYSTEM (CNS).

grief Normal, appropriate emotional response to an external and a consciously recognized loss; it is usually time-limited and subsides gradually. To be distinguished from DEPRESSION. See also MOURNING.

grisi siknis A CULTURE-SPECIFIC SYNDROME that occurs predominantly among the Miskito people of eastern Central America and affects mainly young women ages 15–18 years. It is typically characterized by longer periods of anxiety, nausea, dizziness, irrational anger and fear, interlaced with short periods of rapid frenzy. Traditional Miskito belief holds that *grisi siknis* is the result of evil spirits or black sorcerers. While Western medicine typically has no effect on those afflicted with the disease, the remedies of Miskito herbalists or witch doctors are often successful in curing *grisi siknis*.

group dynamics The interactions and interrelationships among members of a therapy group and between members and the therapist. The effective use of group dynamics is essential in group treatment.

group practice A formal association of three or more physicians, or other health professionals, organized to provide a continuum of broader-based care than is usually provided by a single practitioner. Twenty-four-hour coverage by those within the group, different services, and different specialties may make more services available and management less cumbersome than is possible in larger health care institutions.

group (psycho)therapy Application of psychotherapeutic techniques by a therapist who uses the emotional interactions of the group members to help them get relief from distress and possibly modify their behavior. Other types of psychotherapy (e.g., COGNITIVE-BEHAVIORAL THERAPY) can also be provided in a group setting. Typically, a group is composed of 4–12 persons who meet regularly with the therapist. See GROUP DYNAMICS.

GSR See GALVANIC SKIN RESPONSE (GSR).

guanethidine   An antihypertensive medication that may cause DE-PRESSION and DELIRIUM. The brand name ISMELIN was discontinued by the manufacturer in 2009, and no generics are currently available.

guanfacine   A nonstimulant alpha$_{2A}$-ADRENERGIC RECEPTOR AGONIST originally developed to treat high blood pressure (brand name TENEX). An extended-release formulation (brand name INTUNIV) of guanfacine was approved in 2007 for use in the treatment of ATTENTION-DEFICIT/HYPERAC-TIVITY DISORDER (ADHD). See "Medications Used in Psychiatry."

guardian *ad litem*   See "Legal Terms."

guardianship   See "Legal Terms."

guilt   EMOTION resulting from doing what one conceives of as wrong, thereby violating SUPEREGO precepts; it results in feelings of worthlessness and at times the need for punishment. Also may be a SYMPTOM of several psychiatric disorders, including major DEPRESSION. See SHAME.

gynophobia   The FEAR of women.

H

haan   A term that refers to an individual or collective subconscious emotion in Korean people involving suppressed feelings of anger, rage, despair, frustration, holding of grudges, indignation, and revenge. It is considered an important factor in the development of *HWA-BYUNG*. See also CULTURE-SPECIFIC SYNDROMES.

habeas corpus   See "Legal Terms."

habit reversal training   A behavioral treatment originally developed to address a wide variety of repetitive behavior disorders such as TICS, TRICHOTILLOMANIA, nail biting, thumb sucking, and skin picking (DERMATILLOMANIA). It consists of five components: 1) awareness training, 2) competing response training, 3) contingency management, 4) relaxation training, and 5) generalization training.

hair pulling   See TRICHOTILLOMANIA.

Halcion   Brand name for the BENZODIAZEPINE SEDATIVE-HYPNOTIC drug TRIAZOLAM.

Haldol   Brand name for the CONVENTIONAL ANTIPSYCHOTIC drug HALO-PERIDOL.

halfway house   A specialized residence for patients who do not require full hospitalization but who need an intermediate degree of domiciliary care before returning to independent community living.

Hallervorden-Spatz syndrome   A rare hereditary, degenerative neurological disease, whose onset usually is before ADOLESCENCE. SYMPTOMS include dystonia, spasticity, and a gradually progressive DEMENTIA.

hallucination   A sensory PERCEPTION in the absence of an actual external stimulus; to be distinguished from an ILLUSION, which is a misperception or misinterpretation of an external stimulus. Hallucinations may involve any of the senses.

auditory hallucination   Perception of sound, most frequently of voices but sometimes of clicks or other noises.

olfactory hallucination   Perception of odor, such as of burning rubber or decaying fish.

somatic hallucination   Perception of a physical sensation within the body, such as a feeling of electricity running through one's body.

tactile hallucination   Perception of being touched or of something being under one's skin, such as the sensation of pins being stuck into one's finger. The sensation of something crawling under one's skin is called FORMICATION; it occurs most frequently in ALCOHOL WITHDRAWAL SYNDROME and in COCAINE WITHDRAWAL.

visual hallucination   Perception of an image, such as people (formed) or a flash of light (unformed).

hallucinogen   A chemical agent that produces HALLUCINATIONS. The term is used synonymously with PSYCHOTOMIMETIC.

hallucinogen-related disorders   In DSM-IV-TR, a group of MENTAL DISORDERS that includes hallucinogen DEPENDENCE, hallucinogen ABUSE, hallucinogen INTOXICATION, hallucinogen persisting PERCEPTION disorder (FLASHBACKS), hallucinogen intoxication DELIRIUM, hallucinogen-induced PSYCHOTIC DISORDER, hallucinogen-induced MOOD DISORDER, and hallucinogen-induced ANXIETY DISORDER.

hallucinosis   A condition in which the patient hallucinates in a state of clear consciousness, as in a SUBSTANCE-INDUCED PSYCHOTIC DISORDER.

DSM-IV-TR classifies hallucinosis on the basis of whether REALITY TESTING about the hallucinatory experiences is intact. In patients whose reality testing is impaired, hallucinosis is termed *substance-induced (e.g., alcohol) psychotic disorder, with hallucinations.* In patients whose reality testing is intact, hallucinosis is termed *substance-induced intoxication* (or *withdrawal*), *with perceptual disturbance.*

haloperidol   A CONVENTIONAL ANTIPSYCHOTIC medication (a BUTYROPHE-NONE) used in the treatment of chronic SCHIZOPHRENIA AND OTHER PSY-CHOTIC DISORDERS and often used to manage AGITATION in acutely ill psychiatric patients. Marketed under the brand name HALDOL. See "Medications Used in Psychiatry."

harm avoidance   Term referring to the concept that complete cessation of alcohol and drug ABUSE should not be the only goal of drug and alcohol programs; a decrease in use and the avoidance of harm to the person and others also should be a goal of treatment.

Harm avoidance is also used to describe a PERSONALITY trait characterized by excessive worrying; pessimism; shyness; and being fearful, doubtful, and easily fatigued. In MAGNETIC RESONANCE IMAGING (MRI) studies, harm avoidance has been correlated with reduced GRAY MATTER volume in the orbitofrontal, occipital, and parietal regions.

HCFA   See HEALTH CARE FINANCING ADMINISTRATION (HCFA).

Health and Human Services (HHS)   See DEPARTMENT OF HEALTH AND HUMAN SERVICES (DHHS).

Health Care Financing Administration (HCFA)   A federal agency within the U.S. DEPARTMENT OF HEALTH AND HUMAN SERVICES that in 2001 was renamed CENTERS FOR MEDICARE AND MEDICAID SERVICES (CMS).

health care proxy   See LIVING WILL and "Legal Terms."

Health Insurance Portability and Accountability Act (HIPAA) Enacted by Congress in 1996, this act required the Department of HEALTH AND HUMAN SERVICES to establish national standards for electronic health care transactions and national identifiers for providers, health plans, and employers. It also addressed the security and privacy of health data. Title I of HIPAA protects health insurance coverage for workers and their families when they change or lose their jobs.

health maintenance organization (HMO)   A form of GROUP PRAC-TICE by physicians and supporting personnel to provide comprehensive health services to an enrolled group of subscribers who pay a fixed premium to belong. Emphasis is on maintaining the health of the enrollees as well as treating their illnesses. HMOs must include psychiatric benefits to receive federal support.

hebephrenia   A subtype of SCHIZOPHRENIA characterized especially by incoherence, delusions lacking an underlying theme, and affect that is usually flat or inappropriate. Also known as *disorganized* schizophrenia.

hedonism Pleasure-seeking behavior. Contrast with ANHEDONIA.

helplessness Actual or self-perceived inability to act on one's own behalf; inefficiency in making an impact on one's environment to create change.

hemiballismus A very rare MOVEMENT DISORDER characterized by involuntary flinging motions of the extremities, whose effects can sometimes be severe enough to prevent patients from being able to perform daily functions. It is usually associated with structural BRAIN lesions but can occur with metabolic abnormalities. The symptoms can also decrease while the patient is asleep, unlike some movement disorders.

hemophobia The FEAR of blood.

heritability of psychiatric disorders Family, adoption, and twin studies demonstrate that genetic factors have an important role in certain psychiatric disorders, including SCHIZOPHRENIA, MAJOR DEPRESSIVE DISORDER, and BIPOLAR DISORDER. The heritability of many psychiatric disorders is high compared with that of other complex disorders such as asthma, diabetes, and STROKE. While heritability estimates are high, environmental factors are also critical in determining whether a disorder will develop in a particular individual. For example, the heritability of schizophrenia is estimated to be 82%–85%, yet concordance in monozygotic twins is only 40%–48%.

heroin An illicit (in the United States) OPIOID synthesized from MORPHINE. Heroin, a white or brown powder that is injected intravenously or smoked in glass pipes, is the most commonly abused NARCOTIC.

heterogeneity Dissimilarity in the genotypic structure of individuals originating through sexual reproduction.

HHS See DEPARTMENT OF HEALTH AND HUMAN SERVICES (DHHS).

5-HIAA (5-hydroxyindoleacetic acid) A major metabolite of SEROTONIN, a BIOGENIC AMINE found in the BRAIN and other organs. FUNCTIONAL DEFICITS of serotonin in the CENTRAL NERVOUS SYSTEM (CNS) have been implicated in SUICIDE and impulsivity.

high-risk behavior Actions that put one in danger or render one vulnerable to harmful consequences. Needle sharing by addicted persons, for example, is high-risk behavior because of the likelihood of transmission of HUMAN IMMUNODEFICIENCY VIRUS (HIV) or other pathogens. Also called RISK BEHAVIOR.

HIPAA See HEALTH INSURANCE PORTABILITY AND ACCOUNTABILITY ACT (HIPAA).

hippocampus   A sea horse–shaped structure located within the BRAIN that is an important part of the LIMBIC SYSTEM. The hippocampus is involved in some aspects of MEMORY, in the control of autonomic functions, and in emotional expression.

Hirano bodies   Intracellular aggregates of actin and actin-associated proteins, often occurring as rod shapes in the neurons of individuals affected with certain neurodegenerative disorders, such as ALZHEIMER'S DISEASE and CREUTZFELDT-JAKOB DISEASE. Hirano bodies are frequently seen in hippocampal pyramidal cells.

histamine   An organic nitrogen compound, found in nearly all body cells, that controls local immune responses and regulates physiological function in the gastrointestinal tract; it also acts as a NEUROTRANSMITTER. Histamine triggers the inflammatory response by increasing the permeability of the capillaries to white blood cells and other proteins, allowing them to reach the sites of infection. Four subtypes (designated H_1–H_4) of histamine RECEPTORS have been identified.

histrionic personality disorder   See under PERSONALITY DISORDERS.

HIV   See HUMAN IMMUNODEFICIENCY VIRUS (HIV).

HIV dementia   Also referred to as AIDS DEMENTIA COMPLEX (ADC). A rapidly progressive subcortical DEMENTIA characterized by 1) COGNITIVE DEFICITS such as inattentiveness, impaired concentration and PROBLEM SOLVING, forgetfulness, and impaired reading; 2) motor abnormalities such as TREMORS, slurred speech, ATAXIA, and generalized HYPERREFLEXIA; and 3) behavioral changes such as sluggishness and SOCIAL WITHDRAWAL. COMPUTED TOMOGRAPHY (CT) and MAGNETIC RESONANCE IMAGING (MRI) usually indicate BRAIN atrophy along with an enlargement of the ventricles.

HIV dementia characteristically begins with impaired concentration and mild MEMORY loss. Over a period of several weeks or months, the condition progresses to severe global cognitive impairment.

HIV meningitis   An acute aseptic meningitis that occurs soon after infection with the virus. SYMPTOMS, which are usually mild and self-limited, include headache, fever, painful sensitivity to light, and cranial neuropathy. The symptoms typically disappear in 1–4 weeks.

Cryptococcal meningitis is a more serious form of meningitis that occurs in HIV-infected persons as a result of infection with the common soil fungus *Cryptococcus neoformans.* Symptoms include headache, stiff neck, fever, and painful sensitivity to light.

HMO   See HEALTH MAINTENANCE ORGANIZATION (HMO).

holding environment As conceptualized by D. W. Winnicott (1896–1971), a responsive, nurturing milieu for the developing child, including physical holding as well as the mother's or primary caregiver's preoccupation with the child and her ability to soothe, comfort, and reduce the tension in her infant. Ideally, the mother reflects back the child's worth and value and in other ways responds appropriately to his or her needs. Lack of such responsivity is often termed EMPATHIC FAILURE. In the psychotherapeutic (see PSYCHOTHERAPY) relationship, *holding environment* refers to a therapeutic ambiance or setting that permits the patient to experience safety, thereby facilitating psychotherapeutic work.

hold harmless See "Legal Terms."

holism An approach to the study of the individual in totality rather than as an aggregate of separate physiological, psychological, and social characteristics.

homeostasis Self-regulating biological and psychological processes that maintain the stability and equilibrium of the organism.

homicidal ideation The presence of homicidal thoughts or plans.

homophobia The FEAR of homosexual persons.

homosexuality A primary EROTIC attraction to others of the same sex. Overt homosexual behavior may be inhibited, delayed, or otherwise modified because of family or peer pressure, social bias, or INTRAPSYCHIC CONFLICT caused by the internalization of social prejudice.

homosexual panic An acute and severe attack of ANXIETY based on UNCONSCIOUS CONFLICTS involving GENDER IDENTITY.

homovanillic acid (HVA) A principal metabolite of DOPAMINE, a CATECHOLAMINE found in the BRAIN and other organs.

horizontal split In SELF PSYCHOLOGY, a process by which unwanted qualities of the SELF are warded off by placing them outside of consciousness, while the desirable qualities of the self remain conscious. The primary DEFENSE associated with horizontal split is REPRESSION. Contrast with VERTICAL SPLIT.

hormonal therapies The administration of HORMONES to combat a variety of disorders. In PSYCHIATRY, these therapies may be used to treat early SIGNS and SYMPTOMS of ALZHEIMER'S DISEASE, PARAPHILIAS, HYPOACTIVE SEXUAL DESIRE DISORDER, and PEDOPHILIA.

hormone A discrete chemical substance secreted into the body fluids by an endocrine gland, which has a specific effect on the activities of other organs. See also NEUROHORMONE.

hostility   Actual or threatened aggressive contact, destructive in intent.

hotline   Telephone assistance service for crisis intervention, usually focused on topics such as alcoholic binges, SUICIDE, drugs, and runaways.

HPA axis   See HYPOTHALAMIC-PITUITARY-ADRENAL AXIS (HPA AXIS).

human immunodeficiency virus (HIV)   HIV infection is caused by this retrovirus that becomes incorporated into host cell DEOXYRIBONUCLEIC ACID (DNA) and results in debilitating and fatal disorders. DELIRIUM and DEMENTIA are common psychiatric sequelae.

humiliation   Sense of disgrace and SHAME often experienced in DEPRESSION.

Huntington's disease (chorea)   A rare hereditary and progressive degenerative disease of the CENTRAL NERVOUS SYSTEM (CNS) transmitted as an autosomal dominant trait. Onset is typically in middle adult life with involuntary movements of the face, hands, and shoulders. These movements become more pronounced and often result in a massive jerkiness of the limbs, facial muscles, and diaphragm. Progressive DEMENTIA typically parallels the MOVEMENT DISORDER and results in profound functional impairment. PSYCHOSIS and DEPRESSION are common psychiatric disorders that develop in this condition.

HVA   See HOMOVANILLIC ACID (HVA).

hwa-byung   A Korean CULTURE-SPECIFIC SYNDROME with both somatic and psychological SYMPTOMS, *hwa-byung,* or "anger syndrome," is characterized by sensations of constriction in the chest, palpitations, insomnia, sensations of heat, flushing, headache, dysphoria, ANXIETY, irritability, problems with concentration, and fear of impending death. It is attributed to the suppression of anger.

hydrocephalus   An abnormal increase in the amount of cerebrospinal fluid in the cranium, which causes enlargement of the fluid-filled structures of the BRAIN and deterioration of surrounding brain tissue.

hydroxyzine   An ANTIHISTAMINE medication primarily used in general medicine to treat dermatological conditions (e.g., itching) and cold or allergy SYMPTOMS. It may also be used in PSYCHIATRY to treat mild ANXIETY or to promote SLEEP, especially in children. Marketed under the brand name VISTARIL; may also be known by the discontinued brand name ATARAX. See "Medications Used in Psychiatry."

hyperactive disorder　See ATTENTION-DEFICIT/HYPERACTIVITY DISORDER (ADHD).

hyperactivity　Excessive motor activity that may be purposeful or aimless; movements and utterances usually are more rapid than normal. Hyperactivity is a prominent feature of ATTENTION-DEFICIT/HYPERACTIVITY DISORDER (ADHD).

hyperacusis　Inordinate sensitivity to sounds.

hyperarousal　A state of increased psychological and physiological tension marked by such effects as ANXIETY, exaggeration of the startle response, INSOMNIA, reduced pain tolerance, fatigue, and exacerbation of inherent PERSONALITY traits.

hyperkinetic disorder　See ATTENTION-DEFICIT/HYPERACTIVITY DISORDER (ADHD).

hyperprolactinemia　A pituitary disorder characterized by excessive amounts of the HORMONE PROLACTIN. It is most commonly caused by a pituitary prolactin-secreting tumor or by certain PSYCHOTROPIC medications, such as CONVENTIONAL ANTIPSYCHOTICS (e.g., HALOPERIDOL [HALDOL]). GALACTORRHEA, amenorrhea (failure to menstruate), and decreased LIBIDO in women and gynecomastia (breast enlargement) and decreased SEXUAL DRIVE in men are common manifestations.

hyperreflexia　Overactive or overresponsive reflexes, such as the ankle jerk or the knee jerk, suggestive of upper motor NEURON disease and lessening or LOSS OF CONTROL ordinarily exerted by higher BRAIN centers of lower neural pathways (DISINHIBITION).

hypersexuality　A disturbance of sexuality characterized by excessive sexual activity; known as NYMPHOMANIA in women and SATYRIASIS in men. Hypersexuality has been described as a behavior-addictive disorder, a COMPULSIVE disorder, and an atypical IMPULSE-CONTROL DISORDER. Hypersexuality can also occur in conditions such as ALZHEIMER'S DISEASE, head injury, and KLÜVER-BUCY SYNDROME.

hypersomnia　A DYSSOMNIA consisting of prolonged or daytime SLEEP episodes occurring almost daily. The hypersomnia is called *primary* if it is not related to another MENTAL DISORDER, substance induced, or due to a GENERAL MEDICAL CONDITION.

hypertensive crisis　A sudden and sometimes fatal rise in blood pressure; may occur as a result of combining MONOAMINE OXIDASE INHIBITORS (MAOIs) with food containing high amounts of TYRAMINE (e.g., certain cheeses, fava beans, red wine) or with other SYMPATHOMIMETIC substances (e.g., cough remedies, nose drops).

hyperthyroidism   Excessive activity of the thyroid gland, which may be associated with DEMENTIA, GENERALIZED ANXIETY DISORDER, PANIC DISORDER, HYPOACTIVE SEXUAL DESIRE DISORDER, and INSOMNIA.

hyperventilation   Overbreathing sometimes associated with ANXIETY and marked by reduction of blood carbon dioxide, producing complaints of light-headedness, faintness, tingling of the extremities, palpitations, and respiratory distress.

hypesthesia   Diminished sensitivity to tactile stimuli.

hypnagogic   Referring to the semiconscious state immediately preceding SLEEP; may include HALLUCINATIONS that are of no pathological significance.

hypnophobia   The FEAR of SLEEP.

hypnopompic   Referring to the state immediately preceding awakening; may include HALLUCINATIONS that are of no pathological significance.

hypnosis   A state of decreased general awareness with heightened ATTENTION to a constricted or localized area of stimulation, such as repetitive SUGGESTIONS by another person (the hypnotist) involving consciousness, MEMORY, ANESTHESIA, or paralysis. The state usually is associated with the feeling that the subject is behaving nonvolitionally even though aware of what the behavior is. Factors determining the subject's responsivity include the nature of the preexisting relationship with the hypnotist; prior expectations, beliefs, and motivations concerning hypnosis; and, most important, characterological and individual differences.

hypnotic   Any agent that induces SLEEP. Although SEDATIVES, NARCOTICS, or ANXIOLYTICS in sufficient dosage may produce sleep as an incidental effect, the term *hypnotic* is appropriately reserved for drugs used primarily to produce sleep.

hypnotic use disorder   See SEDATIVE-, HYPNOTIC-, or ANXIOLYTIC-RELATED DISORDERS.

hypoactive sexual desire disorder   See under SEXUAL DESIRE DISORDERS.

hypochondriasis   One of the SOMATOFORM DISORDERS, characterized by persisting worry about health or FEAR of having some disease despite appropriate medical reassurance and lack of findings on physical or laboratory examination.

hypoglycemia   Abnormally low level of blood sugar. See INSULIN COMA TREATMENT.

hypomania   A psychopathological state and ABNORMALITY of MOOD falling somewhere between normal positive mood and MANIA. It is characterized by unrealistic optimism, pressure of speech and activity, and a decreased need for SLEEP. Some people show increased creativity during hypomanic states, whereas others show poor JUDGMENT, irritability, and irascibility. See BIPOLAR DISORDERS.

hypomanic episode   Characteristics are the same as in a MANIC EPISODE but not so severe as to cause marked impairment in social or occupational functioning or to require hospitalization, even though the MOOD change is clearly different from the subject's usual nondepressed mood and is observable to others. See BIPOLAR DISORDERS.

hypomimia   A reduced degree of facial expression, caused by motor impairment, as seen in PARKINSON'S DISEASE.

hyponatremia   A decrease in the serum sodium concentration below the normal range, usually resulting from retention of water by the kidneys. CARBAMAZEPINE, an ANTICONVULSANT medication used as a MOOD STABILIZER, may induce hyponatremia, particularly in older patients.

hypothalamic-pituitary-adrenal axis (HPA axis)   A complex set of interactions between the HYPOTHALAMUS, the pituitary gland, and the adrenal or suprarenal glands. The HPA axis is involved in the regulation of temperature, digestion, immune response, mood, sexuality, and energy usage. The HPA axis is also involved in ANXIETY DISORDERS, BIPOLAR DISORDER, POSTTRAUMATIC STRESS DISORDER (PTSD), and DEPRESSION.

hypothalamus   A complex BRAIN structure composed of many nuclei with various functions. It is the head ganglion of the AUTONOMIC NERVOUS SYSTEM (ANS) and is involved in the control of heat regulation; heart rate, blood pressure, and respiration; sexual activity; water, fat, and carbohydrate metabolism; digestion, appetite, and body weight; wakefulness; FIGHT-OR-FLIGHT RESPONSE; and rage.

hypothyroidism   Decreased activity of the thyroid gland, which may be associated with DEMENTIA, depressed MOOD, HYPOACTIVE SEXUAL DESIRE DISORDER, and SLEEP DISORDERS.

hypoxyphilia   A PARAPHILIA that is a subcategory of sexual masochism, this term refers to a potentially lethal sexual practice in which sexual AROUSAL is produced while reducing the oxygen supply to the BRAIN.

hysteria   A psychiatric SYNDROME first described by the French NEUROLOGIST Jean M. Charcot (1825–1893). The patient with hysteria may show shallow or unmodulated AFFECT, self-absorption, sexual preoccupation or promiscuous sexual behavior, and THOUGHT DISORDER. Hysteria is also referred to as CONVERSION DISORDER because it represents a conversion of ANXIETY related to UNCONSCIOUS CONFLICTS into somatic SYMPTOMS.

hysterical personality   See HISTRIONIC PERSONALITY DISORDER under PERSONALITY DISORDERS.

hysterics   Lay term for uncontrollable emotional outbursts.

I

---

iatrogenic illness   A disorder precipitated, aggravated, or induced by the physician's attitude, examination, comments, or treatment.

ICD-9   The 9th edition of the *INTERNATIONAL CLASSIFICATION OF DISEASES*.

ICD-10   The 10th edition of the *INTERNATIONAL CLASSIFICATION OF DISEASES*.

ICSD   See *INTERNATIONAL CLASSIFICATION OF SLEEP DISORDERS* (ICSD).

id   In Freudian theory, the part of the PERSONALITY that is the UNCONSCIOUS source of unstructured desires and DRIVES. See also EGO; SUPEREGO.

idealization   A mental mechanism in which the person attributes exaggeratedly positive qualities to the self or others. See DEFENSE MECHANISM.

idealized parental imago   In Heinz Kohut's (1913–1981) SELF PSYCHOLOGY, the archaic SELFOBJECT to which the child, as is appropriate for his or her phase of development, needs to admire and feel attached. When development is successful, it becomes transformed into internalized values and ideals that are soothing, DRIVE-channeling structures that maintain and restore internal balance. The idealized parental imago is one pole of the BIPOLAR SELF; the other pole is the GRANDIOSE SELF.

idealizing transference   An attitude in which the therapist is seen in glowing, elevated terms. From a SELF PSYCHOLOGY perspective, this attitude is viewed as an inevitable element in the treatment of narcissistic phenomena. See SELFOBJECT TRANSFERENCE.

ideas of reference   Incorrect interpretations of casual incidents and external events as having direct reference to oneself. May reach sufficient intensity to constitute DELUSIONS.

idée fixe   Fixed idea. Used in PSYCHIATRY to describe a COMPULSIVE DRIVE, an obsessive idea, or a DELUSION.

identification   A DEFENSE MECHANISM, operating unconsciously, by which one patterns oneself after some other person. Identification plays a major ROLE in the development of one's PERSONALITY and specifically of the SUPEREGO, To be differentiated from imitation or role MODELING, which is a CONSCIOUS process.

identity   The sense of self and unity of PERSONALITY over time; one element of identity is GENDER IDENTITY. Identity disturbances are seen in GENDER IDENTITY DISORDER, BORDERLINE PERSONALITY DISORDER, and SCHIZOPHRENIA.

identity crisis   A loss of the sense of the sameness and historical continuity of one's SELF and an inability to accept or adopt the ROLE one perceives as being expected by society. This is often expressed by self-isolation, SOCIAL WITHDRAWAL, extremism, rebelliousness, and negativity and is typically triggered by a sudden increase in the strength of instinctual DRIVES in a milieu of rapid social evolution and technological change. See PSYCHOSOCIAL DEVELOPMENT.

identity diffusion   The lack of a consistent sense of SELF due to a failure of integration of diverse senses of self.

identity problem   This term is applied to adolescents who are in the process of detaching themselves from their families and parental value systems in an attempt to establish their own independent IDENTITIES.

idioms of distress   Ways in which different CULTURES express, experience, and cope with feelings of distress. One example is SOMATIZATION, or the expression of distress through physical SYMPTOMS.

idiopathic   Of unknown cause.

idiopathic recurring stupor   A disturbance of unknown ETIOLOGY characterized by episodic STUPOR that may proceed to coma.

idiot savant   A person with gross INTELLECTUAL DISABILITY who nonetheless is capable of performing certain remarkable feats in sharply circumscribed intellectual areas, such as calendar calculation or puzzle solving.

IED   See INTERMITTENT EXPLOSIVE DISORDER (IED).

ikota   A CULTURE-SPECIFIC SYNDROME. See *DHAT*.

illusion   A misperception of a real external stimulus. For example, a person may misperceive the rustling of leaves as the sound of voices. Contrast with HALLUCINATION.

iloperidone   An ATYPICAL ANTIPSYCHOTIC medication used to treat SCHIZOPHRENIA. Marketed under the brand name FANAPT. See "Medications Used in Psychiatry."

IM   See INTRAMUSCULAR (IM).

imago   In Jungian theory (Carl Gustav Jung, 1875–1961), an UNCONSCIOUS mental image, usually an IDEALIZATION, of an important person in one's early history.

imipramine   A TRICYCLIC ANTIDEPRESSANT medication used to treat DEPRESSION, PANIC DISORDER, and GENERALIZED ANXIETY DISORDER and as ADJUNCTIVE therapy in reducing ENURESIS in children ages 6 years and older. Marketed under the brand name TOFRANIL. See "Medications Used in Psychiatry."

Imitrex   Brand name for the antimigraine drug SUMATRIPTAN.

immediate memory   The RECALL of perceived material within a period of 30 seconds to 25 minutes after presentation.

immunity   See "Legal Terms."

implicit memory   See PROCEDURAL MEMORY.

implosion   See FLOODING.

implosion therapy   A form of behavior therapy involving intensive recollection and review of anxiety-producing situations or events in a patient's life in an attempt to develop more appropriate responses to similar situations in the future.

impotence   1) Inability to achieve or maintain a penile erection of sufficient quality to engage in successful sexual intercourse (i.e., MALE ERECTILE DISORDER; see under SEXUAL AROUSAL DISORDERS).

2) Lacking in masculine sexual power, strength, or vigor; see also CASTRATION; contrast with POTENCY.

imprinting   A term in ETHOLOGY referring to a process similar to rapid learning or behavioral patterning that occurs at critical points in very early stages of animal development. The extent to which imprinting occurs in human development has not been established.

impulse   A desire or propensity to act in a certain way, typically in order to ease tension or gain pleasure.

impulse-control disorders   Disorders characterized by inability to resist an IMPULSE, DRIVE, or temptation to perform some act that is harmful to oneself or to others. The act may be premeditated or unplanned. The person may show regret or GUILT for the action or its consequences. In DSM-IV-TR, this category includes INTERMITTENT EXPLOSIVE DISORDER (IED), KLEPTOMANIA, PATHOLOGICAL GAMBLING, PYRO-

MANIA, TRICHOTILLOMANIA, and IMPULSE-CONTROL DISORDER not otherwise specified [NOS].

imu A CULTURE-SPECIFIC SYNDROME. See *LATAH*.

inappropriate affect A display of EMOTION that is out of harmony with reality or with the verbal or intellectual content that it accompanies. See AFFECT.

incest Sexual activity between close blood relatives, such as father-daughter, mother-son, or between siblings.

incidence The number of new cases of a disorder that occurs during a specified time period.

incoherence Lacking in unity or consistency; often applied to speech or thinking that is not understandable because of any of the following: lack of logical connection between words or phrases; excessive use of incomplete sentences; many irrelevancies or abrupt changes in subject matter; idiosyncratic word usage; or distorted grammar. See also LOOSENING OF ASSOCIATIONS.

incompetence See "Legal Terms."

incompetency Lack of the capacity to understand the nature of, to assess adequately, or to manage effectively a specified transaction or situation that the ordinary person could reasonably be expected to handle. As used in the law, the term refers primarily to COGNITIVE defects that interfere with JUDGMENT.

incorporation A primitive DEFENSE MECHANISM, operating unconsciously, in which the psychic representation of a person, or parts of the person, is figuratively ingested. See INTROJECTION.

Inderal Brand name for the BETA-BLOCKER drug PROPRANOLOL.

individualized education plan Treatment for specific DEVELOPMENTAL DISORDERS in public schools that is mandated by law under the Education for All Handicapped Children Act of 1975 (effective 1978), which calls for special education for all learning-disabled children in the "least restrictive environment." This may include accommodations such as extra time for tests, use of computer, or a specialized setting such as a self-contained classroom.

individual psychology A system of psychiatric theory, research, and therapy developed by Alfred Adler (1870–1937) that emphasizes COMPENSATION and OVERCOMPENSATION for inferiority feelings (inferiority COMPLEX).

individuation A process of DIFFERENTIATION, the end result of which is development of the individual PERSONALITY that is separate and distinct from all others.

indoleamine   One of a group of BIOGENIC AMINES (e.g., SEROTONIN) that contains a five-membered, nitrogen-containing INDOLE ring and an AMINE group within its chemical structure.

indoles   A group of biogenic compounds that include INDOLEAMINES.

industrial psychiatry   See OCCUPATIONAL PSYCHIATRY.

infancy, childhood, and adolescence disorders   In   DSM-IV-TR, the full title for this section is "Disorders Usually First Diagnosed in Infancy, Childhood, or Adolescence." Included are ATTENTION-DEFICIT and DISRUPTIVE BEHAVIOR DISORDERS, COMMUNICATION DISORDERS, ELIMINATION DISORDERS, feeding and EATING DISORDERS of infancy or early childhood, INTELLECTUAL DISABILITY, LEARNING DISORDERS, MOTOR SKILLS DISORDER, PERVASIVE DEVELOPMENTAL DISORDERS, REACTIVE ATTACHMENT DISORDER, SELECTIVE MUTISM, SEPARATION ANXIETY DISORDER, STEREOTYPIC MOVEMENT DISORDER, and TIC DISORDERS.

infantile autism   See AUTISTIC DISORDER.

infantilism   See under SEXUAL MASOCHISM.

infant psychiatry   An aspect of CHILD AND ADOLESCENT PSYCHIATRY that deals with the DIAGNOSIS, treatment, and PREVENTION of maladaptive psychological functioning in the very young.

inferiority complex   See INDIVIDUAL PSYCHOLOGY.

in forma pauperis   See "Legal Terms."

informed consent   Permission by the patient for a medical procedure based on understanding the nature of the procedure, the risks involved, the consequences of withholding permission, and alternative procedures. See also "Legal Terms."

infradian rhythms   See BIOLOGICAL RHYTHMS.

inhalant-related disorders   In DSM-IV-TR, a group of MENTAL DISORDERS that includes inhalant DEPENDENCE; inhalant ABUSE; inhalant INTOXICATION; inhalant intoxication DELIRIUM; inhalant-induced persisting DEMENTIA; inhalant-induced PSYCHOTIC DISORDER, with DELUSIONS or HALLUCINATIONS; inhalant-induced MOOD DISORDER; and inhalant-induced ANXIETY DISORDER.

inhalants   See NITRITE INHALANTS.

inhibited orgasm   See ORGASMIC DISORDERS.

inhibition   Behavioral evidence of an UNCONSCIOUS defense against forbidden instinctual DRIVES (see INSTINCT) that may interfere with or restrict specific activities.

insane   Obsolete term referring to the state of having a MENTAL DISORDER.

insanity An obsolete term for PSYCHOSIS. Still used, however, in strictly legal contexts such as INSANITY DEFENSE. See also "Legal Terms."

insanity defense See "Legal Terms."

insecurity A feeling of HELPLESSNESS against ANXIETY arising from uncertainty about one's goals, ideals, abilities, and/or relationships.

insight Self-understanding; the extent of a person's understanding of the origin, nature, and mechanisms of his or her maladaptive attitudes and behavior. Sometimes used to indicate whether an individual is aware that he or she has a MENTAL DISORDER or that his or her SYMPTOMS have a psychiatric cause.

insight-oriented psychotherapy A form of therapy that is based on the concepts of psychoanalytic theory developed by Sigmund Freud (1856–1939) but uses slightly different techniques and time frames. Treatment involves the therapist assisting patients to gain new or improved understanding and insight into the possible explanations for their feelings, responses, behaviors, and current relationships with other people. Also known as *expressive therapy* or *intensive psychoanalytic psychotherapy*.

insomnia A DYSSOMNIA consisting of difficulty initiating or maintaining SLEEP or of nonrestorative sleep (i.e., sleep is adequate in amount but unrefreshing) associated with daytime fatigue or impaired daytime functioning. The insomnia is called *primary* if it is not related to another MENTAL DISORDER, not substance induced, and not due to a GENERAL MEDICAL CONDITION.

instinct An inborn DRIVE. The primary human instincts include self-preservation, sexuality, and—according to some proponents—the DEATH INSTINCT, of which AGGRESSION is one manifestation.

institutionalization Long-term placement of an individual into a hospital, nursing home, residential center, or other facility where independent living is restricted in varying degrees.

insulin coma treatment Injection of insulin in sufficient quantity to produce profound HYPOGLYCEMIA (low blood sugar) resulting in COMA. First used in 1933 in the treatment of SCHIZOPHRENIA, it is rarely used today.

intake The initial interview between a patient and a member of a psychiatric team in a MENTAL HEALTH facility.

integration The useful organization and incorporation of both new and old data, experience, and emotional capacities into the PERSONALITY. Also refers to the organization and amalgamation of functions at various levels of PSYCHOSEXUAL DEVELOPMENT.

intellectual disability   A disorder characterized by significantly impaired cognitive functioning and deficits in two or more areas of adaptive functioning (conceptual skills, social skills, daily living skills), with onset before 18 years of age. Intellectual disability is usually defined as an INTELLIGENCE QUOTIENT (IQ) of 70 or below. Also referred to as *mental retardation.* Different levels of intellectual disability severity are recognized:

IQ level	Level of severity
50–55 to 70	Mild
35–40 to 50–55	Moderate
20–25 to 35–40	Severe
Below 20–25	Profound

intellectualization   A mental DEFENSE MECHANISM in which the person engages in excessive abstract thinking to avoid CONFRONTATION with CONFLICTS or disturbing feelings. It may be associated with obsessional or PARANOID thinking.

intelligence   The capacity of the mind for abstract thinking, reasoning, problem solving, and learning. May be affected by EMOTIONS.

intelligence quotient (IQ)   A numerical rating determined through PSYCHOLOGICAL TESTING that indicates the approximate relationship of a person's MENTAL AGE (MA) to chronological age (CA). Expressed mathematically as $IQ = [MA/CA] \times 100$. See also INTELLECTUAL DISABILITY.

intentional tort   See "Legal Terms."

inter alia   See "Legal Terms."

interictal behavior syndrome   Sometimes termed *temporal lobe epileptic personality,* this syndrome manifests as PERSONALITY CHANGES in three areas: 1) sexuality, such as sexual PARAPHILIAS, CONFLICTS over sexual preference, or hyposexuality; 2) aggressivity, such as aggressive actions, moral indignation, or plans for retaliation for imagined slights; and 3) EMOTIONS and intellect, such as COMPULSIVE writing or drawing (often related to religious or philosophical speculations), preoccupation with details, and a clinging quality in relationships with others (*social viscosity*). See EPILEPSY.

intermittent explosive disorder (IED) An IMPULSE-CONTROL DISOR-DER consisting of aggressive outbursts (e.g., assaultiveness or destruction of property) that are out of proportion to any evident stressors. Often the behavior is completely uncharacteristic of the person, who does not show this behavior between episodes. In many cases, however, this aggressiveness is expressed in less explosive ways between episodes.

internal capsule See BASAL GANGLIA.

International Classification of Diseases **(ICD)** The official list of disease categories issued by the World Health Organization; subscribed to by all member nations, who may assign their own terms to each ICD category. The ICDA (*International Classification of Diseases, U.S. Public Health Service adaptation*) represents the official list of diagnostic terms to be used for each ICD category in the United States.

International Classification of Sleep Disorders **(ICSD)** Current nosology of SLEEP DISORDERS published by the AMERICAN ACADEMY OF SLEEP MEDICINE (AASM) in association with the European Sleep Research Society, the Japanese Society of Sleep Research, and the Latin American Sleep Society.

internship The first year of graduate medical education, which ordinarily is integrated into a full residency training program in a designated specialty. Currently, *PGY-1* or *PG1* (first postgraduate training year) tends to be the preferred term.

interpersonal (psycho)therapy (IPT) A form of brief (12–15 weeks) PSYCHOTHERAPY originally developed by PSYCHIATRIST Gerald Klerman (1928–1992), PSYCHOLOGIST Myrna Weissman, and colleagues for the treatment of DEPRESSION in which the focus is on four interpersonal problem areas often associated with its onset: GRIEF, ROLE disputes, role transitions, and interpersonal DEFICITS. The focus of the therapy is on current problems, important social relationships, self-evaluation by the patient with ASSESSMENT of his or her current situation, and clarification and modification of maladaptive PERCEPTIONS and current interpersonal relationships. A procedural manual specifies the concept, techniques, and strategies of IPT.

interpersonal skills Effective adaptive behavior in relation to other persons.

interpretation The process by which the therapist helps patients understand a particular aspect of their problems or behavior.

intoxication   The acute effects of overdosage with chemical substances. Characteristically, intoxication with substances of ABUSE produces behavioral or psychological changes because of their effects
on the CENTRAL NERVOUS SYSTEM (CNS). Such changes may be expressed as belligerence, differences in MOOD, or impaired JUDGMENT.

alcohol   Typical SYMPTOMS include maladaptive behavioral changes
such as inappropriate aggressive or sexual behavior, LABILITY of
MOOD, and impaired JUDGMENT. Accompanying physical SIGNS include
slurred speech, incoordination, unsteady gait, and flushed face.

amphetamine   Typical SYMPTOMS include maladaptive psychological or behavioral changes such as EUPHORIA with enhanced vigor
and alertness or GRANDIOSITY; affective blunting with fatigue or sadness; changes in sociability ranging from gregariousness to SOCIAL
WITHDRAWAL; hypervigilance and sensitivity, sometimes leading to
fighting; ANXIETY, tension, or anger; stereotyped, repetitive behavior; and impaired JUDGMENT. Perceptual disturbances also may occur. Accompanying physical SIGNS may include very rapid or very
slow heartbeat, elevated or lowered blood pressure, perspiration
or chills, nausea, evidence of weight loss, muscular weakness,
chest pain, and confusion.

caffeine   Typical SYMPTOMS include restlessness, nervousness, EX-
CITEMENT, INSOMNIA, and PSYCHOMOTOR AGITATION. Accompanying
physical SIGNS include flushed face, muscle twitching, and ram-
bling speech.

cannabis   Maladaptive behavioral or psychological changes include impaired motor coordination, EUPHORIA, ANXIETY, suspiciousness, sensation of slowed time, impaired JUDGMENT, and SOCIAL
WITHDRAWAL. Physical SIGNS may include increased appetite, dry
mouth, and very rapid heartbeat.

cocaine   SIGNS and SYMPTOMS are the same as in AMPHETAMINE intoxication (see above).

hallucinogen   The SYNDROME includes maladaptive behavioral or
psychological changes such as marked ANXIETY or DEPRESSION, FEAR of
losing one's mind, PARANOID IDEATION, and impaired JUDGMENT. Also,
perceptual changes such as intensified PERCEPTIONS, ILLUSIONS, HALLU-
CINATIONS, DEREALIZATION, and DEPERSONALIZATION occur in a state of
full wakefulness. Some physical SIGNS include sweating, very rapid
heartbeat, blurring of vision, TREMORS, and incoordination.

inhalant   Recent use or short-term, high-dose exposure to volatile
inhalants often leads to maladaptive behavioral or psychological

changes such as belligerence, assaultiveness, APATHY, and impaired JUDGMENT. Accompanying physical SIGNS include dizziness, incoordination, slurred speech, unsteady gait, EUPHORIA, lethargy, PSYCHOMOTOR RETARDATION, and blurred vision.

opioid SYMPTOMS include initial EUPHORIA followed by APATHY, PSYCHOMOTOR AGITATION or RETARDATION, and impaired JUDGMENT. Diminished pupil size in the eyes, drowsiness, slurred speech, and impairment in ATTENTION or MEMORY are some of the physical indicators.

phencyclidine (PCP) Recent use of PCP or a related substance may induce belligerence, assaultiveness, impulsiveness, unpredictability, and impaired JUDGMENT. The physical SIGNS may include hypertension or a very rapid heartbeat, numbness or diminished responsiveness to pain, ATAXIA, muscle RIGIDITY, or SEIZURES.

sedative Effects of sedative intoxication are similar to those of alcohol intoxication (see above). SYMPTOMS include inappropriate sexual or aggressive behavior, swings in MOOD, and impaired JUDGMENT. Accompanying physical SIGNS may include slurred speech, incoordination, unsteady gait, and impairment in ATTENTION or MEMORY.

intramuscular (IM) Within or into the muscle.

intrapsychic Taking place within the PSYCHE or mind.

intrapsychic conflict See CONFLICT.

intravenous (IV) Within or into the veins.

introjection A DEFENSE MECHANISM, operating unconsciously (see UNCONSCIOUS), whereby loved or hated external objects are symbolically absorbed within oneself. The converse of PROJECTION. May serve as a defense against CONSCIOUS recognition of intolerable hostile IMPULSES. For example, in severe DEPRESSION, the individual may unconsciously direct unacceptable hatred or AGGRESSION toward herself or himself. Related to the more primitive FANTASY of oral INCORPORATION.

introspection Self-observation or the examination of one's feelings, often as a result of PSYCHOTHERAPY.

introversion Preoccupation with oneself and accompanying reduction of interest in the outside world. Contrast with EXTRAVERSION. Also used to indicate shyness and decreased sociability.

Intuniv Brand name for extended-release formulation of the alpha$_{2A}$-ADRENERGIC RECEPTOR AGONIST drug GUANFACINE.

Invega Brand name for an extended-release formulation of the ATYPICAL ANTIPSYCHOTIC drug PALIPERIDONE.

involuntary commitment The practice of using legal means to commit a person to a psychiatric hospital against his or her will. In the United States, individuals must be exhibiting behavior that is dangerous to themselves or others in order to be committed; the commitment must be for evaluation only, and a court order must be received for more than very short-term treatment or hospitalization (typically no longer than 72 hours). The specifics of the relevant statutes vary from state to state.

IPT See INTERPERSONAL (PSYCHO)THERAPY (IPT).

IQ INTELLIGENCE QUOTIENT.

irkunii A CULTURE-SPECIFIC SYNDROME. See *LATAH*.

irregular sleep-wake pattern See under CIRCADIAN RHYTHM SLEEP DISORDERS.

irresistible impulse test See under INSANITY DEFENSE in "Legal Terms."

Ismelin Former brand name for the discontinued antihypertensive drug GUANETHIDINE.

isocarboxazid A nonselective and irreversible MONOAMINE OXIDASE INHIBITOR (MAOI) ANTIDEPRESSANT medication used for the treatment of DEPRESSION and ANXIETY with or without AGORAPHOBIA. Marketed under the brand name MARPLAN. See "Medications Used in Psychiatry."

isolated sleep paralysis A state of consciousness experienced either while waking up or while falling asleep, characterized by feeling unable to move for several seconds or minutes. The individual who experiences this state is fully aware of the condition and has complete RECALL of the episode. Vivid and terrifying HALLUCINATIONS often accompany this state of consciousness, and a sense of acute danger may be felt. Once the episode of paralysis passes, the individual often sits up with a start and experiences SYMPTOMS of ANXIETY (e.g., tachycardia, HYPERVENTILATION, FEAR) only to realize that the PERCEPTIONS of danger were false. In the African American community, this state of consciousness is also sometimes known as *the witch is riding you* or *the haint has you.* This phenomenon is called *kanashibari* in Japan and *ghost oppression* in China.

isolation An unconscious DEFENSE MECHANISM often used by obsessive-compulsive patients. Isolation separates AFFECT from MEMORY. Thoughts or affects are treated as if they were untouchable, therefore requiring distance. An example is a patient talking about a painful event with a bland expression.

isomers Compounds with the same molecular formula but different structural formulas.

IV See INTRAVENOUS (IV).

J

Jacksonian epilepsy See EPILEPSY.

JCAHO See THE JOINT COMMISSION.

jealousy delusion See DELUSIONAL DISORDER.

jinjinia bemar A CULTURE-SPECIFIC SYNDROME. See *KORO*.

jiryan A CULTURE-SPECIFIC SYNDROME. See *DHAT*.

Joint Commission on Accreditation of Healthcare Organizations (JCAHO) See THE JOINT COMMISSION.

judgment Mental act of comparing choices between a given set of values in order to select a course of action. See also "Legal Terms."

jurisdiction See "Legal Terms."

K

kakorrhaphiophobia The FEAR of failure.

kava kava The active ingredient of this herbal medication is *Piper methysticum,* originally from the South Sea Islands. It is believed to stimulate GABA (GAMMA-AMINOBUTYRIC ACID) RECEPTORS, which may reduce ANXIETY and INSOMNIA.

Kemadrin Former brand name for the discontinued ANTICHOLINERGIC drug PROCYCLIDINE.

keraunophobia The FEAR of thunder.

ketamine An NMDA RECEPTOR ANTAGONIST developed in 1963 as an ANESTHETIC to replace PHENCYCLIDINE (PCP). Although still used as an anesthetic, primarily in veterinary medicine, ketamine has become a street drug, also know as "cat valium," "Kit-Kat," "K," "Vitamin K," and "Special K." Snorted or swallowed, ketamine can cause dream-like states and hallucinations.

kindling   Progressively increasing response of the brain to successive electrical stimuli. In BIPOLAR DISORDER, it is important to prevent the onset of MANIA because with each MANIC EPISODE, there is a tendency for the period until the next episode to become shorter. In this regard, it is believed that the manic episode "kindles" the BRAIN by making it more susceptible to a subsequent manic episode.

kinesics   The study of body posture, movement, and facial expressions.

Kleine-Levin syndrome   Periodic episodes of HYPERSOMNIA accompanied by excessive food intake and (in some cases) HYPERSEXUALITY. The SYNDROME first appears in ADOLESCENCE, usually in boys. It is not classified as either an EATING DISORDER or a SLEEP DISORDER. It is considered a neurological syndrome and is believed to reflect a frontal lobe or hypothalamic disturbance.

kleptomania   The impulsive, COMPULSIVE, addictive stealing of un-needed objects. The person feels an increased sense of tension before and gratification or relief after the theft.

Klinefelter's syndrome   Chromosomal defect in males in which there is an extra X CHROMOSOME. Manifestations may include underdeveloped testes, physical feminization, sterility, and INTELLECTUAL DISABILITY.

klismaphilia   One of the PARAPHILIAS, characterized by marked distress over, or acting on, sexual urges involving enemas.

Klonopin   Brand name for the BENZODIAZEPINE ANXIOLYTIC drug CLONAZEPAM.

Klüver-Bucy syndrome   A SYNDROME following bilateral TEMPORAL LOBE removal consisting of loss of recognition of people, loss of FEAR, unusually low aggression, HYPERSEXUALITY, excessive oral behavior, MEMORY deficits, and overreaction to visual stimuli.

koro   A term, probably of Malaysian origin, that refers to an episode of sudden and intense anxiety that the penis (or the vulva and nipples in females) will recede into the body and possibly cause death. This SYNDROME is reported in South and East Asia, where it is known also as *SHOOK YONG, SHUK YANG, SUK-YEONG,* and *SUO YANG* (China); *JINJINIA BEMAR* (Assam), and *ROK-JOO* (Thailand). It is occasionally found in the West. See CULTURE-SPECIFIC SYNDROMES.

Korsakoff's syndrome   See ALCOHOL AMNESTIC DISORDER (KORSAKOFF'S SYNDROME). See also SUBSTANCE-INDUCED PSYCHOTIC DISORDER; WERNICKE-KORSAKOFF SYNDROME.

Krabbe's disease   A rare GENETIC disorder (also known as LEUKODYS-TROPHY) consisting of a deficiency of the ENZYME beta-galactosidase, which causes the MYELIN sheath surrounding nerves in the BRAIN to degenerate. The disorder is characterized by progressive INTELLECTUAL DISABILITY, paralysis, blindness, deafness, and pseudobulbar palsy.

L

la belle indifférence   Literally, "beautiful indifference." Seen in certain patients with CONVERSION DISORDER who show an inappropriate lack of concern about their disabilities.

labile   Rapidly shifting (as applied to EMOTIONS); unstable.

lability of affect   See AFFECT.

lacrimation   Tearing; it may be a significant SYMPTOM in OPIOID WITHDRAWAL (see WITHDRAWAL SYMPTOMS).

Lamictal   Brand name for the ANTICONVULSANT drug LAMOTRIGINE.

lamotrigine   An ANTICONVULSANT medication sometimes used in PSYCHIATRY to prevent or treat the SYMPTOMS of MANIA and DEPRESSION in BIPOLAR DISORDER. Marketed under the brand name LAMICTAL. See "Medications Used in Psychiatry."

Landau-Kleffner syndrome   A severe form of MIXED RECEPTIVE-EXPRESSIVE LANGUAGE DISORDER (see under COMMUNICATION DISORDERS) accompanied by SEIZURES and other CENTRAL NERVOUS SYSTEM (CNS) dysfunction.

language disorder   See COMMUNICATION DISORDERS.

Lanterman-Petris-Short Act   See "Legal Terms."

lapsus linguae   A slip of the tongue due to UNCONSCIOUS factors.

latah   The term is of Malaysian or Indonesian origin, but the syndrome has been found in many parts of the world. In Malaysia, *latah* is more common in middle-aged women. It presents as hypersensitivity to sudden fright, often with echolalia, echopraxia, command obedience, and dissociative or trancelike behavior. Other terms for this condition are *AMURAKH, IRKUNII, IKOTA, OLAN, MYRIACHIT,* and *MENKEITI* (Siberian groups); *BAH-TSCHI, BAH-TSI,* and *BAAH-JI* (Thailand); *IMU* (Ainu,

Sakhalin, Japan); and *MALI-MALI* and *SILOK* (Philippines). See CULTURE-SPECIFIC SYNDROMES.

late luteal phase dysphoric disorder   See PREMENSTRUAL DYSPHORIC DISORDER.

latency   A developmental phase extending from age 6–7 to age 10–11 years, originally identified by Freud as the period between the oedipal phase and puberty, distinguished by quiescence in regard to libidinal and aggressive drive.

latency period   See PSYCHOSEXUAL DEVELOPMENT.

latent content   The hidden (i.e., UNCONSCIOUS) meaning of thoughts or actions, especially in dreams or FANTASIES. In dreams, it is expressed in distorted, disguised, condensed, and symbolic form. Contrast with MANIFEST CONTENT.

LBD   See LEWY BODY DEMENTIA.

L-deprenyl   See SELEGILINE.

L-dopa   See LEVODOPA.

learned helplessness   A condition in which a person attempts to establish and maintain contact with another by adopting a helpless, powerless stance.

learning disability   A SYNDROME affecting school-aged children of normal or above-normal INTELLIGENCE characterized by specific difficulties in learning to read (DYSLEXIA, WORD BLINDNESS), write (DYSGRAPHIA), and calculate (dyscalculia). The disorder is believed to be related to slow developmental progression of perceptual motor skills. See MINIMAL BRAIN DYSFUNCTION (MBD).

learning disorders   In DSM-IV-TR, this is a major group of INFANCY, CHILDHOOD, AND ADOLESCENCE DISORDERS that includes READING DISORDER, MATHEMATICS DISORDER, and DISORDER OF WRITTEN EXPRESSION. Formerly known as ACADEMIC SKILLS DISORDERS.

Lennox-Gastaut syndrome   A severe form of EPILEPSY with DEVELOPMENTAL DELAYS and behavioral disturbances.

lentiform nucleus   The large, cone-shaped mass of GRAY MATTER that forms the central core of the cerebral hemisphere, whose convex base is formed by the PUTAMEN and whose apical part consists of the GLOBUS PALLIDUS. Also called *lenticular nucleus.*

lesbian   A homosexual woman. See HOMOSEXUALITY.

Lesch-Nyhan syndrome   A rare, GENETIC neurological disorder characterized by self-mutilating behaviors such as head banging and/or lip and finger biting, uncontrolled spastic muscle movements, and involuntary movements of the upper extremities. Moderate INTELLECTUAL DISABILITY is also common.

lethality index   Set of criteria used to predict SUICIDE.

lethologica   Temporary inability to remember a proper noun or name.

leukoaraiosis   A radiological finding of changes in the WHITE MATTER in aged individuals that can be detected with high frequency by COMPUTED TOMOGRAPHY (CT) and MAGNETIC RESONANCE IMAGING (MRI). This white matter pathology is inconsistently associated with COGNITIVE IMPAIRMENT, motor dysfunction, and gait disturbances. Slowed cognitive processing and frontal executive abilities are also common. It may indicate a poorer prognosis and increased risk of stroke and brain hemorrhage.

leukodystrophy   A group of disorders characterized by progressive degeneration of the WHITE MATTER of the BRAIN, caused by GENETIC defects in the growth or development of MYELIN, the fatty covering that acts as an insulator around nerve fibers. Also see KRABBE'S DISEASE.

leukopenia   A decrease below normal levels in the number of white blood cells (leukocytes), most commonly provoked by certain drugs, such as ANTICONVULSANTS. Also known as *neutropenia.*

levodopa (L-dopa)   A precursor of DOPAMINE that readily crosses the BLOOD-BRAIN BARRIER into the CENTRAL NERVOUS SYSTEM (CNS), where it is converted to dopamine. L-dopa is used to treat PARKINSON'S DISEASE in which there is deficiency of dopamine caused by the progressive deterioration of dopamine-producing NEURONS in the SUBSTANTIA NIGRA of the MIDBRAIN.

Lewy bodies   Abnormal aggregates of protein that develop inside nerve cells in PARKINSON'S DISEASE and ALZHEIMER'S DISEASE. Lewy bodies are identified under the microscope when histology is performed on the postmortem BRAIN.

Lewy body dementia (LBD)   A progressive brain disease and the second leading cause of degenerative dementia in the elderly, characterized anatomically by the presence of LEWY BODIES. Core features of LBD include fluctuating COGNITION, recurrent visual hallucinations, and motor features of PARKINSONISM. The loss of CHOLINERGIC neurons is thought to account for the degradation of cognitive functioning, as in ALZHEIMER'S DISEASE, while the loss of DOPAMINERGIC neurons is thought to account for the degradation of motor control, as in

PARKINSON'S DISEASE. The overlap of neuropathologies and presenting symptoms can make an accurate differential diagnosis difficult.

Lexapro   Brand name for the SELECTIVE SEROTONIN REUPTAKE INHIBITOR (SSRI) drug ESCITALOPRAM OXALATE.

lex talionis   See "Legal Terms."

liaison nursing   Consultation by clinical specialists in psychiatric nursing to nursing colleagues on issues of patient management in various clinical settings. See also PSYCHIATRIC NURSE.

liaison psychiatry   See CONSULTATION-LIAISON PSYCHIATRY.

libido   The psychic DRIVE or energy usually associated with the sexual INSTINCT. (*Sexual* is used here in the broad sense to include pleasure and love-object seeking.)

Librium   Brand name for the BENZODIAZEPINE ANXIOLYTIC drug CHLORDIAZEPOXIDE.

light therapy   The use of a balanced-spectrum light box that delivers between 5,000 and 10,000 lux in the treatment of SEASONAL MOOD DISORDER, PREMENSTRUAL DYSPHORIC DISORDER, and some SLEEP DISORDERS (e.g., CIRCADIAN RHYTHM SLEEP DISORDER, jet lag type). Also known as *phototherapy*.

limbic system   Visceral BRAIN; a group of brain structures—including the AMYGDALA, HIPPOCAMPUS, septum, CINGULATE GYRUS, and subcallosal gyrus—that help regulate EMOTION, MEMORY, and certain aspects of movement.

liothyronine   A synthetic form of the thyroid HORMONE L-triiodothyronine (T_3) used primarily for the treatment of hypothyroidism. In psychiatry, liothyronine is used off-label to AUGMENT ANTIDEPRESSANT treatment of REFRACTORY DEPRESSION. Marketed under the brand name CYTOMEL. See "Medications Used in Psychiatry."

lisdexamfetamine   A CENTRAL NERVOUS SYSTEM (CNS) STIMULANT indicated for the treatment of ATTENTION-DEFICIT/HYPERACTIVITY DISORDER (ADHD). Marketed under the brand name VYVANSE. See "Medications Used in Psychiatry."

lithium carbonate   An alkali metal, the carbonate salt of which is used to treat and prevent MANIA and DEPRESSION in BIPOLAR DISORDER. Also may be used as an ADJUVANT treatment for depression. Marketed under the brand name LITHOBID; may also be known by the discontinued brand names ESKALITH, LITHONATE, and LITHOTABS. See "Medications Used in Psychiatry."

lithium citrate   The water-soluble citrate salt of lithium, which is used to treat and prevent MANIA and DEPRESSION in BIPOLAR DISORDER and also sometimes used as an ADJUVANT treatment for depression. See "Medications Used in Psychiatry."

Lithobid   Brand name for LITHIUM CARBONATE.

Lithonate   Brand name (now discontinued) for LITHIUM CARBONATE.

Lithotabs   Brand name (now discontinued) for LITHIUM CARBONATE.

living will   One type of advance directive; a competent person's instructions for medical care, indicating the kind of care that will be consented to or refused. See also "Legal Terms."

lobotomy   A type of PSYCHOSURGERY in which one or more nerve tracts in the CEREBRUM are severed. This procedure is now rarely used in the United States except for intractable OBSESSIVE-COMPULSIVE DISORDER.

locura   A term used by Latinos in the United States and Latin America to refer to a severe form of chronic PSYCHOSIS. The condition is attributed to an inherited vulnerability, to the effect of multiple life difficulties, or to a combination of these factors. Symptoms exhibited include incoherence, agitation, auditory and visual HALLUCINATIONS, inability to follow rules of social interaction, unpredictability, and possibly violence. See CULTURE-SPECIFIC SYNDROMES.

locus coeruleus   A small area in the BRAIN STEM containing NOREPINEPHRINE NEURONS that may play an important role in a person's experience of ANXIETY and FEAR.

Lodosyn   Brand name for the antiparkinsonian agent CARBIDOPA.

logophobia   The FEAR of words.

logorrhea   Uncontrollable, excessive talking.

logotherapy   A form of EXISTENTIAL PSYCHOTHERAPY associated with Viktor Frankl (1905–1997).

long-term memory   The final phase of MEMORY in which information storage may last from hours to a lifetime. Contrast with IMMEDIATE MEMORY.

long-term potentiation (LTP)   The strengthening of connections between two nerve cells that lasts for an extended period of time. Studies of LTP are often carried out with slices of the HIPPOCAMPUS. LTP shares many features with LONG-TERM MEMORY, making it an attractive candidate for a cellular mechanism of learning.

loosening of associations   A disturbance of thinking evident in a person's speech in which the person shifts from one subject to another subject unrelated or minimally related to the first. Statements made by the person that lack a meaningful relationship may be juxtaposed, or speech may shift suddenly from one frame of reference to another. The person gives no indication of being aware of the disconnectedness, contradictions, or illogicality of speech. See also INCOHERENCE.

lorazepam   A BENZODIAZEPINE ANXIOLYTIC medication used to treat various ANXIETY DISORDERS and INSOMNIA. Marketed under the brand name ATIVAN. See "Medications Used in Psychiatry."

loss of control   Failure to restrain IMPULSES, functions, or actions that ordinarily can be regulated consciously (e.g., aggressive actions, sexual impulses, bladder and bowel emptying). In relation to alcohol and other substances, *loss of control* refers to an impaired ability to modulate the amount or frequency of substance intake once any amount of the substance has been administered. Such loss of control, or impaired control, is regarded as one SIGN of DEPENDENCE on the substance used.

Lou Gehrig disease   See AMYOTROPHIC LATERAL SCLEROSIS (ALS).

loxapine   A CONVENTIONAL ANTIPSYCHOTIC medication (a DIBENZOXAZEPINE) used in the treatment of SCHIZOPHRENIA AND OTHER PSYCHOTIC DISORDERS. Now available only as generic but may still be known by the discontinued brand name LOXITANE. See "Medications Used in Psychiatry."

Loxitane   Brand name (now discontinued) for the CONVENTIONAL ANTIPSYCHOTIC drug LOXAPINE.

LSD (lysergic acid diethylamide)   A potent HALLUCINOGEN that produces psychotic SYMPTOMS and behavior such as HALLUCINATIONS, ILLUSIONS, body and time-space distortions, and, less commonly, intense PANIC or mystical experiences.

LTP   See LONG-TERM POTENTIATION (LTP).

lubrication-swelling response   See SEXUAL AROUSAL DISORDERS.

Ludiomil   Brand name (now discontinued) for the TETRACYCLIC ANTIDEPRESSANT drug MAPROTILINE.

lumbar puncture   The insertion of a needle between two lumbar vertebrae and through the meningeal wall to obtain cerebrospinal fluid for diagnostic purposes and to provide ANESTHESIA and paralysis of the lower extremities.

Lunesta   Brand name for the nonbenzodiazepine SEDATIVE-HYPNOTIC drug ESZOPICLONE.

Luria-Nebraska   A neuropsychological battery of tests consisting of 14 scales that assess writing, reading, arithmetic, and RECEPTIVE and

EXPRESSIVE language abilities as well as motor, tactile, auditory (rhythm), visual, MEMORY, and intellectual functioning. The battery may detect both the presence of BRAIN injury or a brain abnormality and its location and may indicate how the injury interferes with functioning.

Luvox Brand name for the SELECTIVE SEROTONIN REUPTAKE INHIBITOR (SSRI) drug FLUVOXAMINE.

Lyrica Brand name for the ANTICONVULSANT drug PREGABALIN.

lysergic acid diethylamide See LSD (LYSERGIC ACID DIETHYLAMIDE).

M

MA See MENTAL AGE (MA).

magical thinking A conviction that thinking equates with doing. Occurs in dreams in children and in patients under a variety of conditions. Characterized by lack of realistic relationship between cause and effect.

magnetic resonance imaging (MRI) A technique for visualizing anatomical structures. It involves placing patients in a strong magnetic field and then, by use of magnetic gradients and brief radio frequency pulses, determining the resonance characteristics at each point in the area to be studied. In PSYCHIATRY, NEUROLOGY, and neurosurgery, it is used to detect structural or anatomical abnormalities. It is better able to differentiate between gray and white matter than is COMPUTED TOMOGRAPHY (CT). See BRAIN IMAGING.

magnetic resonance spectroscopy (MRS) A specialized technique associated with MAGNETIC RESONANCE IMAGING (MRI). MRS allows doctors to obtain biochemical information about the tissues of the human body in a noninvasive way, whereas MRI provides information only about the structure of the body (i.e., the distribution of water and fat).

magnetoencephalography A type of BRAIN IMAGING that measures the magnetic fields created by the electrical activity of nerve cells, both cortical and subcortical.

maintenance drug therapy Continuing a therapeutic drug after it has reached efficacy to prevent an early RELAPSE or a later recurrence of illness. For instance, in clinical trials of ANTIDEPRESSANTS, there are three phases of treatment: the acute phase (which usually lasts 6–8 weeks), the continuation phase (2–6 months), and the maintenance phase (more than 6 months).

major depressive disorder   See under DEPRESSIVE DISORDERS.

major epilepsy (grand mal)   See EPILEPSY.

maladjustment   Unsuccessful attempts at ADAPTATION.

mal de ojo   "Evil eye" is a term widely found in Mediterranean cultures and elsewhere in the world. Children are especially at risk, and also sometimes females. Symptoms include fitful sleep, crying without apparent cause, diarrhea, vomiting, and fever. See CULTURE-SPECIFIC SYNDROMES.

male erectile disorder   See under SEXUAL AROUSAL DISORDERS.

maleness   Anatomical and physiological features that relate to the male's procreative capacity. See MASCULINE.

male orgasmic disorder   See under ORGASMIC DISORDERS.

mali-mali   A CULTURE-SPECIFIC SYNDROME. See *LATAH*.

malingering   Intentional production of false or grossly exaggerated physical or psychological SYMPTOMS motivated by external incentives such as avoiding onerous duties, obtaining financial compensation, evading criminal prosecution, or obtaining drugs. There is often a marked discrepancy between the person's claimed DISABILITY and objective findings. The person may be uncooperative during the diagnostic evaluation or fail to comply with the prescribed treatment.

malitia supplet aetatem   See "Legal Terms."

mal puesto   A CULTURE-SPECIFIC SYNDROME. See ROOTWORK.

managed care   A system organized to create a balance among the use of health care resources, control of health costs, and enhancement of the quality of care. Managed care systems seek to provide care in the most cost-effective manner by closely monitoring the intensity and duration of treatment as well as the settings in which it is provided. Managed care systems also organize physicians and other providers into coordinated networks of care to ensure that those who enroll in the system receive all medically necessary care. A wide array of mechanisms is used to control utilization and reduce costs. Currently, HEALTH MAINTENANCE ORGANIZATIONS (HMOs) are the most frequently used management system for managed care.

mania   A SYNDROME characterized by excessive elation or irritability, inflated self-esteem and GRANDIOSITY, HYPERACTIVITY, AGITATION, accelerated thinking and speaking, and FLIGHT OF IDEAS. The syndrome is found in BIPOLAR DISORDERS and may also occur in certain toxic and drug-induced states.

–mania   Formerly used as a nonspecific term for any type of "madness." Currently used as a suffix to indicate an excessive preoccupation with some kind of idea or activity and/or a COMPULSIVE need to behave in some abnormal way. Examples include DERMATILLOMANIA, EGOMANIA, EROTOMANIA, KLEPTOMANIA, MEGALOMANIA, MONOMANIA, NECROMANIA, NYMPHOMANIA, PYROMANIA, and TRICHOTILLOMANIA.

maniac   An imprecise and misleading term for an emotionally disturbed person. Usually implies violent behavior. Not specifically referable to any psychiatric diagnostic category.

manic-depressive illness   A term often used synonymously with BIPOLAR DISORDER, as defined in DSM-IV-TR.

manic episode   A distinct period (usually lasting at least 1 week) of abnormally and persistently elevated, expansive, or irritable MOOD accompanied by SYMPTOMS such as inflated self-esteem or GRANDIOSITY, decreased need for SLEEP, overtalkativeness or PRESSURED SPEECH, FLIGHT OF IDEAS or feeling that thoughts are racing, inattentiveness and DISTRACTIBILITY, increased goal-directed activity (e.g., at work or school, socially, or sexually), and involvement in pleasurable activities with high potential for painful consequences (e.g., buying sprees, sexual indiscretions, foolish business ventures). See BIPOLAR DISORDERS.

manifest content   The remembered content of a dream or FANTASY, as contrasted with LATENT CONTENT, which is concealed and distorted.

manipulation   A behavior pattern characterized by attempts to exploit interpersonal contact.

MAO   See MONOAMINE OXIDASE (MAO).

MAOIs   See MONOAMINE OXIDASE INHIBITORS (MAOIs).

maprotiline   An older TETRACYCLIC ANTIDEPRESSANT medication infrequently prescribed today because of its association with increased risk of SEIZURES. Now available only as generic but may still be known by the discontinued brand name LUDIOMIL. See "Medications Used in Psychiatry."

Marchiafava-Bignami disease   A SYNDROME in which the corpus callosum shows severe degeneration. Most patients are men with ALCO-

HOLISM, although in rare cases the condition has been seen in nonalcoholic persons.

marijuana   A mixture of the dried leaves, seeds, stems, and flowering tips of CANNABIS SATIVA. The active intoxicating ingredient is delta-9-tetrahydrocannabinol (THC). Marijuana may contain 0.1%–10% THC. The drug is smoked or ingested and produces EUPHORIA, altered PERCEPTIONS, MEMORY impairment, and impaired PSYCHOMOTOR performance.

marital therapy   A treatment whose goal is to ameliorate the problems of married couples. Various psychodynamic, sexual, ethical, and economic aspects of marriage are considered. Husband and wife usually are seen individually or conjointly. A broader term is COUPLES THERAPY, which encompasses unmarried couples.

Marplan   Brand name for the older MONOAMINE OXIDASE INHIBITOR ANTI-DEPRESSANT drug ISOCARBOXAZID.

masculine   Referring to a set of sex-specific social ROLE behaviors that is unrelated to procreative biological function. See GENDER IDEN-TITY; GENDER ROLE; MALENESS.

masculine protest   A term coined by Alfred Adler (1870–1937) to describe a striving to escape IDENTIFICATION with the FEMININE ROLE. Applies primarily to women but also may be noted in men.

masochism   Pleasure derived from physical or psychological pain inflicted on oneself either by oneself or by others. It is called SEXUAL MASOCHISM and classified as a PARAPHILIA when it is consciously sought as a part of the sexual act or as a prerequisite to sexual gratification. It is the converse of SEXUAL SADISM, although the two tend to coexist in the same person.

mass psychogenic illness   See EPIDEMIC HYSTERIA.

maternal deprivation   The result of the premature loss or absence of the mother or the lack of proper mothering.

mathematics disorder   A developmental arithmetic disorder. It is a LEARNING DISORDER characterized by a substantially lower than expected mathematical ability, given the subject's chronological age, measured INTELLIGENCE, and age-appropriate education.

maturational crises   Predictable life events or turning points that occur for most individuals in the course of development.

MBD   See MINIMAL BRAIN DYSFUNCTION (MBD).

MCI   See MILD COGNITIVE IMPAIRMENT (MCI).

MDMA   3,4-Methylenedioxymethamphetamine. See Ecstasy.

medial frontal syndrome   One of the principal FRONTAL LOBE SYN-DROMES. It is characterized by scarcity of movement, sparse verbal output, lower-extremity weakness, and incontinence.

Medicaid   A means-tested ENTITLEMENT program, financed jointly by the state and federal governments, that provides medical services to people with low incomes. States *must* offer certain services, including inpatient and OUTPATIENT hospital services, physicians' (including PSYCHIATRISTS') services, clinical laboratory and X-ray services, and home health services. Additional coverage of persons with mental illnesses is limited.

medical audit   See AUDIT.

medical ethics   The moral code adopted by health professionals in assigning primary value to their patients' needs and interests. The values most commonly applied to medical ethics discussions are autonomy (the patient's right to refuse or choose treatment), beneficence (the best interest of the patient), nonmaleficence ("First, do no harm"), justice (concerns about the distribution of scarce health resources and the decision of who gets what treatment), the right to dignity, and truthfulness and honesty (the concept of INFORMED CONSENT).

medical malpractice   See "Legal Terms."

medical power of attorney   The legal authority given by a competent person to a PROXY or stand-in decision maker to serve in the event of the subject's incapacity. This is one type of ADVANCE DIRECTIVE. See also LIVING WILL and "Legal Terms."

medical record   A written document that contains sufficient information to identify the patient clearly, to justify the DIAGNOSIS and treatment, and to document the results accurately.

medical review   Examination by a team composed of physicians and other appropriate health personnel of the conditions and need for care, including a medical evaluation.

Medicare   An ENTITLEMENT program of health insurance for the elderly and for qualified disabled persons enacted in 1965. Part A, or hospital insurance, usually is earned through employment covered by Social Security. Part B, or supplementary medical insurance, is elected and paid for through a heavily subsidized premium. Covered services include inpatient hospital care, hospital OUTPATIENT services, skilled nursing facility care, home health care, physicians' (including PSYCHIATRISTS') services, laboratory and other diagnostic tests, and hospice care.

medication-induced movement disorders   In DSM-IV-TR, a group of disorders (listed in the section "Other Conditions That May Be a Focus of Clinical Attention") that includes NEUROLEPTIC MALIGNANT SYNDROME, neuroleptic-induced PARKINSONISM, neuroleptic-induced acute AKATHISIA, neuroleptic-induced TARDIVE DYSKINESIA, NEUROLEPTIC-INDUCED ACUTE DYSTONIA, and medication-induced POSTURAL TREMOR.

medulla oblongata   The last part of the vertebrate BRAIN, continuous posteriorly with the SPINAL CORD.

megalomania   Grandiose DELUSIONS of power, wealth, or fame. See also –MANIA.

melancholia   DEPRESSION, typically ENDOGENOUS rather than REACTIVE, and of severe degree. Some authorities use *melancholia* synonymously with DEPRESSION WITH PSYCHOTIC FEATURES. In DSM-IV-TR, melancholia is used as a descriptor for MAJOR DEPRESSIVE DISORDER. In addition to showing loss of pleasure in activities (pervasive ANHEDONIA) and lack of reaction to stimuli that ordinarily would be pleasurable, the patient often has PSYCHOMOTOR RETARDATION or AGITATION, depression that is worse in the morning, early-morning awakening, ANOREXIA NERVOSA and weight loss, and excessive or inappropriate GUILT.

melatonin   A HORMONE produced by the pineal gland in the BRAIN during the early stages of SLEEP. A synthetic form of it is used to reduce the effects of jet lag or to adjust sleep patterns when working rotating shifts.

Mellaril   Brand name (now discontinued) for the CONVENTIONAL ANTIPSYCHOTIC drug THIORIDAZINE.

memantine   An NMDA RECEPTOR ANTAGONIST approved for the treatment of moderate to severe DEMENTIA of the ALZHEIMER's type. Marketed under the brand name NAMENDA. See "Medications Used in Psychiatry."

memory   The ability, process, or act of remembering or recalling; especially the ability to reproduce what has been learned or explained.

memory consolidation   The physical and psychological changes that take place as the BRAIN organizes and restructures information that may become a permanent part of MEMORY.

menarche   The onset of menstruation.

mendacity   Pathological lying.

menkeiti   A CULTURE-SPECIFIC SYNDROME. See *LATAH*.

mens rea   See "Legal Terms."

mental age (MA)   A measure of mental ability as determined by psychological tests.

mental deficiency   See INTELLECTUAL DISABILITY.

mental disease   See MENTAL DISORDER.

mental disorder   A behavioral or psychological SYNDROME that causes significant distress (a painful SYMPTOM) or DISABILITY (impairment in one or more important areas of functioning) or a significantly increased risk for death, pain, or an important loss of freedom. The syndrome is considered to be a manifestation of some behavioral, psychological, or biological dysfunction in the person (and in some cases it is clearly SECONDARY to or due to a GENERAL MEDICAL CONDITION). The term is not applied to behavior or CONFLICTS that arise between the person and society (e.g., political, religious, or sexual preference) unless such conflicts are clearly an outgrowth of a dysfunction within that person. In lay usage, *emotional illness* serves as a term for mental disorder, although it may imply a lesser degree of dysfunction, whereas the term *mental disorder* may be reserved for more severe disturbances.

mental health   A state of being that is relative rather than absolute. The successful performance of mental functions shown by productive activities, fulfilling relationships with other people, and the ability to adapt to change and to cope with adversity.

mental health parity   A health coverage concept in which the scope and limitations of MENTAL HEALTH services included in a health insurance plan are identical to those provided for medical health care services. Usually, the "parity" is restricted to disorders that are considered BRAIN or neurobiologically based disorders such as SCHIZOPHRENIA, BIPOLAR DISORDER, MAJOR DEPRESSIVE DISORDER, AUTISTIC DISORDER, PANIC DISORDER, and OBSESSIVE-COMPULSIVE DISORDER. Under the California Mental Health Parity Legislation (AB88), health plans must provide equal coverage for nine severe MENTAL DISORDERS: schizophrenia, SCHIZOAFFECTIVE DISORDER, obsessive-compulsive disorder, bipolar disorder, panic disorder, ANOREXIA NERVOSA, BULIMIA NERVOSA, major depressive disorder, and PERVASIVE DEVELOPMENTAL DISORDERS. As neuroscience research into the causes of MENTAL DISORDERS becomes more advanced, the distinction between neurobiological disorders and those with a psychological basis will continue to diminish.

mental health problems   SIGNS and SYMPTOMS of insufficient intensity or duration to meet the criteria for any MENTAL DISORDER.

mental illness   See MENTAL DISORDER.

mental retardation   See INTELLECTUAL DISABILITY.

mental status   The level and style of functioning of the PSYCHE, including a person's intellectual functioning and emotional, attitudinal, psychological, and PERSONALITY aspects and the relationships between them. The term is commonly used to refer to the results of the examination of the patient's mental state. See ASSOCIATION.

mental status examination   The process of estimating psychological and behavioral function by observing the patient, eliciting his or her self-description, and using formal questioning. Included in the examination are 1) ASSESSMENT of any psychiatric condition present, including provisional DIAGNOSIS and PROGNOSIS, determination of degree of impairment, suitability for treatment, and indications for particular types of therapeutic intervention; 2) formulation of the PERSONALITY structure of the subject, which may suggest the historical and developmental antecedents of whatever psychiatric condition exists; and 3) estimation of the subject's ability and willingness to participate appropriately in treatment. The MENTAL STATUS is reported in a series of narrative statements describing things such as AFFECT, speech, thought content, PERCEPTION, and COGNITIVE functions. The mental status examination is part of the general examination of all patients, although it may be markedly abbreviated in the absence of PSYCHOPATHOLOGY.

meprobamate   A nonbenzodiazepine SEDATIVE-HYPNOTIC medication used to treat ANXIETY DISORDERS or for the short-term relief of ANXIETY symptoms. Now available only as generic but may still be known by the discontinued brand names EQUANIL and MILTOWN. See "Medications Used in Psychiatry."

Meridia   Former brand name for the withdrawn appetite suppressant drug SIBUTRAMINE.

mescaline   An alkaloid originally derived from the peyote cactus, resembling AMPHETAMINE and adrenaline (EPINEPHRINE) chemically; used to induce altered PERCEPTIONS. Also used by Native Americans of the Southwest in religious rites.

mesmerism   Early term for HYPNOSIS. Named after German physician Franz Anton Mesmer (1734–1815).

mesomorphic   See CONSTITUTIONAL TYPES.

mesoridazine   An older CONVENTIONAL ANTIPSYCHOTIC medication used to treat SCHIZOPHRENIA AND OTHER PSYCHOTIC DISORDERS. Mesoridazine (including all generic and brand [SERENTIL] products) was withdrawn from the U.S. market in 2004 because of its association with dangerous cardiac effects.

MET See MOTIVATIONAL ENHANCEMENT THERAPY (MET).

Metadate Brand name for the CENTRAL NERVOUS SYSTEM (CNS) STIMU-LANT drug METHYLPHENIDATE.

metapsychiatry The interface between PSYCHIATRY and psychic phenomena such as PARAPSYCHOLOGY, mysticism, altered states of consciousness, and nonmedical healing.

metapsychology The branch of theoretical or speculative PSYCHOLOGY that deals with the significance of mental processes; the nature of the mind-body relationship; the origin, purpose, and structure of the mind; and similar hypotheses that are beyond the realm of empirical verification.

methadone A synthetic NARCOTIC that is used as an ANALGESIC in pain management and in the treatment of OPIOID DEPENDENCE. For opioid dependence, because of methadone's long duration of effect, it is used as a substitute for shorter-acting NARCOTICS such as HEROIN or MORPHINE, producing a less socially disabling ADDICTION or aiding in WITHDRAWAL from opioids. Methadone may itself be abused, however. See NARCOTIC-BLOCKING DRUGS.

methamphetamine A longer-acting, legally produced form of the psychostimulant drug, marketed under the brand name DESOXYN. Although it is approved for the treatment of ATTENTION-DEFICIT/HYPERACTIVITY DISORDER (ADHD), methamphetamine is infrequently prescribed because of its abuse potential. See "Medications Used in Psychiatry."

3-methoxy-4-hydroxyphenylglycol (MHPG) See MHPG (3-METHOXY-4-HYDROXYPHENYLGLYCOL).

3,4-methylenedioxymethamphetamine (MDMA) See ECSTASY.

Methylin Brand name for the CENTRAL NERVOUS SYSTEM (CNS) STIMU-LANT drug METHYLPHENIDATE.

methylnaltrexone A newer OPIOID ANTAGONIST medication that blocks some of the side effects of opioid drugs, such as the constipating effects on the gastrointestinal tract, without affecting analgesia or precipitating withdrawal. It is available only as an injection (marketed under the brand name RELISTOR). See "Medications Used in Psychiatry."

methylphenidate A longer-acting CENTRAL NERVOUS SYSTEM (CNS) STIMULANT used in the treatment of ATTENTION-DEFICIT/HYPERACTIVITY DISORDER (ADHD). Methylphenidate is available in immediate-release (brand names METHYLIN and RITALIN) and extended-release (brand names CONCERTA, METADATE CD, RITALIN LA, and RITALIN SR) formulations. See "Medications Used in Psychiatry."

methylphenidate transdermal system   A transdermal patch form of methylphenidate, a mild CENTRAL NERVOUS SYSTEM (CNS) STIMULANT used in the treatment of ATTENTION-DEFICIT/HYPERACTIVITY DISORDER (ADHD). Marketed under the brand name DAYTRANA. See "Medications Used in Psychiatry."

MHPG (3-methoxy-4-hydroxyphenylglycol)   A major metabolite of BRAIN NOREPINEPHRINE excreted in urine.

microaggression   Offensive mechanisms or actions by a person that are designed to keep other individuals in an inferior, dependent, or helpless ROLE. These actions are nonverbal and kinetic, and they are well suited to control space, time, energy, and mobility of an individual (usually nonwhite or female) while producing feelings of degradation. See also MICROINSULT.

micrographia   A term used to describe abnormally small, cramped handwriting and/or the progression to continually smaller handwriting. Micrographia is one of the symptoms of PARKINSON'S DISEASE.

microinsult   Offensive mechanisms or actions by a person that are designed to keep other individuals in an inferior, dependent, or helpless ROLE. Microinsults usually are verbal exchanges that involve stereotyping of individuals (e.g., assuming that a female physician is a nurse or that the African American attending physician is the resident and the European-American resident is the attending).

midbrain   The part of the brain—also called the *mesencephalon*—that contains the tectum, the tegmentum, the ventricular mesocoelia, and the cerebral peduncles. The midbrain adjoins the pons caudally and the DIENCEPHALON rostrally.

middle age   Conventionally considered to occur between ages 40 and 60–65 years and primarily defined by psychosocial rather than by physiological events.

midlife crisis   The set of problems that arise when individuals discover visible SIGNS that they are AGING and become preoccupied with the realization.

migraine   A SYNDROME characterized by recurrent, severe, and usually one-sided headaches; often associated with nausea, vomiting, and visual disturbances.

mild cognitive impairment (MCI)   A DIAGNOSIS given to individuals who have cognitive impairment that is beyond what would be expected for their age and education but that does not interfere significantly with their daily activities. MCI is considered to represent the transitional stage between normal aging and DEMENTIA.

milieu therapy   Socioenvironmental therapy in which the attitudes and behavior of the staff of a treatment service and the activities prescribed for the patients are determined by the patients' emotional and interpersonal needs. This therapy is an essential part of all inpatient treatment.

milnacipran   A SEROTONIN-NOREPINEPHRINE REUPTAKE INHIBITOR (SNRI) ANTIDEPRESSANT medication approved to treat MAJOR DEPRESSIVE DISORDER and FIBROMYALGIA. Marketed under the brand name SAVELLA. See "Medications Used in Psychiatry."

Miltown   Brand name (now discontinued) for the nonbenzodiazepine SEDATIVE-HYPNOTIC drug MEPROBAMATE.

minimal brain dysfunction (MBD)   An older term, currently out of favor, for ATTENTION-DEFICIT/HYPERACTIVITY DISORDER (ADHD).

Mini-Mental State Examination (MMSE)   A screening test for COGNITIVE dysfunction that is frequently used by consultation PSYCHIATRISTS when assessing patients hospitalized in a general hospital who develop psychiatric disorders.

Minipress   Brand name for the antihypertensive drug PRAZOSIN.

Minnesota Multiphasic Personality Inventory (MMPI)   A PERSONALITY questionnaire of 567 true or false statements that is frequently used to assess personality styles and types. It was developed at the University of Minnesota in 1940 and revised in the early 1990s; hence, now it is known as the *MMPI-2*. Its primary use is to understand the psychiatric SYMPTOMS and personality characteristics of the patient. It is also used to correlate personality variables to types of illness, critical life events, habitual behaviors, or other psychological variables.

minor depressive disorder   A proposed disorder (listed in DSM-IV-TR Appendix B, "Criteria Sets and Axes Provided for Further Study") characterized by one or more periods of depressive SYMPTOMS that are identical to MAJOR DEPRESSIVE EPISODES in duration but that involve fewer symptoms and less impairment. Contrast with RECURRENT BRIEF DEPRESSIVE DISORDER.

minor epilepsy (petit mal)   See EPILEPSY.

Miranda warning   See "Legal Terms."

Mirapex   Brand name for the antiparkinsonian drug PRAMIPEXOLE.

mirroring 1) As conceptualized by Heinz Kohut (1913–1981), the empathic responsiveness of the parent to the developing child's activities. The parental response teaches the child which of his or her potential qualities are most highly valued. Mirroring validates the child as to who he or she is and affirms his or her worth. The content of the SUPEREGO is the residue of the mirroring experience. See GRANDIOSE SELF.

2) A technique in PSYCHODRAMA in which another person in the group plays the ROLE of the patient, who watches the enactment as if gazing into a mirror. The first person may exaggerate one or more aspects of the patient's behavior. Following the portrayal, the patient is usually encouraged to comment on what he or she has observed.

mirtazapine An ATYPICAL ANTIDEPRESSANT medication believed to exert its effects through antagonism of central presynaptic alpha$_2$-ADRENERGIC RECEPTORS of both NORADRENERGIC and SEROTONERGIC neurons. It has been characterized as a NORADRENERGIC AND SPECIFIC SEROTONERGIC ANTIDEPRESSANT (NaSSA). Marketed under the brand name REMERON. See "Medications Used in Psychiatry."

mixed anxiety-depressive disorder A proposed disorder (listed in DSM-IV-TR Appendix B, "Criteria Sets and Axes Provided for Further Study") featuring symptoms of ANXIETY and DEPRESSION that cause significant impairment or distress but do not meet the criteria for an ANXIETY DISORDER or a MOOD DISORDER.

mixed receptive-expressive language disorder See under COMMUNICATION DISORDERS.

MMPI See MINNESOTA MULTIPHASIC PERSONALITY INVENTORY (MMPI).

MMSE See MINI-MENTAL STATE EXAM (MMSE).

M'Naghten **rule** See under INSANITY DEFENSE in "Legal Terms."

Moban Former brand name for the discontinued CONVENTIONAL ANTIPSYCHOTIC drug MOLINDONE.

modafinil An atypical STIMULANT (unrelated to the AMPHETAMINES) used to improve wakefulness in patients with excessive daytime sleepiness associated with OBSTRUCTIVE SLEEP APNEA; NARCOLEPSY; and CIRCADIAN RHYTHM SLEEP DISORDER, shift work type. Marketed under the brand name PROVIGIL. See "Medications Used in Psychiatry."

modeling Learning by imitation; a form of BEHAVIOR THERAPY based on social learning in which the model (e.g., the therapist, an actor, or someone else the patient views as competent) displays the desired behavior, the patient repeats it, and successful repetitions are reinforced.

molecular biology   The type of biology concerned with the study of structures and processes at the cellular level and particularly of intracellular responses such as the role of a protein, an ENZYME, and other chemicals in a metabolic pathway; how nucleic acid stores information affecting cellular structure and function; and how metabolites in one cell may affect the function of other cells.

molindone   A CONVENTIONAL ANTIPSYCHOTIC medication (a DIHYDROINDOLONE) used to treat SCHIZOPHRENIA AND OTHER PSYCHOTIC DISORDERS. The brand name MOBAN was discontinued by the manufacturer in 2010, and no generics are currently available.

mongolism   See DOWN SYNDROME.

monoamine   An AMINE containing only one amino group.

monoamine oxidase (MAO)   An ENZYME found in the CENTRAL NERVOUS SYSTEM (CNS) and peripheral organs, including the BRAIN, gastrointestinal tract, and liver, that breaks down BIOGENIC AMINES (NEUROTRANSMITTERS) and other MONOAMINES (e.g., TYRAMINE), rendering them inactive. Inhibition of this enzyme (for which there are two forms, MAO-A and MAO-B) by certain ANTIDEPRESSANT drugs (MONOAMINE OXIDASE INHIBITORS [MAOIs]) may alleviate depressed states by increasing the levels of biogenic amines in the brain.

monoamine oxidase inhibitors (MAOIs)   A group of ANTIDEPRESSANT medications that exert their ANTIDEPRESSANT and ANXIOLYTIC effects through inhibition of the ENZYME MONOAMINE OXIDASE (MAO) in the BRAIN, resulting in elevated levels of NEUROTRANSMITTERS. MAOIs are infrequently prescribed because of the risk of HYPERTENSIVE CRISIS if dietary restrictions are not followed and because of the potential for dangerous drug-DRUG INTERACTIONS. See "Medications Used in Psychiatry."

monocultural ethnocentrism   An assumption that an individual's cultural way of doing things is the only correct way and all other ways have no value.

monomania   Pathological preoccupation with a single subject. See also –MANIA.

monotherapy   Use of a single medication or therapy to treat a disease or disorder. Contrast with COMBINATION TREATMENT.

monozygotic twins   Twins who develop from a single fertilized ovum; identical twins. Often referred to as MZ twins, in contrast to DZ twins (DIZYGOTIC TWINS).

mood   Pervasive and sustained EMOTION. See AFFECT.

mood-congruent psychotic features   See DEPRESSION WITH PSYCHOTIC FEATURES; MANIC EPISODE.

mood disorder due to a general medical condition   SECONDARY MOOD DISORDER; prominent and persistent DEPRESSION (with depressed mood or loss of interest or pleasure) or MANIA (elevated, expansive, or irritable mood), or both, associated with a medical condition classified outside the ICD-10 list of MENTAL DISORDERS.

mood disorders   In DSM-IV-TR, this category includes DEPRESSIVE DISORDERS, BIPOLAR DISORDERS, MOOD DISORDER DUE TO A GENERAL MEDICAL CONDITION, and substance-induced (INTOXICATION or WITHDRAWAL) mood disorder.

mood-incongruent psychotic features   See DEPRESSION WITH PSYCHOTIC FEATURES; MANIC EPISODE.

mood stabilizers   A group of medications that includes LITHIUM CARBONATE, certain ANTICONVULSANTS, and the ATYPICAL ANTIPSYCHOTICS. Mood stabilizers are believed to function at the RECEPTOR or intracellular level to prevent the onset of MANIA or DEPRESSION in BIPOLAR DISORDER and are effective in treating the SYMPTOMS of mania. See "Medications Used in Psychiatry."

mood swing   Fluctuation of a person's emotional tone between periods of elation and periods of DEPRESSION.

moral reconation therapy (MRT)   Developed in 1985 by Gregory Little and Kenneth Robinson, this systematic treatment strategy seeks to decrease recidivism among juvenile and adult criminal and substance ABUSE offenders by increasing moral reasoning. It is a long-term approach focused on changing the criminal thought processes of convicted felons.

moral treatment   A philosophy and technique of treating mental patients that began to prevail in the first half of the nineteenth century that emphasized removal of restraints, humane and kindly care, attention to religion, and performance by the patients of useful tasks in the hospital.

morbidity   In PSYCHIATRY, the term is used to describe associated adverse effects of a mental or physical disorder or treatment in physical or mental terms.

morphine   A potent OPIOID ANALGESIC used in medicine to control pain. As with other OPIATES, morphine's analgesic effect is exerted directly on the CENTRAL NERVOUS SYSTEM (CNS), where the drug interacts with OPIOID RECEPTORS. Tolerance develops with chronic use or abuse, and morphine has a high potential for addiction, leading to physical and psychological dependence. With addiction, withdrawal symptoms ensue with cessation of dosing. Acute WITHDRAWAL from morphine requires medical management. Morphine addiction may be treated with substitution and subsequent withdrawal of METHADONE under a physician's supervision.

motivational enhancement therapy (MET) A time-limited therapy that has been found useful in the treatment of ALCOHOLISM; it encourages patients to talk about the positive and negative aspect of use, emphasizing ABSTINENCE.

motivational interviewing A client-centered, nonjudgmental, nonconfrontational, and nonadversarial method of engaging intrinsic motivation to change behavior by developing discrepancy and exploring and resolving ambivalence within the client. The approach attempts to increase the client's awareness of the potential problems caused, consequences experienced, and risks faced as a result of the behavior in question.

motor skills disorder Includes DEVELOPMENTAL COORDINATION DISORDER, which is characterized by poor performance in activities requiring motor coordination. Performance is below that expected given the subject's age and INTELLIGENCE. Examples are delays in achieving motor milestones such as walking, crawling, or sitting; clumsiness; lack of expected proficiency in sports; or poor handwriting.

motor tic disorder See TIC DISORDERS.

mourning GRIEF; reaction to the loss of a love object (i.e., important person, object, ROLE, status, or anything considered an important and positive part of one's life) consisting of a process of emotional DETACHMENT from that object, which frees the person to find other interests and enjoyments.

movement disorders Disorders affecting motor behavior or body movements, characterized by SYMPTOMS such as TREMOR, CHOREA, DYSTONIA, BRADYKINESIA, BALLISMUS, ATAXIA, AKATHISIA, and AKINESIA. Neurological conditions associated with movement disorders include PARKINSON'S DISEASE, HUNTINGTON'S DISEASE, and HEMIBALLISMUS. Movement disorders may also be the result of medication effects (see MEDICATION-INDUCED MOVEMENT DISORDERS).

MPD MULTIPLE PERSONALITY DISORDER. See DISSOCIATIVE IDENTITY DISORDER (DID).

MRI See MAGNETIC RESONANCE IMAGING (MRI).

MRS See MAGNETIC RESONANCE SPECTROSCOPY (MRS).

MRT See MORAL RECONATION THERAPY (MRT).

MST   See MULTISYSTEMIC THERAPY (MST).

muina   A CULTURE-SPECIFIC SYNDROME whose symptoms include acute nervous tension, headache, trembling, screaming, stomach disturbances, and in more severe cases, loss of consciousness. The underlying cause is thought to be strongly experienced anger or rage. Also known as *BILIS* or *COLERA*.

multiaxial system   The system used in PSYCHIATRY to evaluate various aspects of a patient's mental, physical, psychosocial, and global functioning. DSM-IV-TR lists five axes:

Axis I   Clinical disorders. Used to indicate the major disorders, such as SCHIZOPHRENIA, BIPOLAR DISORDER, and PANIC DISORDER.

Axis II   PERSONALITY DISORDERS or mental retardation (INTELLECTUAL DISABILITY). A separate axis is used to ensure that consideration is given to the possible presence of these conditions, which may otherwise be overlooked.

Axis III   GENERAL MEDICAL CONDITIONS. Used to code major medical disorders that may be relevant to the patient's care (e.g., thyroid disease, diabetes, hypertension).

Axis IV   Psychosocial and environmental problems. Used to indicate problems that might interact with the psychiatric and medical diagnoses (e.g., homelessness, substance ABUSE) and treatment.

Axis V   GLOBAL ASSESSMENT OF FUNCTIONING. Also known as the **GAF SCALE**, Axis V provides a global assessment of the level of functioning and MENTAL HEALTH of a patient, including psychological, social, and occupational functioning on a hypothetical continuum of mental illness to mental health, from 1 to 100, with 100 being the highest functioning.

multidimensional impairment   A condition that includes a variety of impairing psychiatric SYMPTOMS, including poor REALITY TESTING, perceptual disturbances, neuropsychological DEFICITS, affective instability, and an inability to relate to peers despite attempts to do so.

multi-infarct dementia   See VASCULAR DEMENTIA.

multiple personality disorder (MPD)   See DISSOCIATIVE IDENTITY DISORDER (DID).

multisystemic therapy (MST)   An intensive, family-focused, home-based service used in the treatment of CONDUCT DISORDER. The primary objective is to assist parents and community organizations in developing skills for intervening with risk factors for ANTISOCIAL BEHAVIOR in children.

Munchausen syndrome (pathomimicry) In DSM-IV-TR, a chronic form of FACTITIOUS DISORDER with physical SYMPTOMS that may be totally fabricated, self-inflicted, or intentional exaggerations of preexisting physical conditions. Much of the person's life may consist of seeking admission to or staying in hospitals (often under different names). Multiple invasive procedures and operations are eagerly solicited. The need is to assume the SICK ROLE rather than to reap any economic benefit or ensure better care or physical well-being.

muscarinic receptors A subtype of CHOLINERGIC RECEPTOR specifically responsive to muscarine. See also ANTIMUSCARINICS.

mutation A change in GENETIC structure that produces transmissible, permanent differences. May occur spontaneously or may be induced by agents such as high-energy radiation. See GENES.

mutism Refusal to speak; may be for CONSCIOUS or UNCONSCIOUS reasons.

myelin The insulating sheath that surrounds nerve cells, enabling them to conduct impulses between the BRAIN and other parts of the body. When myelin becomes damaged, neurodegenerative autoimmune diseases, such as MULTIPLE SCLEROSIS, can develop.

myoclonus A brief, involuntary twitching of a muscle or a group of muscles. Myoclonus is one of several SIGNS in a wide variety of nervous system disorders such as MULTIPLE SCLEROSIS, PARKINSON'S DISEASE, ALZHEIMER'S DISEASE, CREUTZFELDT-JAKOB DISEASE, and some forms of EPILEPSY. In almost all instances in which myoclonus is caused by CENTRAL NERVOUS SYSTEM (CNS) disease, it is preceded by other symptoms; for instance, in CREUTZFELDT-JAKOB DISEASE myoclonus is generally a late-stage clinical feature that appears after the patient has already started to exhibit gross neurological deficits. Anatomically, myoclonus may originate from lesions of the CEREBRAL CORTEX, subcortex, or SPINAL CORD.

myriacit A CULTURE-SPECIFIC SYNDROME. See *LATAH*.

mysophobia The FEAR of dirt and germs.

N

naloxone A potent, short-acting competitive ANTAGONIST of mu-OPIOID RECEPTORS in the CENTRAL NERVOUS SYSTEM (CNS) with no agonistic effects of its own; the drug of choice in the treatment of NARCOTIC overdose. Naloxone rapidly reverses the toxic and clinical effects of OPIATES, including respiratory depression, hypotension, and sedation, but it also produces rapid withdrawal symptoms. Its short duration of action (2–4 hours) makes it generally inappropriate for chronic treatment of NARCOTIC ADDICTION. Now available only as generic but may still be known by the discontinued brand name NARCAN. See "Medications Used in Psychiatry."

naltrexone   An OPIOID ANTAGONIST medication used to facilitate maintenance of ABSTINENCE after HEROIN or alcohol DETOXIFICATION. Marketed under the brand names ReVia and Vivitrol; may also be known by the discontinued brand name Depade. See "Medications Used in Psychiatry."

Namenda   Brand name for the NMDA RECEPTOR ANTAGONIST drug MEMANTINE.

NAMI   See National Alliance on Mental Illness (NAMI).

Narcan   Brand name (now discontinued) for the OPIOID ANTAGONIST drug NALOXONE.

narcissism   Self-love as opposed to object-love (love of another person). To be distinguished from egotism, which carries the connotation of self-centeredness, selfishness, and conceit. Egotism is but one expression of narcissism. Revisions in psychoanalytic theory (SELF PSYCHOLOGY) have viewed the concept of narcissism in less pathological terms.

narcissistic personality disorder   See under PERSONALITY DISORDERS.

narcissistic rage   In Heinz Kohut's (1913–1981) SELF PSYCHOLOGY, AGGRESSION in a person reacting to breakdowns in crucial self-serving mental images that have been revealed to be false. Two examples of conditions that can provoke such behavior are deflation of infantile GRANDIOSITY or traumatic disappointment in idealized figures. The aggression may range from mild annoyance to intense and violent destruction. See FRAGMENTATION; GRANDIOSE SELF; IDEALIZED PARENTAL IMAGO.

narcoanalysis   See NARCOSYNTHESIS.

narcolepsy   A DYSSOMNIA consisting of irresistible attacks of refreshing SLEEP during the day, CATAPLEXY (sudden bilateral loss of muscle tone) typically associated with intense EMOTION, and recurrent intrusions of REM SLEEP into the transition between sleep and wakefulness.

narcosis Stupor of varying depth induced by certain drugs.

narcosynthesis Psychotherapeutic treatment occurring under partial ANESTHESIA, such as that induced by BARBITURATES, which is now rarely used. Originally used to treat acute MENTAL DISORDERS occurring in a military combat setting.

narcotic Any OPIOID-derived drug, natural or synthetic, that relieves pain or alters MOOD. May cause ADDICTION. See also DRUG DEPENDENCE; HYPNOTIC; SEDATIVE.

narcotic antagonists See NARCOTIC-BLOCKING DRUGS.

narcotic-blocking drugs (narcotic antagonists) Agents structurally similar to the OPIOIDS and probably occupying the same RECEPTOR sites in the CENTRAL NERVOUS SYSTEM (CNS). In sufficient doses, they block the effects of OPIATE drugs by competing for the OPIOID RECEPTOR sites. If given after OPIATE DEPENDENCE has developed, these agents will precipitate an acute ABSTINENCE SYNDROME. See NALOXONE; NALTREXONE.

Nardil Brand name for the MONOAMINE OXIDASE INHIBITOR (MAOI) ANTIDEPRESSANT PHENELZINE.

NaSSAs See NORADRENERGIC AND SPECIFIC SEROTONERGIC ANTIDEPRESSANTS (NaSSAs).

National Alliance on Mental Illness (NAMI) An organization whose members are parents and relatives of mentally ill patients and former patients whose main objective is for better and more sustained care. Its trustees and chapter officers engage in active lobbying and in education projects.

National Comorbidity Survey Conducted from September 1990 through February 1992; the first nationally representative MENTAL HEALTH survey in the United States to use a fully structured research diagnostic interview to assess the PREVALENCE of psychiatric disorders in a community setting.

National Institute of Mental Health (NIMH) One of the 27 institutes and centers that constitute the NATIONAL INSTITUTES OF HEALTH (NIH). NIMH is responsible for research on the causes and treatments of MENTAL DISORDERS.

National Institute on Alcohol Abuse and Alcoholism (NIAAA) One of the 27 institutes and centers that constitute the NATIONAL INSTITUTES OF HEALTH (NIH). NIAAA supports and conducts biomedical and behavioral research on the causes, consequences, treatment, and PREVENTION of ALCOHOLISM and alcohol-related problems.

National Institute on Drug Abuse (NIDA)   One of the 27 institutes and centers that constitute the NATIONAL INSTITUTES OF HEALTH (NIH). NIDA's mission is to lead the fight on drug ABUSE and ADDICTION.

National Institutes of Health (NIH)   An agency of the U.S. Department of HEALTH AND HUMAN SERVICES that is a world-renowned institution supporting biomedical and behavioral research; the principal biomedical research agency of the federal government. Its components are the National Cancer Institute; the National Eye Institute; the National Heart, Lung, and Blood Institute; the National Human Genome Research Institute; the National Institute on Aging; the NATIONAL INSTITUTE ON ALCOHOL ABUSE AND ALCOHOLISM (NIAAA); the National Institute of Allergy and Infectious Diseases; the National Institute of Arthritis and Musculoskeletal and Skin Diseases; the National Institute of Biomedical Imaging and Bioengineering; the National Institute of Child Health and Human Development; the National Institute on Deafness and Other Communication Disorders; the National Institute of Dental and Craniofacial Research; the National Institute of Diabetes and Digestive and Kidney Diseases; the NATIONAL INSTITUTE ON DRUG ABUSE (NIDA); the National Institute of Environmental Health Sciences; the National Institute of General Medical Sciences; the NATIONAL INSTITUTE OF MENTAL HEALTH (NIMH); the National Institute of Neurological Disorders and Stroke; the National Institute of Nursing Research; the National Library of Medicine; the Center for Information Technology; the Center for Scientific Review; the John E. Fogarty International Center; the National Center for Complementary and Alternative Medicine; the National Center on Minority Health and Health Disparities; the National Center for Research Resources; and the Warren Grant Magnuson Clinical Center.

National Mental Health Association (NMHA)   Now called Mental Health America (see "Mental Health Resources"). The oldest and largest nonprofit organization addressing all aspects of mental health and mental illness. Founded by Clifford W. Beers in 1909 as the National Committee for Mental Hygiene.

Navane   Brand name for the CONVENTIONAL ANTIPSYCHOTIC drug THIOTHIXENE.

NCSE   See NEUROBEHAVIORAL COGNITIVE STATUS EXAMINATION (NCSE).

NDRIs   See NOREPINEPHRINE-DOPAMINE REUPTAKE INHIBITORS (NDRIs).

necromania   Pathological preoccupation with dead bodies. See also −MANIA.

necrophilia   One of the PARAPHILIAS, characterized by marked distress over, or acting on, urges involving sexual activity with corpses.

nefazodone   An ATYPICAL ANTIDEPRESSANT (characterized as a SEROTONIN ANTAGONIST AND REUPTAKE INHIBITOR [SARI]) used to treat DEPRESSION and certain ANXIETY DISORDERS. Nefazodone is infrequently prescribed today because of its association with life-threatening liver failure. Although available only as generic, it may still be known by the discontinued brand name SERZONE. See "Medications Used in Psychiatry."

negative symptoms (of schizophrenia)   A group of SYMPTOMS characteristic of SCHIZOPHRENIA that include loss of fluency and spontaneity of verbal expression, impaired ability to focus or sustain ATTENTION on a particular task, difficulty in initiating or following through on tasks, impaired ability to experience pleasure or form emotional ATTACHMENT to others, and blunted AFFECT.

negative therapeutic reaction   In Freudian theory, resistance to change in psychoanalytic therapy. The worsening of symptoms in response to the therapist's effort to foster INSIGHT. The patient's neurotic behavior increases after first improving with therapy, and he or she gets worse instead of improving as would be expected. Because such a reaction seemed to defy the PLEASURE PRINCIPLE, Freud related the reaction to UNCONSCIOUS GUILT and MASOCHISM and to the workings of the DEATH INSTINCT.

negativism   Opposition or resistance, either covert or overt, to the SUGGESTIONS or advice of others.

neglect syndrome   The result of lesions of the right PARIETAL LOBE that leave a patient inattentive to stimuli to the left side of the body after a STROKE or an accident. It sometimes occurs after similar damage to the left hemisphere but much less frequently and in milder form. The patient appears to behave as if the whole left side of space, and sometimes even the left side of his or her own body, does not exist.

negligence   See "Legal Terms."

neocortex   The part of the CEREBRAL CORTEX involved in higher functions such as sensory perception, generation of motor commands, spatial reasoning, conscious thought, and language.

neologism   In PSYCHIATRY, a new word or condensed combination of several words coined by a person to express a highly complex idea not readily understood by others; seen in SCHIZOPHRENIA and DEMENTIA.

neostriatum   The most recently evolved part of the CORPUS STRIATUM, consisting of the CAUDATE NUCLEUS and PUTAMEN.

nervios   A common idiom of distress among Latinos in the United States and Latin America. A number of other ethnic groups have related, though often somewhat distinctive, ideas of "nerves" (such as *nevra* among Greeks and *nervi* among Italians). *Nervios* refers both to a general state of vulnerability to stressful life experiences and to a syndrome brought on by difficult life circumstances. Symptoms include emotional distress, irritability, sleep disturbances, inability to concentrate, and *mareos* (dizziness with occasional vertigo-like manifestations). It is a very broad syndrome that ranges from cases free of a mental disorder to presentations resembling adjustment, anxiety, depressive, dissociative, somatoform, or psychotic disorders. See CULTURE-SPECIFIC SYNDROMES.

nervous breakdown   A nonmedical, nonspecific euphemism for a MENTAL DISORDER.

network therapy   A treatment modality designed to allow the therapist to treat addictive disorders in the ambulatory setting. Family members and friends are enlisted to provide ongoing support.

neurasthenia   A disorder in ICD-10, characterized by persisting complaints of mental or physical fatigue or weakness after performing daily activities and inability to recover with normal periods of rest or entertainment. Typical SYMPTOMS include muscular aches and pains, dizziness, tension headaches, SLEEP disturbance, and irritability.

neuregulin 1 (*NRG1*) gene   The GENE responsible for encoding NRG1, a protein known to be involved in the development of the nervous system. *NRG1* is currently one of the most studied candidate genes for SCHIZOPHRENIA. Altered expression of the *NRG1* gene has been found in the dorsolateral prefrontal CORTEX in schizophrenia, and it has been proposed that *NRG1* might influence disease susceptibility by altering the expression of GLUTAMATERGIC NMDA (N-METHYL-D-ASPARTIC ACID) RECEPTORS.

neuritic plaques   Characteristic structural abnormalities found in the brains of people with ALZHEIMER'S DISEASE. These deposits are made of a protein called BETA-AMYLOID, which accumulates outside of neurons and other brain cells in a space known as the extracellular space.

Neurobehavioral Cognitive Status Examination (NCSE)   An examination that assesses a broader range of COGNITIVE functioning than the MINI-MENTAL STATE EXAM (MMSE) but is brief enough to be given at the bedside in clinical settings.

neurochemistry   The branch of chemistry that deals with the nervous system, including its chemical components and the passage of the nerve impulse through the nerve cell and its transmission across SYNAPSES.

neuroendocrinology   The science of the relationships between the nervous system (particularly the BRAIN) and the endocrine system. Of particular importance is the action of the HYPOTHALAMUS, which stimulates or inhibits the pituitary's secretion of HORMONES. See also PSYCHOENDOCRINOLOGY.

neurofibrillary tangles   Nonsoluble twisted fibers found inside the brain's cells. These tangles consist primarily of a protein called TAU, which forms part of a structure called a microtubule. The microtubule helps transport nutrients and other important substances from one part of the nerve cell to another. In ALZHEIMER'S DISEASE, however, the tau protein is abnormal and the microtubule structures collapse.

neurohormone   A chemical messenger usually produced within the HYPOTHALAMUS, carried to the pituitary and then to other cells within the CENTRAL NERVOUS SYSTEM (CNS). Neurohormones are similar to NEUROTRANSMITTERS except that they interact with a variety of cells, whereas neurotransmitters interact only with other NEURONS.

neuroimaging   A general term used to refer to rapidly developing technologies such as COMPUTED TOMOGRAPHY (CT), MAGNETIC RESONANCE IMAGING (MRI), SINGLE-PHOTON EMISSION COMPUTED TOMOGRAPHY (SPECT), and POSITRON EMISSION TOMOGRAPHY (PET) used to assess BRAIN disorders.

neuroleptic   An older term for the first ANTIPSYCHOTIC medications, such as CHLORPROMAZINE, which produced notable PSYCHOMOTOR RETARDATION, APATHY, and emotional detachment. With the introduction of newer ATYPICAL ANTIPSYCHOTIC drugs with less propensity to cause these side effects, the term became outdated as a general synonym for *antipsychotic,* although it is still used to refer to the older CONVENTIONAL ANTIPSYCHOTICS.

neuroleptic-induced acute dystonia   Abnormal positioning or spasm of the muscles of the head, neck, limbs, or trunk; the dystonia develops within a few days of starting or raising the dose of a NEUROLEPTIC (ANTIPSYCHOTIC) medication because of dysfunction of the EXTRAPYRAMIDAL SYSTEM. See also MEDICATION-INDUCED MOVEMENT DISORDERS.

neuroleptic-induced disorders   See MEDICATION-INDUCED MOVEMENT DISORDERS.

neuroleptic malignant syndrome   A severe MEDICATION-INDUCED MOVEMENT DISORDER associated with the use of a NEUROLEPTIC (ANTIPSYCHOTIC) medication. SYMPTOMS include muscle RIGIDITY, high fever, and related findings such as DYSPHAGIA, incontinence, confusion, and MUTISM.

neurologist   A physician with postgraduate training and experience in the field of ORGANIC DISEASES of the nervous system whose professional work focuses primarily on this area. Neurologists also receive training in PSYCHIATRY.

neurology   The branch of medicine that studies the organization, function, and treatment of diseases of the nervous system.

neuron   A nerve cell.

neuronal plasticity   The ability of the nervous system to adapt its structural organization to new situations emerging from changes of developmental and environmental situations, as well as other factors (e.g., injuries) affecting the condition of the nervous system.

Neurontin   Brand name for the ANTICONVULSANT/MOOD STABILIZER drug GABAPENTIN.

neuropathic pain   Pain of unknown cause that results when special nerve endings, called *nociceptors,* are stimulated. Neuropathic pain is possible whenever nerves are damaged by trauma; by diseases such as diabetes, herpes zoster, and late-stage cancer; or by chemical injury (e.g., toxic doses of drugs). The most dramatic and mysterious example of neuropathic pain is called PHANTOM LIMB SYNDROME. This occurs when an arm or a leg has been removed because of illness or injury but the BRAIN still gets pain messages from the nerves that originally carried impulses from the missing limb. These nerves now seem to misfire and cause troubling pain.

neurophysiology   The study of the relation between the structure of the nervous system and its function.

neuropsychiatry   The medical specialty that combines NEUROLOGY and PSYCHIATRY, emphasizing the somatic substructure on which EMOTIONS are based and the ORGANIC disturbances of the CENTRAL NERVOUS SYSTEM (CNS) that give rise to MENTAL DISORDERS.

neuropsychological testing   A series of tests administered to assess various aspects of COGNITIVE functioning, including MEMORY, ATTENTION, language, and EXECUTIVE FUNCTIONING. The ultimate goal of the

ASSESSMENT is to clarify how changes in BRAIN structure and function are affecting behavior.

neuroreceptors   Binding sites in the CENTRAL NERVOUS SYSTEM (CNS) for psychoactive drugs, NEUROTRANSMITTERS, and HORMONES.

neuroscience   The study of BRAIN function and the neural substrates of behavior. This interdisciplinary field includes investigation in areas such as anatomy, GENETICS, BIOCHEMISTRY, PSYCHIATRY, and computer science.

neurosis   An older term for emotional disturbances of all kinds other than PSYCHOSIS. It implies subjective psychological pain or discomfort beyond what is appropriate to the conditions of one's life. The meaning of the term has changed since it was first introduced into standard nomenclature. In regard to current usage, some clinicians limit the term to its descriptive meaning, NEUROTIC DISORDER, whereas others include the concept of a specific etiological process (see ETIOLOGY). Common neuroses are as follows:

anxiety neurosis   Chronic and persistent apprehension manifested by autonomic HYPERACTIVITY (e.g., sweating, palpitations, dizziness), musculoskeletal tension, and irritability. Somatic SYMPTOMS may be prominent.

depersonalization neurosis   Feelings of unreality and of estrangement from the self, body, or surroundings. Different from the process of DEPERSONALIZATION, which may be a manifestation of ANXIETY or of another MENTAL DISORDER.

depressive neurosis   An outmoded term for excessive reaction of DEPRESSION due to an internal CONFLICT or to an identifiable event such as loss of a loved one or of a cherished possession.

hysterical neurosis, conversion type   Disorders of the special senses or the voluntary nervous system, such as blindness, deafness, ANESTHESIA, PARESTHESIA, pain, paralysis, and impaired muscle coordination for which no organic cause is found. A patient with this disorder may manifest *LA BELLE INDIFFÉRENCE* in regard to the SYMPTOMS, which may actually provide SECONDARY GAIN by winning the patient SYMPATHY or relief from unpleasant responsibilities. See also CONVERSION.

hysterical neurosis, dissociative type   Alterations in the state of consciousness or in IDENTITY, producing SYMPTOMS such as AMNESIA.

obsessive-compulsive neurosis   Persistent intrusion of unwanted and uncontrollable EGO-DYSTONIC thoughts, urges, or actions. The thoughts may consist of single words, ruminations, or trains of thought that are seen as nonsensical. The actions may vary from simple movements to complex RITUALS, such as repeated hand washing. See also COMPULSION.

phobic neurosis   An intense FEAR of an object or a situation that the person consciously recognizes as harmless. Apprehension may be experienced as faintness, fatigue, palpitations, perspiration, nausea, TREMOR, and even PANIC. See also PHOBIA.

neurotic disorder   An older term for a MENTAL DISORDER in which the predominant disturbance is a distressing SYMPTOM or group of symptoms that one considers unacceptable to one's PERSONALITY. There is no marked loss of REALITY TESTING; behavior does not actively violate social norms, although it may be quite disabling. The disturbance is relatively enduring or recurrent without treatment and is not limited to a mild transitory reaction to stress. There is no demonstrable ORGANIC ETIOLOGY. See also NEUROTIC PROCESS.

neuroticism   An enduring tendency to experience negative emotional states. Individuals who score high on measures of neuroticism are more likely than the average person to experience such feelings as ANXIETY, anger, GUILT, and DEPRESSION. They respond more poorly to environmental stress and are more likely to interpret ordinary situations as threatening and minor frustrations as hopelessly difficult.

neurotic process   A specific etiological process involving the following sequence: UNCONSCIOUS CONFLICTS between opposing wishes or between wishes and prohibitions lead to unconscious PERCEPTION of anticipated danger or DYSPHORIA, which leads to use of DEFENSE MECHANISMS that result in either SYMPTOMS, PERSONALITY disturbance, or both. See also NEUROSIS; NEUROTIC DISORDER.

neurotoxin   A substance that is poisonous or destructive to nerve tissue.

neurotransmitter   A chemical (e.g., ACETYLCHOLINE, GABA [GAMMA-AMINOBUTYRIC ACID], DOPAMINE, NOREPINEPHRINE, SEROTONIN) found in the nervous system that facilitates the transmission of IMPULSES across SYNAPSES between NEURONS. Disorders in the BRAIN physiology of neurotransmitters have helped us to understand the actions of drugs used to treat several psychiatric illnesses, particularly MOOD DISORDERS and SCHIZOPHRENIA.

neutropenia   See LEUKOPENIA.

NGRI (not guilty by reason of insanity)   See "Legal Terms."

NIAAA See National Institute on Alcohol Abuse and Alcoholism (NIAAA).

nicotine-related disorders In DSM-IV-TR, a group of MENTAL DISORDERS that includes nicotine DEPENDENCE and nicotine WITHDRAWAL.

nicotinic receptors A subtype of CHOLINERGIC RECEPTOR specifically responsive to nicotine. See also ANTINICOTINICS.

NIDA See National Institute on Drug Abuse (NIDA).

night hospital See PARTIAL HOSPITALIZATION.

nightmare disorder Dream anxiety disorder; a PARASOMNIA consisting of repeated awakenings from SLEEP with detailed RECALL of extended and extremely frightening dreams, usually involving threats to survival, security, or self-esteem. On awakening from the frightening dream, the person rapidly becomes oriented and alert. This contrasts with the confusion and DISORIENTATION characteristic of SLEEP TERROR DISORDER and some forms of EPILEPSY. Nightmares generally occur during the second half of the sleep period.

night terror (*pavor nocturnus*) See SLEEP TERROR DISORDER.

NIH See National Institutes of Health (NIH).

nihilistic delusion The DELUSION of nonexistence of the self or part of the self, or of some object in external reality.

NIMH See National Institute of Mental Health (NIMH).

nitrite inhalants Inhaled substances (street name: "POPPERS"), including amyl, butyl, and isobutyl nitrite, that produce an INTOXICATION characterized by a feeling of fullness in the head, mild EUPHORIA, a change in the PERCEPTION of time, relaxation of smooth muscles, and possibly an increase in sexual feelings. The nitrites may produce psychological DEPENDENCE and may impair immune functioning, irritate the respiratory system, and induce a toxic reaction involving vomiting, severe headache, and dizziness.

nitrous oxide Laughing gas; it rapidly produces INTOXICATION, with light-headedness and a floating sensation. SYMPTOMS disappear within minutes after discontinuation of the substance; however, temporary but clinically relevant confusion and reversible PARANOID states have followed regular use.

NMDA (*N*-methyl-D-aspartic acid) A compound that acts as a specific AGONIST at the NMDA RECEPTOR, mimicking the effects of the NEUROTRANSMITTER GLUTAMATE.

NMDA receptor antagonists   A class of drugs that inhibit the action of the NMDA (N-METHYL-D-ASPARTIC ACID) RECEPTOR. Examples include KETAMINE and PHENCYCLIDINE (PCP) (often used illicitly for recreational purposes), MEMANTINE (used to treat the SYMPTOMS of ALZHEIMER'S DISEASE), and AMANTADINE (used to treat SIDE EFFECTS of CONVENTIONAL ANTIPSYCHOTIC medications, especially DYSTONIA and AKATHISIA).

NMHA   See NATIONAL MENTAL HEALTH ASSOCIATION (NMHA).

NMR   See NUCLEAR MAGNETIC RESONANCE (NMR); MAGNETIC RESONANCE IMAGING (MRI).

nocturnal myoclonus   See DYSSOMNIAS.

nolle prosequi   See "Legal Terms."

nolo contendere   See "Legal Terms."

nominal damages   See "Legal Terms."

non compos mentis   See "Legal Terms."

non-24-hour sleep-wake pattern   See under CIRCADIAN RHYTHM SLEEP DISORDERS.

Noonan syndrome   A congenital (present at birth) genetic condition whose principal features include congenital heart defect, short stature, indentation of the chest, impaired blood clotting, and a characteristic configuration of facial features. Cognitive deficits, social problems, attention deficits, and ANXIETY are also present.

noradrenergic   Referring to the NEUROTRANSMITTER NOREPINEPHRINE (noradrenaline).

noradrenergic and specific serotonergic antidepressants (NaSSAs)   A class of ATYPICAL ANTIDEPRESSANTS that exert their effects by antagonizing presynaptic alpha$_2$ receptors of both NORADRENERGIC and SEROTONERGIC neurons, resulting in enhanced neurotransmission of NOREPINEPHRINE and SEROTONIN. NaSSAs are used primarily for the treatment of DEPRESSION and ANXIETY DISORDERS. An example of an NaSSA is MIRTAZAPINE (REMERON).

norepinephrine   A CATECHOLAMINE NEUROTRANSMITTER related to EPINEPHRINE that is found in both the peripheral nervous system and the CENTRAL NERVOUS SYSTEM (CNS). FUNCTIONAL excesses of norepinephrine in the BRAIN have been implicated in the pathogenesis of manic states (see MANIA); functional DEFICITS have been implicated in the pathogenesis of certain depressive states. Also called *noradrenaline.* See also BIOGENIC AMINES.

norepinephrine-dopamine reuptake inhibitors (NDRIs)   A class of medications that increase the levels of both NOREPINEPHRINE and

DOPAMINE, inhibiting their reabsorption back into presynaptic neurons. Examples of NDRIs include the mild CENTRAL NERVOUS SYSTEM (CNS) STIMULANTS DEXMETHYLPHENIDATE and METHYLPHENIDATE.

norepinephrine reuptake inhibitors (NRIs)   A class of medications (also called *selective norepinephrine reuptake inhibitors* or *norepinephrine specific reuptake inhibitors*) that increase levels of the NEUROTRANSMITTERS NOREPINEPHRINE and EPINEPHRINE by blocking the action of the norepinephrine transporter and hence the reuptake of neurotransmitters back into neurons. NRIs may be used in the clinical treatment of ATTENTION-DEFICIT/HYPERACTIVITY DISORDER (ADHD) and NARCOLEPSY (e.g., ATOMOXETINE [STRATTERA]) as well as MOOD DISORDERS such as MAJOR DEPRESSIVE DISORDER (e.g., the TETRACYCLIC agent MAPROTILINE [LUDIOMIL]).

Norpramin   Brand name for the TRICYCLIC ANTIDEPRESSANT drug DESIPRAMINE.

nortriptyline   A TRICYCLIC ANTIDEPRESSANT medication used to treat DEPRESSION and certain ANXIETY DISORDERS. Marketed under the brand names AVENTYL and PAMELOR. See "Medications Used in Psychiatry."

nosology   Science of the classification of disorders.

not guilty by reason of insanity (NGRI)   See "Legal Terms."

NREM sleep   Non-rapid eye movement SLEEP.

NRG1   See NEUREGULIN 1 (NRG1) GENE.

NRIs   See NOREPINEPHRINE REUPTAKE INHIBITORS (NRIS).

nuclear family   Immediate members of a family.

nuclear magnetic resonance (NMR)   See MAGNETIC RESONANCE IMAGING (MRI). See also BRAIN IMAGING.

nuclear self   See BIPOLAR SELF.

nucleus accumbens   A collection of NEURONS within the subcortical part of the FOREBRAIN, called the *striatum,* which receives input from the BASAL GANGLIA and the CEREBRAL CORTEX. The nucleus accumbens is thought to play an important role in reward, laughter, pleasure, addiction, fear, and the PLACEBO EFFECT.

nucleus basalis of Meynert   See BASAL NUCLEUS OF MEYNERT.

null hypothesis   The assumption that any difference found between two samples or populations is due to chance rather than to a systematic variation.

nursing care plan   A means of providing nursing personnel with information about the needs of and therapeutic strategy for each patient.

Nuvigil Brand name for the atypical STIMULANT drug ARMODAFINIL.

nyctophobia The FEAR of night.

nymphomania Abnormal and excessive need or desire in a woman for sexual intercourse; known as SATYRIASIS in men. May be of psychological or ORGANIC ETIOLOGY. See also HYPERSEXUALITY; –MANIA.

nystagmus Abnormal movements of the eyeballs; side to side (horizontal), up and down (vertical), or circular (rotary). Such movements suggest ORGANIC pathology of the CENTRAL NERVOUS SYSTEM (CNS) or of the oculomotor, trochlear, or abducens cranial nerves. Seen in toxic states such as INTOXICATION with alcohol, SEDATIVE-HYPNOTICS, ANXIOLYTICS, or PHENCYCLIDINE (PCP).

O

object constancy The final step in the process of SEPARATION-INDIVIDUATION as described by Margaret Mahler (1897–1985). The child is able to maintain an internal representation of the mother and is therefore able to tolerate separation from the mother. Object constancy develops between ages 24 and 36 months.

object permanence A part of the sensorimotor stage of COGNITIVE DEVELOPMENT as described by Jean Piaget (1896–1980). Object permanence develops during the second year of life. The child is able to maintain a mental image of the object. For example, the child will look for a toy after it disappears.

object relations The emotional bonds between one person and another, as contrasted with interest in and love for the self; usually described in terms of capacity for loving and reacting appropriately to others. Melanie Klein (1882–1960) is generally credited with founding the British object relations school.

obsession Recurrent and persistent thought, IMPULSE, or image experienced as intrusive and distressing. Recognized as being excessive and unreasonable even though it is the product of one's mind. This thought, impulse, or image cannot be expunged through logic or reasoning.

obsessive-compulsive disorder An ANXIETY DISORDER characterized by OBSESSIONS, COMPULSIONS, or both that are time-consuming, are distressing, or interfere significantly with normal routine, occupational functioning, usual social activities, or relationships with others.

obsessive-compulsive personality disorder See under PERSONALITY DISORDERS.

obsessive-compulsive spectrum disorders Conditions that have obsessive-compulsive qualities and show similarities to OBSESSIVE-COMPULSIVE DISORDER. Disorders proposed as belonging to this spectrum include HYPOCHONDRIASIS, BODY DYSMORPHIC DISORDER (BDD), and TRICHOTILLOMANIA.

obstructive sleep apnea A common BREATHING-RELATED SLEEP DISORDER characterized by pauses in breathing during sleep. It is caused by obstruction of the airway, despite the effort to breathe. The episodes of breathing cessation occur repeatedly throughout sleep and last long enough that one or more breaths are missed. See also CENTRAL ALVEOLAR HYPOVENTILATION SYNDROME; CENTRAL SLEEP APNEA.

occupational problem Job or work difficulty that is not due to a MENTAL DISORDER. Examples are job dissatisfaction or uncertainty about career choices.

occupational psychiatry (industrial psychiatry) A field of PSYCHIATRY concerned with the DIAGNOSIS and PREVENTION of MENTAL ILLNESS in industry, with the return of the psychiatric patient to work, and with psychiatric aspects of absenteeism, ABUSE, retirement, and related phenomena. A PSYCHIATRIST in this field often works in consultation with an EMPLOYEE ASSISTANCE PROGRAM (EAP).

occupational therapy An ADJUNCTIVE therapy that uses purposeful activities as a means of altering the course of illness. The patient's relationship to staff and to other patients in the occupational therapy setting is often more therapeutic than the activity itself.

odynophobia The FEAR of pain.

Oedipus complex ATTACHMENT of the child to the parent of the opposite sex, accompanied by envious and aggressive feelings toward the parent of the same sex. These feelings are largely repressed (i.e., made UNCONSCIOUS) because of the FEAR of displeasure or punishment by the parent of the same sex. In its original use, the term applied only to the boy or man.

olan A CULTURE-SPECIFIC SYNDROME. See *LATAH*.

olanzapine   An ATYPICAL ANTIPSYCHOTIC medication approved for the treatment of SCHIZOPHRENIA and for acute and maintenance treatment of BIPOLAR DISORDER. Marketed under the brand name ZYPREXA. See "Medications Used in Psychiatry."

olanzapine–fluoxetine combination   A compound medication—consisting of OLANZAPINE (an ATYPICAL ANTIPSYCHOTIC) and FLUOXETINE (a SELECTIVE SEROTONIN REUPTAKE INHIBITOR)—indicated for the acute treatment of depressive episodes associated with treatment-resistant DEPRESSION and BIPOLAR I DISORDER in adults. Marketed under the brand name SYMBYAX. See "Medications Used in Psychiatry."

onanism   Coitus interruptus. The term is sometimes incorrectly used interchangeably with masturbation.

ontogenetic   Pertaining to the development of the individual. Contrast with PHYLOGENETIC.

operant conditioning (instrumental conditioning)   A form of behaviorism and behavior modification in which the likelihood of a specific behavior is increased or decreased based on positive or negative reinforcement when the behavior is exhibited. See also RESPONDENT CONDITIONING; SHAPING.

ophidiophobia   The FEAR of snakes.

opiate   Any chemical derived from opium; it relieves pain and produces a sense of well-being.

opiate dependence   The ADDICTION to HEROIN and other related substances, such as codeine, MORPHINE, meperidine (Demerol), or hydromorphone (Dilaudid).

opioid   A drug, an endogenous chemical produced in the BRAIN, or a naturally occurring substance that resembles opium or one or more of its alkaloid derivatives that binds to OPIOID RECEPTORS in the brain to modulate pain.

opioid antagonists   Substances such as NALOXONE and NALTREXONE, which occupy OPIOID RECEPTORS but do not activate them. Opioid ANTAGONISTS are used in the treatment of OPIATE overdose and ALCOHOLISM.

opioid receptors   Receptors located in the BRAIN and spinal cord, as well the intestinal tract, that bind with endogenous OPIOIDS (ENDORPHINS) and OPIATE drugs. There are four major opioid receptor types—mu (μ), delta (δ), kappa (κ) and nociceptin (ORL-1)—and numerous subtypes (e.g., μ_1, μ_2, μ_3). The opioid system is known primarily for its role in pain modulation, but it may have other functions as well.

opioid-related disorders   In DSM-IV-TR, a group of MENTAL DISOR-
DERS that includes opioid DEPENDENCE; opioid ABUSE; opioid INTOXICA-
TION; opioid WITHDRAWAL; opioid intoxication DELIRIUM; opioid-
induced PSYCHOTIC DISORDER, with DELUSIONS or HALLUCINATIONS; opioid-
induced MOOD DISORDER; opioid-induced SEXUAL DYSFUNCTION; and opioid-induced SLEEP DISORDER.

oppositional defiant disorder   A pattern of negativistic and hostile
behavior in a child that lasts at least 6 months. SYMPTOMS may include
losing one's temper; arguing with adults or actively refusing their requests; deliberately annoying others; being easily annoyed, angry,
and resentful; and being spiteful or vindictive.

oral phase   See PSYCHOSEXUAL DEVELOPMENT.

Orap   Brand name for the CONVENTIONAL ANTIPSYCHOTIC drug PIMOZIDE.

orbitofrontal syndrome   One of the principal FRONTAL LOBE SYN-
DROMES. It is characterized by disinhibited, impulsive behavior; emo-
tional lability; inappropriate jocular AFFECT; and poor JUDGMENT and
INSIGHT.

organic   Obsolete term denoting a clear biological—as opposed to
psychological ("FUNCTIONAL")—cause of an illness or symptom. See
also ORGANIC MENTAL DISORDER.

organic brain syndrome   See ORGANIC MENTAL DISORDER.

organic disease   In older terminology, a disease characterized by a
demonstrable structural or biochemical abnormality in an organ or
a tissue (i.e., an EXOGENOUS ETIOLOGY) Sometimes imprecisely used as
an antonym for FUNCTIONAL DISORDER.

organic mental disorder   An older and nearly obsolete category
originally created to distinguish physiological (termed EXOGENOUS or
ORGANIC) causes of mental impairment from psychiatric (termed EN-
DOGENOUS or FUNCTIONAL) causes. The term was abandoned in DSM-
IV because it was judged to incorrectly imply that "nonorganic" men-
tal disorders did *not* have a biological basis.

orgasm   Sexual climax; peak psychophysiological response to sexual
stimulation.

orgasmic disorders   A subcategory of SEXUAL DYSFUNCTIONS that includes FEMALE ORGASMIC DISORDER, MALE ORGASMIC DISORDER, and PREMA-
TURE EJACULATION.

  female orgasmic disorder   Refers to absence of, or delay in attaining, ORGASM following a normal sexual excitement phase. The

orgasmic capacity is less than would be expected for the woman's age, sexual experience, and the degree or type of sexual stimulation. It is frequently severe enough to cause marked distress or interpersonal difficulty. The disorder is termed *generalized* if it is present in all situations and *situational* if the woman is less orgasmic under some conditions or with some partners.

male orgasmic disorder   Refers to absence of, or delay in attaining, ORGASM following a normal sexual excitement phase during sexual activity that is adequate in focus, intensity, and duration.

premature ejaculation   Refers to ejaculation following minimal sexual stimulation before, at the point of, or shortly after entry and before the man wishes it.

orgasmic dysfunction   FEMALE ORGASMIC DISORDER (see under ORGASMIC DISORDERS).

orientation   Awareness of one's SELF in relation to time, place, and person.

orphan drugs   Drugs that the pharmaceutical companies do not wish to develop either because they cannot be patented, because they are used only in rare conditions by very few people, or because of a variety of economic reasons. In such cases, the federal government may work with the companies to make the drugs available to those persons who need them.

orthopsychiatry   An approach that involves the collaborative efforts of PSYCHIATRY, PSYCHOLOGY, PSYCHIATRIC SOCIAL WORK, and other behavioral, medical, and social sciences in the study and treatment of human behavior in the clinical setting. Emphasis is placed on preventive techniques to promote healthy emotional growth and development, particularly of children.

outpatient   A patient who is receiving ambulatory care at a hospital or other health facility without being admitted to the facility.

overanxious disorder   An ANXIETY DISORDER of childhood and ADOLESCENCE, sometimes considered equivalent to the adult DIAGNOSIS of GENERALIZED ANXIETY DISORDER (GAD). SYMPTOMS include multiple unrealistic anxieties concerning the quality of one's performance in school and in sports, hobbies, money matters, punctuality, health, appearance, or other issues. The patient is tense and unable to relax and has recurrent somatic complaints for which no physical cause can be found.

overcompensation   A CONSCIOUS or an UNCONSCIOUS process in which a real or an imagined physical or psychological DEFICIT generates exaggerated correction. Concept introduced by the Austrian PSYCHIA-TRIST Alfred Adler (1870–1937).

overdetermination   The concept of multiple UNCONSCIOUS causes of an emotional reaction or SYMPTOM.

overstimulation   Excitation that exceeds the subject's or the system's ability to master it or to discharge it. In accordance with the ECONOMIC VIEWPOINT, the PSYCHE has a finite capacity for tension. When that capacity is exceeded, the psyche feels pain (ANXIETY), and the excessive stimulation constitutes a trauma. Eventually, anxiety becomes a signal that danger is approaching, and defenses against being overwhelmed are brought forth (see SIGNAL ANXIETY). The adult is able to master more stimulation than the child, but even the mature psyche cannot cope with an unlimited amount of increasing or repeated overstimulation.

oxazepam   A BENZODIAZEPINE ANXIOLYTIC medication most commonly used to treat various ANXIETY DISORDERS, alcohol WITHDRAWAL SYMPTOMS, and sometimes (together with an ANTIDEPRESSANT) ANXIETY associated with DEPRESSION. Now available only as generic but may still be known by the discontinued brand name SERAX. See "Medications Used in Psychiatry."

oxcarbazepine   An ANTICONVULSANT medication used in NEUROLOGY as an ADJUNCTIVE treatment or as MONOTHERAPY for partial SEIZURES in adults and children with EPILEPSY and used in PSYCHIATRY to treat BIPO-LAR DISORDER that has not responded to standard treatments. Marketed under the brand name TRILEPTAL. See "Medications Used in Psychiatry."

oyako-shinju   A CULTURE-SPECIFIC SYNDROME, unique to Japan and not listed in DSM-IV-TR, in which the parent kills the child before committing suicide. The parent kills the child because that is considered preferable to leaving the child to make its way in the world without a family.

P

pain disorder   One of the SOMATOFORM DISORDERS, characterized by pain in one or more sites that causes marked distress or impairs occupational or social functioning. The pain may occur in the absence of any physical finding that might explain it (psychological type), or it may be related to an existing GENERAL MEDICAL CONDITION.

palilalia   A neurological condition characterized by the repetition of a phrase or word with increasing rapidity. It can be a SYMPTOM of TOURETTE'S DISORDER, ASPERGER'S DISORDER, or AUTISTIC DISORDER.

palinopsia   Perceptual distortion in which an image persists after removal of the stimulus.

paliperidone   An ATYPICAL ANTIPSYCHOTIC medication indicated for the acute and maintenance treatment of SCHIZOPHRENIA. Marketed under the brand name INVEGA. See "Medications Used in Psychiatry."

pallidotomy   A procedure in which a tiny electrical probe is placed in the GLOBUS PALLIDUS and heated to 80° Celsius in order to destroy a small area of brain cells. Pallidotomy is used to treat DYSKINESIAS in patients with PARKINSON'S DISEASE. Creating a scar in the globus pallidus reduces the brain activity in that area, which may help relieve movement symptoms such as tremor and rigidity.

Pamelor   Brand name for the TRICYCLIC ANTIDEPRESSANT drug NORTRIPTYLINE.

PANDAS   See PEDIATRIC AUTOIMMUNE NEUROPSYCHIATRIC DISORDERS ASSOCIATED WITH STREPTOCOCCAL INFECTIONS (PANDAS).

pandemic   See under EPIDEMIOLOGY.

panic   Sudden, overwhelming ANXIETY of such intensity that it produces terror and physiological changes.

panic attack   A period of intense FEAR or discomfort, with the abrupt development of a variety of physical SYMPTOMS and fears of dying, going crazy, or losing control that reach a crescendo within 10 minutes. The symptoms may include shortness of breath or smothering sensations; dizziness, faintness, or feelings of unsteadiness; trembling or shaking; sweating; choking; nausea or abdominal distress; flushes or chills; and chest pain or discomfort.

   Panic attacks occur in several ANXIETY DISORDERS. In PANIC DISORDER, they are typically unexpected and happen "out of the blue." In disorders such as SOCIAL PHOBIA, SPECIFIC PHOBIA, OBSESSIVE-COMPULSIVE DISORDER, and BODY DYSMORPHIC DISORDER (BDD), they are cued and occur when exposed to or in anticipation of a situational trigger. These attacks occur also in POSTTRAUMATIC STRESS DISORDER (PTSD).

panic disorder   Recurrent, unexpected PANIC ATTACKS, at least one of which is followed by a month or more of persisting concern about having these attacks. Panic disorder is categorized as with or without AGORAPHOBIA, depending on whether criteria for that condition are also met.

panphobia   The FEAR of everything.

paradoxical intention   A technique used in BEHAVIOR THERAPY in which individuals are encouraged to engage in whatever behavior they are trying to stop. For example, a person with COMPULSIVE hand washing might be instructed to wash even more frequently.

parahippocampal gyrus   A GRAY MATTER cortical region of the BRAIN that surrounds the HIPPOCAMPUS. This region plays an important role in MEMORY encoding and retrieval.

paralysis agitans   See PARKINSONISM.

paramnesia   Distortion of MEMORY with confusion of fact and FANTASY.

paranoia   A condition characterized by the gradual development of an intricate, complex, and elaborate system of thinking based on (and often proceeding logically from) misinterpretation of an actual event; it may meet criteria for a type of DELUSIONAL DISORDER. Despite its often CHRONIC course, this condition does not seem to interfere with other aspects of thinking and PERSONALITY. To be distinguished from SCHIZOPHRENIA, PARANOID type.

paranoid   A lay term commonly used to describe an overly suspicious person. The technical use of the term refers to persons with PARANOID IDEATION or to a type of SCHIZOPHRENIA. See also DELUSIONAL DISORDER.

paranoid ideation   Suspiciousness or a nondelusional belief that one is being harassed, persecuted, or unfairly treated.

paranoid personality disorder   See under PERSONALITY DISORDERS.

paranoid schizophrenia   See SCHIZOPHRENIA.

paraphasia   A notable feature of APHASIA in which one loses the ability to speak correctly, substitutes one word for another, and changes words and sentences in an inappropriate way. Three types of paraphasia have been described:

literal/phonological paraphasia   More than half of the intended word is produced correctly. For example, a patient may say "pun" instead of "spun." In addition, transpositions of sounds can occur (e.g., "tevilision" for "television").

neologistic paraphasia   Less than half of the intended word is produced correctly. In some cases, the entire word is produced incorrectly. Neologisms may occur in the speech of people with SCHIZOPHRENIA.

verbal paraphasia   Another word is substituted for the target word. (The substitution must be a real word. If it is not, the paraphasia is classified as neologistic.)

paraphilias   One of the major groups of SEXUAL DISORDERS; in DSM-IV-TR, this group includes EXHIBITIONISM, FETISHISM, FROTTEURISM, PEDO-PHILIA, SEXUAL MASOCHISM, SEXUAL SADISM, TRANSVESTIC FETISHISM, VOYEUR-ISM, and paraphilia not otherwise specified (including KLISMAPHILIA and NECROPHILIA). The paraphilias (also called PERVERSIONS or sexual deviations) are recurrent, intense sexual urges and sexually arousing FANTA-SIES that involve nonhuman objects, children or other nonconsenting persons, or the suffering or HUMILIATION of oneself or the sexual partner.

parapraxis   A faulty act, blunder, or lapse of MEMORY such as a slip of the tongue or misplacement of an article. According to Freud, these acts are caused by UNCONSCIOUS motives.

paraprofessional   A trained aide who assists a professional person, usually in a medical setting.

parapsychology   The study of sensory and motor phenomena shown by some human beings (and some animals) that are posited to occur without the mediation of the known sensory and motor organs. The data of parapsychology are not accounted for by the tenets of conventional science. See EXTRASENSORY PERCEPTION (ESP); TELEPATHY.

parasomnias   One of two major subgroups of SLEEP DISORDERS (DYSSOM-NIAS are the other major subgroup). Parasomnias are disorders characterized by abnormal behavioral or physiological events occurring in association with sleep, specific sleep stages, or sleep-wake transitions. In DSM-IV-TR, this group includes NIGHTMARE DISORDER, SLEEP TERROR DISORDER, and SLEEPWALKING DISORDER.

parasympathetic nervous system   The part of the AUTONOMIC NER-VOUS SYSTEM (ANS) that controls the life-sustaining organs of the body under normal, danger-free conditions. The parasympathetic nervous system uses chiefly ACETYLCHOLINE as its NEUROTRANSMITTER. Contrast with SYMPATHETIC NERVOUS SYSTEM.

parataxic distortion   A term for inaccuracies in JUDGMENT and PER-CEPTION, particularly in interpersonal relationships, based on the observer's need to perceive subjects and relationships in accordance with a pattern set by earlier experience. Parataxic distortions develop as a defense against ANXIETY.

paratonia   The reduced ability of a muscle to stretch during passive movement that develops during the course of DEMENTIA.

parens patriae   See "Legal Terms."

parent-child relational problem   See RELATIONAL PROBLEMS.

parenteral   Route of drug or nutrition administration other than by way of the intestines (i.e., oral or rectal). Examples of parenteral administration include INTRAVENOUS, subcutaneous, and INTRAMUSCULAR injection. Inhalation of medication is not considered parenteral, nor is topical administration.

paresis   Muscle weakness; incomplete paralysis; term often used instead of GENERAL PARALYSIS.

paresthesia   Abnormal tactile sensation, often described as burning, pricking, tickling, tingling, or creeping.

parietal lobe   The part of the BRAIN that integrates sensory information from different modalities, particularly determining spatial sense and navigation. BALINT SYNDROME is associated with bilateral lesions of the parietal lobe.

parkinsonism (Parkinson's disease, paralysis agitans)   One of the MEDICATION-INDUCED MOVEMENT DISORDERS, consisting of a rapid, coarse TREMOR; muscular RIGIDITY; masklike FACIES; or AKINESIA developing within a few weeks of starting or raising the dose of NEUROLEPTIC (ANTIPSYCHOTIC) medication or of reducing medication used to treat EXTRAPYRAMIDAL SYMPTOMS (EPS).

Parkinson's disease   A slowly progressive disease of the CENTRAL NERVOUS SYSTEM (CNS), more frequent in males than in females, characterized by TREMOR at rest, AKINESIA, and BRADYKINESIA, as well as cognitive, emotional, and behavioral symptoms and signs. The SYMPTOMS are due to the destruction of the DOPAMINE-producing cells in the SUBSTANTIA NIGRA and a subsequent reduction in the amount of DOPAMINE in the BRAIN.

"Parkinson's Plus" syndromes   The atypical parkinsonian syndromes—DEMENTIA WITH LEWY BODIES, MULTIPLE SYSTEM ATROPHY, PROGRESSIVE SUPRANUCLEAR PALSY, and CORTICOBASAL GANGLIONIC DEGENERATION—are often difficult to differentiate from PARKINSON'S DISEASE and each other. Although these syndromes are clinically distinct, modern immunocytochemical techniques and new GENETIC findings have revealed intriguing interconnections at a basic molecular level, providing a scientific rationale for lumping these diseases into two groups, the SYNUCLEINOPATHIES and the TAUOPATHIES.

Parlodel   Brand name for the mixed DOPAMINE AGONIST-ANTAGONIST drug BROMOCRIPTINE.

Parnate   Brand name for the MONOAMINE OXIDASE INHIBITOR (MAOI) ANTIDEPRESSANT TRANYLCYPROMINE.

paroxetine hydrochloride   A SELECTIVE SEROTONIN REUPTAKE INHIBITOR (SSRI) ANTIDEPRESSANT medication used to treat DEPRESSION, GENERALIZED ANXIETY DISORDER, OBSESSIVE-COMPULSIVE DISORDER, PANIC DISORDER, POST-TRAUMATIC STRESS DISORDER (PTSD), and SOCIAL PHOBIA. Marketed under the brand name PAXIL. See "Medications Used in Psychiatry."

paroxetine mesylate   A SELECTIVE SEROTONIN REUPTAKE INHIBITOR (SSRI) ANTIDEPRESSANT medication related to PAROXETINE HYDROCHLORIDE (PAXIL) and indicated for the treatment of MAJOR DEPRESSIVE DISORDER, OBSESSIVE-COMPULSIVE DISORDER, PANIC DISORDER, and GENERALIZED ANXIETY DISORDER. Marketed under the brand name PEXEVA. See "Medications Used in Psychiatry."

partial hospitalization   A psychiatric treatment program for patients who require hospitalization only during the day, overnight, or on weekends.

partner relational problem   See RELATIONAL PROBLEMS.

pasmo   A CULTURE-SPECIFIC SYNDROME. See *susto*.

passive-aggressive personality disorder   A proposed disorder (listed in DSM-IV-TR Appendix B, "Criteria Sets and Axes Provided for Further Study") characterized by a pervasive pattern of negativistic attitudes and passive resistance to others' expectations of and demands for adequate performance in social and occupational situations. Behavioral tactics include procrastination; postponement of completion of routine tasks; sulkiness, irritability, or argumentativeness if asked to do something he or she does not want to do, and then working unreasonably slowly and inefficiently; and avoidance of obligations by claiming to have forgotten. Also known as *negativistic personality disorder.*

pastoral counseling   The use of psychological principles by clergy trained to assist members of their congregation who seek help with emotional problems.

pathognomonic   A SYMPTOM or group of symptoms that are specifically diagnostic or typical of a disease.

pathological gambling   An IMPULSE-CONTROL DISORDER whose pathological and maladaptive nature is suggested by the following: preoccupation with gambling; handicapping or planning the next venture with scheming to get money to gamble with; a need to gamble with more and more money in order to achieve the desired excitement; restlessness or irritability when attempting to reduce or stop gambling, or failure to stop; concealment of the extent of involvement in gambling from others; illegal activity used to finance gambling; or negative effects on significant relationships or career opportunities.

pathomimicry   See MUNCHAUSEN SYNDROME.

Pavlovian conditioning   See RESPONDENT CONDITIONING.

pavor nocturnus   See SLEEP TERROR DISORDER.

Paxil   Brand name for the SELECTIVE SEROTONIN REUPTAKE INHIBITOR (SSRI) ANTIDEPRESSANT drug PAROXETINE HYDROCHLORIDE.

PCP   See PHENCYCLIDINE (PCP).

PDD   PERVASIVE DEVELOPMENTAL DISORDER; also primary degenerative DEMENTIA (see ALZHEIMER'S DISEASE).

PDR (*Physicians' Desk Reference*)   The compendium of all drugs that have been approved by the FOOD AND DRUG ADMINISTRATION (FDA), including dosage, SIDE EFFECTS, and contraindications.

pederasty   Homosexual anal intercourse between men and boys with the latter as the passive partners. The term is used less precisely to denote male homosexual anal intercourse.

pediatric autoimmune neuropsychiatric disorders associated with streptococcal infections (PANDAS)   This term is used to describe a subset of disorders in children who have OBSESSIVE-COMPULSIVE DISORDER and/or TIC DISORDERS such as TOURETTE'S DISORDER, and in whom symptoms worsen following streptococcal infections (e.g., strep throat/scarlet fever). The children usually have dramatic, "overnight" onset of symptoms, including motor or vocal tics, OBSESSIONS, and/or COMPULSIONS. In addition to these symptoms, children may also become moody or irritable or show concerns about separating from parents or loved ones.

pedophilia   One of the PARAPHILIAS, characterized by marked distress over, or acting on, urges involving sexual activity with a prepubescent child who, more often than not, is of the same sex.

pedophobia   The FEAR of children.

peeping   See VOYEURISM.

peer review   Review by panels of physicians, and sometimes allied health professionals, of services rendered by other physicians. Also refers to the process whereby publications have been independently reviewed by anonymous professionals who are experts in the context area. See also PEER REVIEW ORGANIZATION (PRO); PROFESSIONAL STANDARDS REVIEW ORGANIZATION (PSRO); UTILIZATION REVIEW COMMITTEE.

peer review organization (PRO)   A system that determines the appropriateness and reasonableness of medical care under the MEDICARE or MEDICAID programs.

Pelizaeus-Merzbacher disease   An inherited condition that rarely affects females and involves the BRAIN and the CENTRAL NERVOUS SYSTEM (CNS). This disease is one of a group of GENETIC disorders called LEUKODYSTROPHIES. Pelizaeus-Merzbacher disease is caused by an inability to form MYELIN. As a result, individuals with this condition have impaired intellectual functions, such as language and memory, and delayed motor skills, such as coordination and walking.

pellagra   A vitamin B_3 (nicotinamide) deficiency that may be a cause of major mental SYMPTOMS such as DELUSIONS and impaired thinking, as well as physical symptoms such as dermatitis.

pemoline   A STIMULANT medication used in the treatment of ATTENTION-DEFICIT/HYPERACTIVITY DISORDER (ADHD). Pemoline (including all generic and brand [CYLERT] products) was withdrawn from the U.S. market in 2005 because of its association with life-threatening liver failure.

penis envy   In psychoanalytic theory (see PSYCHOANALYSIS), envy by the female child of the male child's genitals and presumably associated powers or privileges.

pentazocine   An OPIOID partial AGONIST used to treat moderate to severe pain. Marketed under the brand name TALWIN. See "Medications Used in Psychiatry."

perception   Mental processes by which intellectual, sensory, and emotional data are organized logically or meaningfully.

perdida del alma   A CULTURE-SPECIFIC SYNDROME. See *SUSTO*.

pergolide   A DOPAMINE AGONIST used as an ADJUNCTIVE treatment with CARBIDOPA-LEVODOPA therapy in the management of signs and symptoms of PARKINSON'S DISEASE. Pergolide (including all generic and brand [PERMAX] products) was withdrawn from the U.S. market in 2007 after several published studies revealed a link between the drug and increased rates of valvular dysfunction.

Periactin   Brand name (now discontinued) for CYPROHEPTADINE.

periaqueductal gray area   A cluster of NEURONS lying in the THALAMUS and PONS. It contains ENDORPHIN-producing neurons and OPIOID RECEPTOR sites and thus can affect the sensation of pain.

peripheral neuropathy A SYNDROME of sensory loss, muscle weakness and atrophy, decreased deep tendon reflexes, and vasomotor SYMPTOMS. May be caused by CARBAMAZEPINE or MONOAMINE OXIDASE INHIBITORS (MAOIs).

Permax Former brand name for the withdrawn antiparkinsonian drug PERGOLIDE.

perphenazine A CONVENTIONAL ANTIPSYCHOTIC medication (a PHENOTHIAZINE of the piperazine class) used to treat SCHIZOPHRENIA AND OTHER PSYCHOTIC DISORDERS. Now available only as generic but may still be known by the discontinued brand name TRILAFON. See "Medications Used in Psychiatry."

perphenazine–amitriptyline combination A compound medication—consisting of PERPHENAZINE (a CONVENTIONAL ANTIPSYCHOTIC) and AMITRIPTYLINE (a TRICYCLIC ANTIDEPRESSANT)—used to treat ANXIETY, AGITATION, and DEPRESSION. Now available only as generic but may still be known by the discontinued brand names ETRAFON and TRIAVIL. See "Medications Used in Psychiatry."

persecutory delusion See DELUSIONAL DISORDER.

perseveration Tendency to emit the same verbal or motor response again and again to varied stimuli.

persona In Jungian theory (Carl Gustav Jung, 1875–1961), the PERSONALITY mask or facade that each person presents to the outside world, as distinguished from the person's inner being, or ANIMA (animus).

personality The characteristic way in which a person thinks, feels, and behaves; the ingrained pattern of behavior that each person evolves, both consciously and unconsciously, as his or her style of life or way of being.

personality change Alterations in characteristic patterns of relating to the environment and the self that occur from social, psychological, or physical stressors such as having catastrophic experiences, having a MENTAL DISORDER, or having a GENERAL MEDICAL CONDITION (e.g., BRAIN trauma). The PERSONALITY shows a definite change from the preexisting personality; in children, there is a significant change from usual behavior patterns or a disruption in development. Features appear that were not present earlier, such as a hostile, mistrustful, or suspicious attitude; SOCIAL WITHDRAWAL; feelings of emptiness or hopelessness; or poor IMPULSE control or aggressive behavior.

personality disorders Enduring patterns of perceiving, relating to, and thinking about the environment and oneself that begin by early adulthood and are exhibited in a wide range of important social and personal contexts. These patterns are inflexible and maladaptive, causing either significant functional impairment or subjective distress.

Many types of PERSONALITY or personality disorders have been described. The following are those specified in DSM-IV-TR, which groups them into three clusters:

Cluster A   Paranoid, schizoid, schizotypal

Cluster B   Antisocial, borderline, histrionic, narcissistic

Cluster C   Avoidant, dependent, obsessive-compulsive

antisocial personality disorder   Characterized by a pattern of disregard for and violation of the rights of others. Manifestations may include superficiality; lack of EMPATHY or remorse, with callous unconcern for the feelings of others; disregard for social norms; poor behavioral control, with irritability, impulsivity, and low frustration tolerance; and inability to feel GUILT or to learn from experience or punishment. Often, there is evidence of CONDUCT DISORDER in childhood or of overtly irresponsible and antisocial behavior in adulthood, such as inability to sustain consistent work behavior, conflicts with the law, repeated failure to meet financial obligations, and repeated lying to, "conning," and/or exploitation of others.

avoidant personality disorder   Characterized by social discomfort and reticence, low self-esteem, and hypersensitivity to negative evaluation. Manifestations may include avoiding activities that involve contact with others because of FEARS of criticism or disapproval; experiencing inhibited development of relationships with others because of fears of being foolish or being shamed; having few friends despite the desire to relate to others; or being unusually reluctant to take personal risks or engage in new activities because they may prove embarrassing.

borderline personality disorder   Characterized by instability of interpersonal relationships, self-image, AFFECTS, and control over IMPULSES. Manifestations may include frantic efforts to avoid real or imagined abandonment; unstable, intense relationships that alternate between extremes of IDEALIZATION and DEVALUATION; REPETITIVE SELF-MUTILATION or SUICIDE threats; and inappropriate, intense, or uncontrolled anger.

dependent personality disorder   Characterized by an excessive need to be taken care of, resulting in submissive and clinging behavior and FEARS of separation. Manifestations may include excessive need for advice and reassurance about everyday decisions, encouragement of others to assume responsibility for major areas of his or her life, inability to express disagreement because of possible anger or lack of support from others, and preoccupation with fears of being left to take care of himself or herself.

histrionic personality disorder   Characterized by excessive emotional instability and attention seeking. Behavior includes discomfort if not the center of attention; excessive attention to physical attractiveness; rapidly shifting and shallow EMOTIONS; speech that is excessively impressionistic and lacking in detail; viewing relationships as being more intimate than they actually are; and seeking immediate gratification.

narcissistic personality disorder   Characterized by a pervasive pattern of GRANDIOSITY in FANTASY or behavior and an excessive need for admiration. Manifestations may include having an exaggerated sense of self-importance, having a feeling of being so special that one should associate only with other special people, exploiting others to advance one's own ends, lacking EMPATHY, and believing that others envy him or her.

obsessive-compulsive personality disorder   Also known as *compulsive personality*; characterized by preoccupation with perfectionism, mental and interpersonal control, and orderliness, all at the expense of flexibility, openness, and efficiency. Some of the manifestations are preoccupation with rules, lists, or similar items; excessive devotion to work, with little attention paid to recreation and friendships; limited expression of warm EMOTIONS; reluctance to delegate work and the demand that others submit exactly to one's way of doing things; and miserliness.

paranoid personality disorder   Characterized by a pervasive distrust and suspiciousness of others such that their motives are interpreted as malevolent. This distrust is shown in many ways, including unreasonable expectation of exploitation or harm by others; questioning without justification the loyalty or trustworthiness of friends or associates; reading demeaning or threatening meanings into benign remarks or events; having a tendency to bear grudges and be unforgiving of insults or injuries; or experiencing unfounded, recurrent suspiciousness about the fidelity of one's sexual partner.

schizoid personality disorder   Characterized by DETACHMENT from social relationships and restricted emotional range in interper-

sonal settings. The individual tends not to desire or enjoy close relationships, prefers solitary activities, appears indifferent to praise
or criticism, has no (or only one) close friends or confidants, and
is emotionally cold or detached.

schizotypal personality disorder   Characterized by a combination of discomfort with, and reduced capacity for, close relationships and COGNITIVE or perceptual distortions and eccentricities of
behavior. Possible manifestations include odd beliefs or MAGICAL
THINKING inconsistent with cultural norms; unusual perceptual experiences including bodily ILLUSIONS; odd thinking and speech; no
(or only one) close friends because of lack of desire, discomfort
with others, or eccentricities; and persisting, excessive social ANX-
IETY that tends to be associated with PARANOID FEARS rather than negative JUDGMENTS about oneself. The ICD-10 lists schizotypal
personality disorder as an AXIS I disorder (schizotypal disorder) associated with schizophrenia, not as a personality disorder (AXIS II).

persuasion   A therapeutic approach based on direct SUGGESTION and
guidance intended to influence favorably patients' attitudes, behaviors, and goals.

pervasive developmental disorders   In DSM-IV-TR, this group includes AUTISTIC DISORDER, RETT'S DISORDER, CHILDHOOD DISINTEGRATIVE
DISORDER, and ASPERGER'S DISORDER.

perversion   An imprecise term used to designate sexual variance.
See PARAPHILIA.

PET   See POSITRON EMISSION TOMOGRAPHY (PET).

petit mal   See EPILEPSY.

pet therapy   The use of tranquil domestic animals (e.g., dogs and
cats) to provide comfort and solace to patients with DEMENTIA or major psychiatric disorders during visits conducted by a person over-
seeing the animals.

Pexeva   Brand name for the SELECTIVE SEROTONIN REUPTAKE INHIBITOR
(SSRI) ANTIDEPRESSANT drug PAROXETINE MESYLATE.

PG1   See INTERNSHIP.

PGY-1   See INTERNSHIP.

phallic phase   See PSYCHOSEXUAL DEVELOPMENT.

phantom limb   A phenomenon frequently experienced by ampu-
tees in which sensations, often painful, appear to originate in the
amputated extremity.

pharmacodynamics   The study of the biochemical and physiological effects of drugs and their mechanisms of action.

pharmacogenetics   The interaction between genetic factors and therapeutic drugs. Generally, the term is used to describe the study of the genetic bases for individual responses to drugs.

Psychiatric pharmacogenetics is a burgeoning area, which constitutes a major arm of current psychiatric research. Ultimately, the goal is to use the patient's genotype to predict both the response to treatment and the development of side effects. Specific genes linked to the efficacy of psychotropic drugs have already been identified; however, these studies still need to be replicated in different populations. See also PHARMACOGENOMICS.

pharmacogenomics   The interaction between GENETIC factors and therapeutic drugs. This term applies to the study of variability in the genetic basis of disease susceptibility and drug responses at a population level. See also PHARMACOGENETICS.

pharmacokinetics   The study of the process and rates of drug distribution, metabolism, and disposition in the organism.

pharmacotherapy   The treatment of a disease through the use of pharmaceutical agents.

phase-of-life problem   Difficulty in adapting to a particular developmental phase that is not due to a MENTAL DISORDER. Some examples are entering school, leaving parental control, and starting a new career. Other examples are the changes involved in marriage, divorce, or retirement.

phencyclidine (PCP)   An NMDA RECEPTOR ANTAGONIST developed in the 1950s as an INTRAVENOUS anesthetic. PCP is capable of inducing hallucinogenic and PSYCHOTOMIMETIC reactions, and its use was discontinued because patients often became agitated, delusional, and irrational while recovering from anesthesia. Today, PCP is illegally manufactured in laboratories and is sold on the street under names such as "ANGEL DUST," "ozone," "wack," and "rocket fuel." PCP is addictive, and its use often leads to psychological DEPENDENCE, craving, and COMPULSIVE drug-seeking behavior. PCP users can become violent or suicidal and can be very dangerous to themselves and to others.

phencyclidine-related disorders   In DSM-IV-TR, a group of MENTAL DISORDERS that includes PHENCYCLIDINE (PCP) (or related substance) DEPENDENCE; PCP ABUSE; PCP INTOXICATION; PCP intoxication DELIRIUM; PCP-induced PSYCHOTIC DISORDER, with DELUSIONS or HALLUCINATIONS; PCP-induced MOOD DISORDER; and PCP-induced ANXIETY DISORDER.

phenelzine   An ANTIDEPRESSANT that is a potent inhibitor of MONOAMINE OXIDASE; used in the treatment of DEPRESSION, especially in patients with atypical SYMPTOMS, such as rejection sensitivity, ANXIETY, and HYPERSOMNIA. Also used to treat certain ANXIETY DISORDERS. Marketed under the brand name NARDIL. See "Medications Used in Psychiatry."

phenobarbital   A BARBITURATE (a class of CENTRAL NERVOUS SYSTEM [CNS] depressants with potent sedative and hypnotic properties) that is potentially addictive and lethal in overdose. For this reason, phenobarbital is seldom prescribed for treatment of ANXIETY or INSOMNIA; however, it is still used as an ANTICONVULSANT to control seizures.

phenomenology   The study of occurrences or happenings in their own right rather than from the point of view of inferred causes; specifically, the theory that behavior is determined not by external reality as it can be described objectively in physical terms but rather by the way in which the subject perceives that reality at any moment. See also EXISTENTIAL PSYCHIATRY.

phenothiazines   A subgroup of CONVENTIONAL ANTIPSYCHOTIC drugs that, chemically, have in common a phenothiazine configuration (i.e., phenyl rings and heterocyclic ring containing nitrogen and sulfur) but differ from one another through variations in side chains. Based on the side chain attached to the nitrogen atom in the middle ring, the phenothiazines are subdivided into three subgroups: *aliphatic* (e.g., CHLORPROMAZINE), *piperazine* (e.g., FLUPHENAZINE, TRIFLUOPERAZINE, PERPHENAZINE), and *piperidine* (e.g., MESORIDAZINE, THIORIDAZINE).

phenotype   The observable attributes of an individual; the physical manifestations of the GENOTYPE.

phenylketonuria (PKU)   A GENETIC metabolic disturbance characterized by an inability to convert phenylalanine to tyrosine. It is treatable by diet when detected in early infancy; if untreated, INTELLECTUAL DISABILITY results. Also known as *phenylpyruvic oligophrenia.*

phenytoin (diphenylhydantoin)   An ANTICONVULSANT medication used to treat grand mal SEIZURES and seizures occurring during or following neurosurgery. Marketed under the brand name DILANTIN. See "Medications Used in Psychiatry."

phobia   FEAR cued by the presence or anticipation of a specific object or situation, exposure to which almost invariably provokes an immediate ANXIETY response or PANIC ATTACK even though the subject recognizes that the fear is excessive or unreasonable. The phobic stimulus is avoided or endured with marked distress. Two types of phobia have been differentiated:

specific phobia Formerly called *simple phobia,* specific phobia is subtyped on the basis of the object feared: animals; the natural environment (e.g., heights, storms, water); blood, injection, or injury; certain situations (e.g., cars, airplanes, heights, tunnels); and other stimuli (e.g., fear of choking, vomiting, or contracting an illness).

social phobia Also called *social anxiety disorder,* social phobia is the persistent fear of social situations that might expose one to scrutiny by others and induce one to act in a way or show anxiety SYMPTOMS that will be humiliating or embarrassing. Avoidance may be limited to one or only a few situations, or it may extend to most social situations. Performing in front of others or interacting socially may be the focus of concern. It is sometimes difficult to distinguish between social phobia and AGORAPHOBIA when social avoidance accompanies PANIC ATTACKS. Social phobia occurring in childhood and adolescence has been termed AVOIDANT DISORDER.

phonological disorder See under COMMUNICATION DISORDERS.

phonophobia The FEAR of or increased sensitivity to loud noises.

photophobia The FEAR of light or sensitivity to light (e.g., in MIGRAINE).

phototherapy See LIGHT THERAPY.

phrenology A discredited theory positing a relationship between the structure of the skull and mental traits.

phylogenetic Pertaining to the development of the species. Contrast with ONTOGENETIC.

Physicians' Desk Reference See PDR (*PHYSICIANS' DESK REFERENCE*)

pia mater The innermost of the meninges; a delicate fibrous membrane closely enveloping the BRAIN and SPINAL CORD.

piblokto Observed primarily among Eskimo communities, *piblokto* is an abrupt dissociative episode accompanied by extreme excitement of up to 30 minutes' duration and frequently followed by convulsive seizures and COMA lasting up to 12 hours. Also referred to as *arctic hysteria.* See CULTURE-SPECIFIC SYNDROMES.

pica A feeding and EATING DISORDER of infancy or early childhood characterized by developmentally inappropriate, persistent, or recurring eating of nonnutritive substances (e.g., dirt).

Pick's disease A presenile degenerative disease of the BRAIN, possibly hereditary, that affects the CEREBRAL CORTEX focally, particularly the frontal lobes. SYMPTOMS include intellectual deterioration, emotional instability, and loss of social ADJUSTMENT. See also ALZHEIMER'S DISEASE.

piloerection   Gooseflesh, or the diffuse erection of hair follicles in the skin in response to cold, fright, OPIOID WITHDRAWAL, or other conditions.

pimozide   A CONVENTIONAL ANTIPSYCHOTIC medication (a DIPHENYLBUTYLPIPERIDINE) used to treat SCHIZOPHRENIA AND OTHER PSYCHOTIC DISORDERS as well as the motor and phonic TICS of TOURETTE'S DISORDER. Marketed under the brand name ORAP. See "Medications Used in Psychiatry."

PKU   See PHENYLKETONURIA (PKU).

placebo   A material without pharmacological activity but identical in appearance to an active drug. Used in pharmacological research as a method of determining the actual effects of the drug being tested.

placebo effect   The production or enhancement of psychological or physical effects with the use of pharmacologically inactive substances administered under circumstances in which SUGGESTION or expectation leads the subject to believe a particular effect will occur.

plaintiff   See "Legal Terms."

plaques   Certain areas of the BRAIN that have undergone a specific form of degeneration. Senile plaques (NEURITIC PLAQUES) consist of a central AMYLOID core surrounded by a less densely staining zone composed of abnormal NEURONS, with many axonal and dendritic processes and masses of paired helical filaments (NEUROFIBRILLARY TANGLES). In ALZHEIMER'S DISEASE, plaques are particularly dense in the amygdaloid complex and the HIPPOCAMPUS. The relation between the abnormal protein fibers inside neurons (the paired helical filaments) and those outside the cells (i.e., amyloid) is currently under investigation.

plasma level   See BLOOD LEVELS.

play therapy   A treatment technique using the child's play as a medium for expression and communication between patient and therapist.

pleasure principle   The psychoanalytic concept (see PSYCHOANALYSIS) that people instinctually seek to avoid pain and discomfort and strive for gratification and pleasure. In PERSONALITY development theory, the pleasure principle antedates and subsequently comes in CONFLICT with the REALITY PRINCIPLE.

PMDD   See PREMENSTRUAL DYSPHORIC DISORDER (PMDD).

poinephobia   The FEAR of punishment.

police power   See "Legal Terms."

polydipsia Excessive or abnormal thirst. Patients with OBSESSIVE-COMPULSIVE DISORDER and other psychiatric disorders, such as SCHIZO-PHRENIA, may have polydipsia, which may produce a type of diabetes insipidus.

polyphagia Pathological overeating. Also known as BULIMIA NERVOSA.

polypharmacy The term is used when too many forms of medication are used by a patient, when more drugs are prescribed than is clinically warranted, or even when all prescribed medications are clinically indicated but there are too many pills to take (pill burden). Furthermore, a portion of the treatments may not be evidence-based. The most common results of polypharmacy are increased adverse drug reactions and drug-drug interactions. Polypharmacy is most common in the elderly but is also widespread in the general population.

polysomnography The all-night recording of a variety of physiological parameters (e.g., BRAIN waves, eye movements, muscle tonus, respiration, heart rate, penile tumescence) in order to diagnose SLEEP-related disorders.

polysubstance dependence In DSM-IV-TR, defined as use of at least three different substances (not including nicotine or caffeine) for 6 months or more, during which time no single substance has predominated.

polyuria Excessive urination, which can be induced by LITHIUM CARBONATE as well as many other medications and clinical conditions.

pons A broad mass of nerve fibers on the ventral surface of the BRAIN.

"poppers" A street name for NITRITE INHALANTS that are sometimes abused.

porphyria A metabolic disorder characterized by the excretion of porphyrins in the urine and accompanied by attacks of abdominal pain, PERIPHERAL NEUROPATHY, and a variety of mental SYMPTOMS. Some types are precipitated by BARBITURATES and alcohol.

positive symptoms (of schizophrenia) A group of SYMPTOMS characteristic of SCHIZOPHRENIA that include DELUSIONS, which may be bizarre in nature; HALLUCINATIONS, especially auditory; disorganized speech; INAPPROPRIATE AFFECT; and disorganized behavior. Also see SCHIZOPHRENIA.

positron emission tomography (PET) A BRAIN IMAGING technique that permits evaluation of regional metabolic differences by looking at radioisotope distribution. By using positron-emitting isotopes of glucose, oxygen, NEUROTRANSMITTERS, or drugs, one can localize sites of increased (or decreased) metabolic turnover or blood flow in a wide variety of neurological or psychiatric conditions. The visual display is similar to that in COMPUTED TOMOGRAPHY (CT).

possession   See DISSOCIATIVE TRANCE DISORDER.

postconcussional disorder   A proposed disorder (listed in DSM-IV-TR Appendix B, "Criteria Sets and Axes Provided for Further Study") whose essential features are acquired cognitive impairment and behavioral disturbance that develop after head trauma. The cognitive and neurobehavioral sequelae appear within 4 weeks of experiencing the trauma and are accompanied by somatic complaints (headache, dizziness, noise intolerance), emotional changes (irritability, DEPRESSION, ANXIETY), difficulty in concentration, INSOMNIA, and reduced TOLERANCE to alcohol. Physical examination and laboratory tests give evidence of cerebral damage.

posthallucinogen perception disorder   Reexperiencing one or more of the perceptual SYMPTOMS that had been experienced while using the HALLUCINOGEN, following cessation of its use. Some examples are the ILLUSION of objects changing shape, false PERCEPTIONS of movement in the peripheral field of vision, flashes or intensification of colors, or trails of images of moving objects. See also INTOXICATION.

postpartum depression (PPD)   Moderate to severe depression that affects between 8% and 20% of women after pregnancy. Most of the time, it occurs within the first 4 weeks after delivery, although it may occur soon after delivery or up to a year later. Women with postpartum depression have such strong feelings of sadness, anxiety, or despair that they have trouble coping with their daily tasks, including caring for their infants and other children.

postpartum psychosis   An inexact, general term for any type of PSYCHOSIS occurring within 90 days after childbirth.

posttraumatic stress disorder (PTSD)   An ANXIETY DISORDER in which exposure to an exceptional mental or physical stressor is followed, sometimes immediately and sometimes not until 6 months or more after the stress, by persistent reexperiencing of the event, avoidance of stimuli associated with the trauma or numbing of general responsiveness, and manifestations of HYPERAROUSAL. The trauma typically includes experiencing, witnessing, or confronting an event that involves actual or threatened death or injury, or a threat to the physical integrity of oneself or others, with an immediate reaction of intense FEAR, HELPLESSNESS, or horror.

postural (orthostatic) hypotension   A form of hypotension in which a person's blood pressure suddenly falls when the person stands up from a seated or recumbent position.

postural instability   A loss of balance that causes someone to feel unsteady. Postural instability is one of the most common causes of falls in people with PARKINSON'S DISEASE. This symptom must be taken seriously, as it can result in head injury or bone fractures.

postural tremor, medication-induced   Fine shaking when attempting to maintain a posture that develops in association with the use of medications such as LITHIUM CARBONATE, ANTIDEPRESSANTS, and VALPROATE.

posturing   See CATATONIC BEHAVIOR.

potency   The male's ability to carry out sexual relations. Often refers specifically to the male's capacity to achieve and maintain adequate erection of the penis during sexual intercourse. Also used metaphorically to denote masculine power, strength, or vigor. Contrast with IMPOTENCE.

poverty of speech   Restriction in the amount of speech; spontaneous speech and replies to questions range from brief and unelaborated to monosyllabic or no response at all. When the amount of speech is adequate, there may be a poverty of content if the answer is vague or if there is a substitution of stereotyped or obscure phrases for meaningful responses.

power of attorney   See "Legal Terms."

PPD   See POSTPARTUM DEPRESSION (PPD).

practice guidelines   According to the Institute of Medicine, practice guidelines are "systematically developed statements to assist practitioners and patient decisions about appropriate health care for specific clinical circumstances." The AMERICAN PSYCHIATRIC ASSOCIATION (APA) practice guidelines provide evidence-based recommendations for the assessment and treatment of PSYCHIATRIC DISORDERS.

Prader-Willi syndrome   A developmental DISABILITY caused by GENETIC changes on CHROMOSOME 15. Between ages 1 and 4, children with this SYNDROME develop an increased interest in food, which may become an insatiable OBSESSION and is often associated with compact body build, underdeveloped sexual characteristics, and poor muscle tone. Most patients have mild INTELLECTUAL DISABILITY and delays in language and motor development.

pramipexole   A medication indicated for the treatment of the signs and symptoms of IDIOPATHIC PARKINSON'S DISEASE and of moderate to severe primary RESTLESS LEGS SYNDROME. Marketed under the brand name MIRAPEX.

prazosin   An alpha$_1$-ADRENERGIC RECEPTOR blocker originally developed to treat hypertension but also effective in treating various other conditions, such as POSTTRAUMATIC STRESS DISORDER (PTSD) symptoms, including increased startle response, recurrent nightmares and sleep disturbance related to PTSD, and reexperiencing of past traumas. In recent clinical studies, prazosin has also shown some effectiveness in treatment of ALCOHOL DEPENDENCE. Marketed under the brand name MINIPRESS. See "Medications Used in Psychiatry."

preconscious   Thoughts that are not in immediate awareness but that can be recalled by CONSCIOUS effort. One's own telephone number would be an example.

pregabalin   An ANTICONVULSANT medication approved for treatment of neuropathic pain, FIBROMYALGIA, and GENERALIZED ANXIETY DISORDER (Europe only). Marketed under the brand name LYRICA. See "Medications Used in Psychiatry."

pregenital   In PSYCHOANALYSIS, refers to the period of early childhood before the genitals have begun to exert the predominant influence in the organization or patterning of sexual behavior. Oral and anal influences predominate during this period. See also PSYCHOSEXUAL DEVELOPMENT.

premature ejaculation   Undesired ejaculation occurring immediately before or very early in sexual intercourse. See under ORGASMIC DISORDERS.

premenstrual dysphoric disorder (PMDD)   A proposed disorder (listed in DSM-IV-TR Appendix B, "Criteria Sets and Axes Provided for Further Study") characterized by rapidly changing feelings or persistent and marked anger, ANXIETY, or tension; depressed MOOD with feelings of hopelessness or self-deprecating thoughts; and many other SYMPTOMS, such as lethargy, difficulty in concentrating, overeating or food cravings, INSOMNIA or HYPERSOMNIA, breast tenderness or swelling, headaches, weight gain, increased sensitivity to rejection and avoidance of social activities, or increased interpersonal CONFLICTS. The SYNDROME occurs in as many as 5% of menstruating women, with symptoms concentrated in the week before and a few days after the onset of menses.

preoperational thought   See COGNITIVE DEVELOPMENT.

preponderance of the evidence   See "Legal Terms."

presenile dementia   A DEMENTIA of the ALZHEIMER'S type beginning before age 65. See also ALZHEIMER'S DISEASE; PICK'S DISEASE.

pressured speech   Rapid, accelerated, frenzied speech. Sometimes it exceeds the ability of the vocal musculature to articulate, leading to jumbled and cluttered speech; at other times, it exceeds the ability of the listener to comprehend because the speech expresses a FLIGHT OF IDEAS (as in MANIA) or unintelligible jargon. See also LOGORRHEA.

prevalence   The total number of cases of any mental disorder that exist within a unit of population.

prevention (preventive psychiatry)   In traditional medical usage, the prevention or prophylaxis of a disorder. In COMMUNITY PSYCHIATRY, the meaning of prevention encompasses the amelioration, control, and limitation of a MENTAL DISORDER. Prevention of mental disorders is often categorized as follows:

primary prevention   Measures implemented to prevent the occurrence of a MENTAL DISORDER (e.g., by nutrition, substitute parents).

secondary prevention   Measures implemented to limit an existing disease process (e.g., through early case-finding and treatment).

tertiary prevention   Measures implemented to reduce impairment or DISABILITY following development of a disorder (e.g., through REHABILITATION programs).

primal scene   In psychoanalytic theory (see PSYCHOANALYSIS), the real or fancied observation by the child of parental or other heterosexual intercourse and the meaning the child attaches to it.

primal scream therapy   See EXPERIENTIAL THERAPY.

primary care physician   Usually a general practitioner or specialist in family practice, internal medicine, pediatrics, or, occasionally, obstetrics and gynecology who serves as an initial contact for patients in MANAGED CARE systems.

primary degenerative dementia   See ALZHEIMER'S DISEASE.

primary diagnosis   The condition established as the primary reason for the patient seeking treatment from a health or MENTAL HEALTH provider. See also PRINCIPAL DIAGNOSIS.

primary gain   The relief from emotional CONFLICT and the freedom from ANXIETY achieved by a DEFENSE MECHANISM. Contrast with SECONDARY GAIN.

primary identification   The earliest form of IDENTIFICATION with an OBJECT, which occurs before the infant can distinguish the SELF from the object.

primary process In psychoanalytic theory (see PSYCHOANALYSIS), the generally unorganized mental activity characteristic of the UNCONSCIOUS. This activity is marked by the free discharge of energy and excitation without regard to the demands of environment, reality, or logic. Contrast with SECONDARY PROCESS.

principal diagnosis The condition established as the primary reason for the admission of the patient to the hospital or for OUTPATIENT treatment. See also PRIMARY DIAGNOSIS.

prion A small protein particle that can transmit an infectious disease. Prion diseases are often referred to as SPONGIFORM ENCEPHALOPATHIES because of the postmortem appearance of the BRAIN, with large vacuoles in the CEREBRAL CORTEX and CEREBELLUM. Most mammalian species can develop these diseases. CREUTZFELDT-JAKOB DISEASE is the most common of the prion diseases.

prison psychosis See GANSER SYNDROME.

Pristiq Brand name for an extended-release formulation of the SEROTONIN-NOREPINEPHRINE REUPTAKE INHIBITOR (SNRI) ANTIDEPRESSANT drug DESVENLAFAXINE.

privilege See "Legal Terms."

privileged communication Information imparted by a patient or client within the context of a professional relationship with a practitioner (i.e., physician, lawyer) that is immune to disclosure without the patient's or client's expressed permission. See also "Legal Terms."

PRO See PEER REVIEW ORGANIZATION (PRO).

problem-oriented record A simple conceptual framework to expedite and improve MEDICAL RECORDS. It contains four logically sequenced sections: the database, the problem list, plans, and follow-up.

problem solving A specific form of intellectual activity used when a person faces a situation that cannot be handled in terms of past learning. Problem-solving strategies are considered crucial in any psychotherapeutic endeavor.

procedural memory A memory that is not readily available in words or images, is not conscious, and is revealed by behavioral and emotional patterns that are elicited without the subject's awareness. Contrast with DECLARATIVE MEMORY.

procyclidine An ANTICHOLINERGIC medication used to treat PARKINSON'S DISEASE and to control medication-induced EXTRAPYRAMIDAL SYMPTOMS (EPS). The brand name KEMADRIN was discontinued by the manufacturer in 2008, and no generics are currently available.

prodrome (precursor) An early or premonitory SYMPTOM or set of symptoms of a disease or a disorder.

professional standards review organization (PSRO) A physician-sponsored organization charged with comprehensive and ongoing review of services provided under MEDICARE, MEDICAID, and maternal and child health programs. The object of this review is to determine for purposes of reimbursement under these programs whether services are medically necessary; are provided in accordance with professional criteria, norms, and standards; and, in the case of institutional services, are rendered in appropriate settings. See also PEER REVIEW ORGANIZATION (PRO).

prognosis The prediction of the future course of an illness.

progressive nonfluent aphasia One of three clinical syndromes associated with FRONTOTEMPORAL LOBAR DEGENERATION (FTLD), characterized by progressive difficulties with the production of speech.

progressive supranuclear palsy A degenerative disease of the CENTRAL NERVOUS SYSTEM (CNS) characterized by balance difficulties and the inability to aim the eyes. Patients often show MOOD alteration, DEPRESSION, APATHY, and progressive mild DEMENTIA. Also known as *Steele-Richardson-Olszewski syndrome.*

projection A DEFENSE MECHANISM, operating unconsciously (see UNCONSCIOUS), in which an individual attributes to another person an unacceptable thought, feeling, or attribute, such as an aggressive or sexual impulse, that in fact is his or her own.

projective identification A term introduced by PSYCHOANALYST Melanie Klein (1882–1960) to refer to the UNCONSCIOUS process of PROJECTION of one or more parts of the SELF or of the internal object onto another person (such as the mother). What is projected may be an intolerable, painful, or dangerous part of the self or object (the BAD OBJECT). It also may be a valued aspect of the self or object (the good object) that is projected into the other person for safekeeping. The other person is changed by the projection and is dealt with as though he or she is in fact characterized by the aspects of the self that have been projected.

projective tests Psychological diagnostic tests in which the test material is amorphous or unstructured so that any response will reflect a PROJECTION of some aspect of the subject's underlying PERSONALITY and PSYCHOPATHOLOGY.

prolactin A HORMONE secreted by the anterior pituitary that promotes lactation in the female and may stimulate testosterone secretion in the male. Inhibiting and releasing factors in the BRAIN in part control prolactin secretion. Because DOPAMINE is involved in the brain's inhibition of prolactin secretion, the measurement of serum prolactin has been proposed as a way of judging the efficacy of specific ANTIPSY-CHOTIC medications that act by blocking DOPAMINE RECEPTORS.

Prolixin   Brand name (now discontinued) for FLUPHENAZINE.

promiscuity   Indiscriminately engaging in sexual activity with many people.

propranolol   A nonselective beta-ADRENERGIC RECEPTOR–blocking agent (i.e., BETA-BLOCKER) used in general medical practice to treat hypertension and used "off label" in PSYCHIATRY to treat performance ANXIETY and AGITATION and AGGRESSION, especially in patients who have experienced a brain injury. Marketed under the brand name INDERAL. See "Medications Used in Psychiatry."

pro se   See "Legal Terms."

ProSom   Brand name (now discontinued) for the BENZODIAZEPINE SEDA-TIVE-HYPNOTIC drug ESTAZOLAM.

prosopagnosia   A neurological condition that renders a person incapable of recognizing faces. It arises when the part of the BRAIN dedicated to face recognition is damaged or unable to perform its function.

protriptyline   An older TRICYCLIC ANTIDEPRESSANT medication seldom prescribed today. Marketed under the brand name VIVACTIL. See "Medications Used in Psychiatry."

Provigil   Brand name for the atypical STIMULANT drug MODAFINIL.

proximate cause   See "Legal Terms."

proxy   See "Legal Terms."

Prozac   Brand name for the SELECTIVE SEROTONIN REUPTAKE INHIBITOR (SSRI) ANTIDEPRESSANT drug FLUOXETINE.

pseudocyesis   Included in DSM-IV-TR as a SOMATOFORM DISORDER not otherwise specified. Pseudocyesis is characterized by a false belief of being pregnant and by the occurrence of SIGNS of being pregnant, such as abdominal enlargement, breast engorgement, and labor pains.

pseudodementia   A SYNDROME in which DEMENTIA is mimicked or caricatured by a psychiatric disorder such as DEPRESSION. SYMPTOMS and response to MENTAL STATUS EXAMINATION questions are similar to those found in verified cases of dementia. In pseudodementia, the chief DIAGNOSIS to be considered in the differential is depression in an older person versus COGNITIVE deterioration on the basis of ORGANIC DISEASE in the BRAIN. See also GANSER SYNDROME.

pseudologia fantastica   One of several terms applied to the behavior of habitual or compulsive lying. The stories are not entirely improbable and often have some element of truth. They are not a manifestation of DELUSIONS or some wider form of PSYCHOSIS: upon confrontation, the person can acknowledge them to be untrue, even if unwillingly.

pseudoseizure   An attack that resembles an epileptic SEIZURE but has psychological causes and lacks electroencephalographic dysrhythmia.

PSRO   See PROFESSIONAL STANDARDS REVIEW ORGANIZATION (PSRO).

psyche   The realm of the mind, as distinguished from the realm of the body, or SOMA.

psychedelic   A term applied to any of several drugs that may induce HALLUCINATIONS and altered mental states, including the production of distortions of time, sound, color, and so forth. Among the more commonly used psychedelics are LSD (LYSERGIC ACID DIETHYLAMIDE), MARIJUANA, MESCALINE, and psilocybin.

psychiatric illness   See MENTAL DISORDER.

psychiatric nurse   Any nurse employed in a psychiatric hospital or other psychiatric setting who has special training and experience in the management of psychiatric patients. Sometimes the term is used to denote only those nurses who have a master's degree in psychiatric nursing.

psychiatric social work   A specialty of SOCIAL WORK that is concerned with the PREVENTION of mental illness, the treatment and REHABILITATION of mentally ill patients, and the prevention of RELAPSE. Particular attention is given to familial, environmental, cultural, and other social factors that may be involved in the development, continuation, or recurrence of mental illness and in the patient's response to treatment.

psychiatrist   A licensed physician who specializes in the DIAGNOSIS, treatment, and PREVENTION of MENTAL DISORDERS. Training encompasses a medical degree and 4 years or more of approved training after medical school. For those who wish to enter a subspecialty such as CHILD PSYCHIATRY, FORENSIC PSYCHIATRY, GERIATRIC PSYCHIATRY, PSYCHOANALYSIS, administration, or ADDICTION PSYCHIATRY, additional training is required.

psychiatry   The science and medical specialty that deals with the origin, DIAGNOSIS, PREVENTION, and treatment of MENTAL DISORDERS.

psychic defense   See DEFENSE MECHANISM.

psychic determinism   See DETERMINISM.

psychic trauma   An INTRAPSYCHIC event brought on by exposure to an unanticipated danger. The acute SYNDROME is characterized by psychological shock; HELPLESSNESS; numbness of feelings; disturbances of speech, eating, and sleeping (nightmares); and SOCIAL WITHDRAWAL. Persistence of the helpless state may result in death. The long-term effects are usually persistent preoccupation with the self; somatic concerns; depressive and ANXIETY SYMPTOMS; and FEAR of being further victimized. See POSTTRAUMATIC STRESS DISORDER (PTSD).

psychoactive substance   A chemical agent that alters MOOD or behavior. Includes prescribed medications and other substances with mood-, cognition-, or behavior-altering effects, as well as toxins, industrial solvents, and other agents to which one may be exposed unintentionally and whose effects on the nervous system may lead to behavioral or COGNITIVE disturbances.

psychoactive substance use disorders   See DRUG DEPENDENCE.

psychoanalysis   A theory of the PSYCHOLOGY of human development and behavior, a method of research, and a system of PSYCHOTHERAPY, originally developed by Sigmund Freud (1856–1939). Through analysis of FREE ASSOCIATIONS and INTERPRETATION of dreams, EMOTIONS and behavior are traced to the influence of repressed instinctual DRIVES and defenses against them in the UNCONSCIOUS. Psychoanalytic treatment seeks to eliminate or diminish the undesirable effects of unconscious CONFLICTS by helping the ANALYSAND become aware of their existence, origin, and inappropriate expression in current emotions and behavior.

psychoanalyst   A person, often a PSYCHIATRIST, who has had training in PSYCHOANALYSIS and who uses the techniques of psychoanalytic theory in the treatment of patients.

psychoanalytically oriented psychotherapy   A form of PSYCHOTHERAPY that uses a variety of psychotherapeutic techniques, some of which are used in PSYCHOANALYSIS (e.g., use of clarification and INTERPRETATION), as well as other techniques (e.g., the use of SUGGESTION, reassurance, and advice giving). This form of therapy is now generally seen as existing on a continuum with psychoanalysis and is often termed *psychoanalytic* or PSYCHODYNAMIC PSYCHOTHERAPY.

psychobiology   A school of psychiatric thought that views biological, psychological, and social life experiences of a person as an integrated unit. Associated with the psychiatrist Adolf Meyer (1866–1950), who introduced the term in the United States in 1915.

psychodrama   A technique of group PSYCHOTHERAPY conceived and practiced by Jacob L. Moreno (1889–1974), in which individuals express their own or assigned emotional problems through dramatization.

psychodynamic psychotherapy   A form of therapy whose goal is to provide greater insights into UNCONSCIOUS CONFLICTS and other sources of signs and symptoms which lead to changes in emotional, cognitive, and behavioral problems. Psychodynamic treatments are among the most widely used PSYCHOTHERAPIES, and many of the principles of psychodynamic therapy have been incorporated into other therapeutic approaches.

psychodynamics   The systematized knowledge and theory of human behavior and its motivation, the study of which depends largely on the FUNCTIONAL significance of EMOTION. Psychodynamics recognizes the ROLE of UNCONSCIOUS motivation in human behavior. The science of psychodynamics assumes that one's behavior is determined by past experience, GENETIC ENDOWMENT, and current reality.

psychoendocrinology   The study of the psychological effects of neuroendocrinological activity. For example, it is known that the release and inhibition of pituitary HORMONES are mediated in part by BRAIN MONOAMINES, disorders of which have been implicated in the pathogenesis of various psychiatric illnesses. See also NEUROENDOCRINOLOGY.

psychogenesis   Production or causation of a SYMPTOM or illness by mental or psychic factors as opposed to organic ones.

psychogenic amnesia   See DISSOCIATIVE AMNESIA.

psychogenic excoriation   See DERMATILLOMANIA.

psychogenic fugue   See DISSOCIATIVE FUGUE.

psychogenic pain disorder   See PAIN DISORDER.

psychohistory   An approach to history that examines events within a psychological framework.

psychoimmunology   The study of the connection between the BRAIN and EMOTIONS and the immune system.

psycholinguistics   The study of mental factors that affect communication and the comprehension of verbal information. See also KINESICS.

psychological autopsy   Postmortem evaluation of the PSYCHODYNAMICS contributing to a person's SUICIDE.

psychological testing ASSESSMENTS that measure characteristics, abilities, and skills related to mental functioning. See "Psychiatric Measures."

psychologist A person who holds a degree in PSYCHOLOGY from an accredited program. Providers of psychological services are licensed under applicable state law, whereas those psychologists who teach or do research are usually exempt from licensure requirements.

psychology An academic discipline, a profession, and a science dealing with the study of mental processes, COGNITION, emotions, and behavior of people and animals.

psychometry The science of testing and measuring mental and psychological ability, efficiency potentials, and functioning, including psychopathological components (see PSYCHOPATHOLOGY).

psychomotor Referring to combined physical and mental activity.

psychomotor agitation Excessive motor activity associated with a feeling of inner tension. When severe, AGITATION may also involve shouting and loud complaining. The activity is usually nonproductive and repetitious and consists of behavior such as pacing, wringing of hands, and inability to sit still.

psychomotor retardation A generalized slowing of physical, cognitive, and emotional responses. Specifically, the slowing of movements such as eye blinking; frequently seen in DEPRESSION.

psychoneuroimmunology The study of the interaction between psychological processes and the nervous and immune systems.

psychopathic personality ANTISOCIAL PERSONALITY DISORDER (see under PERSONALITY DISORDERS).

psychopathology The study of the significant causes and processes in the development of MENTAL DISORDERS. Also the manifestations of mental disorders.

psychopharmacology The study of the effects of PSYCHOACTIVE SUBSTANCES on behavior, mood, sensation, and COGNITION. Clinical psychopharmacology includes both the study of medication effects in patients and the expert use of medications in the treatment of psychiatric disorders.

psychophysiological disorders A group of disorders characterized by physical SYMPTOMS that are affected by emotional factors and involve a single organ system, usually under AUTONOMIC NERVOUS SYSTEM (ANS) control. Symptoms are caused by physiological changes that normally accompany certain emotional states, but the changes are more intense and sustained. Frequently called PSYCHOSOMATIC disorders. These disorders are usually named and classified according to the organ system involved (e.g., gastrointestinal, respiratory). In DSM-IV-TR, such cases would be diagnosed as psychological factors affecting a GENERAL MEDICAL CONDITION. The specific physical condition is diagnosed and recorded separately. When there is no diagnosable physical condition, some other disorder may be cited. See AUTONOMIC AROUSAL DISORDER.

psychosexual development   A series of stages from infancy to adulthood, relatively fixed in time, determined by the interaction between a person's biological DRIVES and the environment. With resolution of this interaction, a balanced, reality-oriented development takes place; with disturbance, FIXATION and CONFLICT ensue. This disturbance may remain latent or give rise to mental disorders. In the theory of classical psychoanalytic PSYCHOLOGY, the stages of development are as follows:

oral   The earliest of the stages of infantile psychosexual development, lasting from birth to 12 months or longer. Usually subdivided into two stages: the oral EROTIC, relating to the pleasurable experience of sucking; and the oral sadistic, associated with aggressive biting. Both oral eroticism and oral sadism continue into adult life in disguised and sublimated forms, such as the CHARACTER traits of demandingness or pessimism. Oral CONFLICT, as a general and pervasive influence, has been hypothesized to underlie the psychological determinants of addictive disorders, DEPRESSION, and some FUNCTIONAL psychotic disorders.

anal   The period of PREGENITAL psychosexual development, usually from 1 to 3 years, in which the child has particular interest in and concern with the process of defecation and the sensations connected with the anus. The pleasurable part of the experience is termed *anal eroticism*. See also ANAL CHARACTER.

phallic   The period, from about ages 2½ to 6 years, during which sexual interest, curiosity, and pleasurable experience in boys center on the penis and in girls, to a lesser extent, the clitoris.

oedipal   Overlapping to some extent with the phallic stage, this phase (ages 4–6 years) represents a time of inevitable CONFLICT between the child and parents. The child must desexualize the relationship to both parents in order to retain affectionate kinship with both of them. The process is accomplished by the internalization of the images of both parents, thereby giving more definite shape to the child's PERSONALITY. With this internalization largely completed, the regulation of self-esteem and moral behavior comes about.

psychosexual therapy   A form of therapy that deals with a range of sexual problems including SEXUAL AROUSAL DISORDERS, ORGASMIC DISORDERS, and loss of sexual desire.

psychosis   A severe MENTAL DISORDER characterized by gross impairment in REALITY TESTING, typically manifested by DELUSIONS, HALLUCINATIONS, disorganized speech, or disorganized or CATATONIC BEHAVIOR. Psychosis can be caused by psychiatric illnesses such as SCHIZOPHRENIA, DELUSIONAL DISORDERS, and some MOOD DISORDERS; by medical and neurological diseases; by brain injury; and by substances of abuse.

psychosocial development   Progressive interaction between a person and the environment through stages beginning in infancy, as described by Erik Erikson (1902–1994). A person at phase-specific developmental points faces specific developmental tasks involving social relations and the role of social reality. The early stages parallel those of PSYCHOSEXUAL DEVELOPMENT; the later stages extend through adulthood. Successful and unsuccessful outcomes at each stage are listed below with the corresponding chronological period and psychosexual stage where applicable. See also COGNITIVE DEVELOPMENT.

Successful vs. unsuccessful outcomes of developmental tasks	Chronological period	Psychosexual stage
Trust vs. mistrust	Infancy	Oral
Autonomy vs. shame, doubt	Early childhood (toddler)	Anal
Initiative vs. guilt	Preschool	Phallic (oedipal)
Industry vs. inferiority	School-age	Latency
Identity vs. identity diffusion	Adolescence	
Intimacy vs. isolation	Young adulthood	Genital
Generativity vs. self-absorption	Adulthood	
Integrity vs. despair	Mature age	

psychosocial history An evaluation of the patient that includes a history of psychiatric illness, developmental history, educational history, marital and family life, and employment history.

psychosomatic Referring to the constant and inseparable interaction of the PSYCHE (mind) and the SOMA (body). Most commonly used to refer to illnesses in which the manifestations are primarily physical but with at least a partial emotional ETIOLOGY. See SOMATOFORM DISORDERS.

psychosomatic medicine An AMERICAN BOARD OF PSYCHIATRY AND NEUROLOGY (ABPN) subspecialization in the diagnosis and treatment of psychiatric disorders and symptoms in medically ill patients. This includes treatment of patients with acute or chronic medical, neurological, obstetrical, or surgical illness in which psychiatric illness is affecting their medical care and/or quality of life such as HIV infection, organ transplantation, heart disease, renal failure, cancer, stroke, traumatic brain injury, high-risk pregnancy, and chronic obstructive pulmonary disease, among others. Patients also may be those who have a psychiatric disorder that is the direct consequence of a primary medical condition, or a SOMATOFORM DISORDER or psychological factors affecting a GENERAL MEDICAL CONDITION. Psychiatrists specializing in psychosomatic medicine provide consultation-liaison services in general medical hospitals, attend on medical psychiatry inpatient units, and provide collaborative care in primary care and other outpatient settings.

psychosurgery The treatment of MENTAL DISORDERS by means of BRAIN surgery. The first consistent technique for psychosurgery, called LOBOTOMY, consisted of severing fiber tracts between the THALAMUS and the frontal lobes and was a radical attempt to reduce PSYCHOSIS, severe DEPRESSION, or violent behavior in treatment-REFRACTORY patients. With the advance of minimally invasive surgical techniques, such as FUNCTIONAL stereotactic neurosurgery and radiosurgery, physicians are now able to lesion with high precision much smaller areas of the brain involved in emotional control. These small surgically created lesions have little effect on other intellectual or emotional spheres and may be quite effective in controlling violent behavior caused by intracranial tumors, untreatable severe depression, severe ANXIETY DISORDERS (including OBSESSIVE-COMPULSIVE DISORDER), or chronic pain.

psychotherapist A person trained to practice PSYCHOTHERAPY.

psychotherapy A form of treatment in which a person who wishes to relieve SYMPTOMS or resolve problems through verbal interaction seeks help from a qualified MENTAL HEALTH professional and enters into an implicit or explicit contract to interact in a prescribed way with a PSYCHOTHERAPIST. See also BRIEF PSYCHOTHERAPY.

psychotic depression   See DEPRESSION WITH PSYCHOTIC FEATURES; MELAN-CHOLIA.

psychotic disorder due to a general medical condition   Prominent HALLUCINATIONS or DELUSIONS that develop in relation to some GENERAL MEDICAL CONDITION. In older classifications, such disorders were termed ORGANIC BRAIN SYNDROMES or SECONDARY psychotic disorders (see SECONDARY DISORDER).

psychotomimetic   Literally, mimicking a PSYCHOSIS. Used to refer to certain drugs, such as LSD (LYSERGIC ACID DIETHYLAMIDE) or MESCALINE, that may produce psychotic-like states.

psychotropic   A term used to describe medications that have a special action on mental function.

PTSD   See POSTTRAUMATIC STRESS DISORDER (PTSD).

punitive damages   See "Legal Terms."

putamen   A round structure, located at the base of the FOREBRAIN, whose main function is to regulate movements and influence various types of learning. It does so employing DOPAMINE to perform its functions. The putamen plays a role in degenerative neurological disorders, such as PARKINSON'S DISEASE. Also, the putamen may decrease in size as a result of damage in HUNTINGTON'S DISEASE.

pyromania   Fire setting; an IMPULSE-CONTROL DISORDER consisting of deliberate and purposeful fire setting on more than one occasion. As in other disorders of impulse control, an increasing sense of tension or affective AROUSAL immediately precedes the action, and its completion brings a sense of intense pleasure, gratification, or relief. See also −MANIA.

pyrophobia   The FEAR of fire.

Q

qi-gong psychotic reaction   A term describing an acute, time-limited episode characterized by dissociative, PARANOID, or other psychotic or nonpsychotic symptoms that may occur after participation in the Chinese folk health-enhancing practice of *qi-gong* ("exercise of vital energy"). See CULTURE-SPECIFIC SYNDROMES.

Q-sort A PERSONALITY ASSESSMENT technique in which the subject (or an observer) indicates the degree to which a standardized set of descriptive statements actually describes the subject. The term reflects the "sorting" procedures occasionally used with this technique.

quality assurance Activities and programs intended to ensure the STANDARD OF CARE (see "Legal Terms") in a defined medical setting or program. Such programs must include educational components intended to remedy identified deficiencies in quality.

quazepam A BENZODIAZEPINE SEDATIVE-HYPNOTIC medication indicated for the treatment of INSOMNIA. Marketed under the brand name DORAL. See "Medications Used in Psychiatry."

quetiapine An ATYPICAL ANTIPSYCHOTIC medication approved for the treatment of SCHIZOPHRENIA and for acute and maintenance treatment of BIPOLAR DISORDER. Marketed under the brand name SEROQUEL. See "Medications Used in Psychiatry."

R

race Most people think of "race" as a biological category or as a way to label different groups according to a set of common, inborn biological traits (e.g., skin color, or shape of eyes, nose, and face). Despite this popular view, there are no biological criteria for dividing races into distinct categories. Race is not a biological category, but it can have meaning as a social category. Different CULTURES classify people into racial groups according to a set of characteristics that are socially significant. The concept of race is especially potent when certain social groups are separated, treated as inferior or superior, and given differential access to power and opportunities.

racism The practice of racial discrimination, segregation, persecution, and domination based on a feeling of racial differences or antagonisms, especially with reference to supposed racial superiority, inferiority, or purity.

ramelteon A nonbenzodiazepine SEDATIVE-HYPNOTIC medication approved for long-term use in the treatment of INSOMNIA. Marketed under the brand name ROZEREM. See "Medications Used in Psychiatry."

random   A statistical term that denotes accuracy by chance or without attention to selection or planning.

rape   Sexual assault; forced sexual intercourse without the partner's consent.

raphe nuclei   A moderate-sized cluster of nuclei found in the BRAIN STEM, whose main function is to release SEROTONIN to the rest of the brain. SELECTIVE SEROTONIN REUPTAKE INHIBITOR (SSRI) ANTIDEPRESSANTS are believed to act in these nuclei, as well as at their targets.

rapid cycling   Referring to BIPOLAR DISORDER in which four or more episodes of MOOD disturbance (MANIC, HYPOMANIC, or MAJOR DEPRESSIVE EPISODE) occur within 1 year.

rapid eye movement (REM)   See REM SLEEP.

rapport   The feeling of harmonious accord and mutual responsiveness that contributes to the patient's confidence in the therapist and willingness to work cooperatively. To be distinguished from TRANSFERENCE, which is UNCONSCIOUS.

rasagiline   An irreversible inhibitor of MONOAMINE OXIDASE used as MONOTHERAPY in early PARKINSON'S DISEASE or as ADJUNCTIVE therapy in more advanced cases. Marketed under the brand name AZILECT.

rational-emotive psychotherapy (RET)   See EXPERIENTIAL THERAPY.

rationalization   A DEFENSE MECHANISM, operating unconsciously, in which an individual attempts to justify or make consciously tolerable by plausible means feelings or behavior that otherwise would be intolerable. Not to be confused with CONSCIOUS evasion or dissimulation. See also PROJECTION.

Razadyne   Brand name for the ACETYLCHOLINESTERASE INHIBITOR drug GALANTAMINE.

rCBF   See REGIONAL CEREBRAL BLOOD FLOW (rCBF).

reaction formation   A DEFENSE MECHANISM, operating unconsciously, in which a person adopts AFFECTS, ideas, and behaviors that are the opposites of IMPULSES harbored either consciously or unconsciously (see CONSCIOUS; UNCONSCIOUS). For example, excessive moral zeal may be a reaction to strong but repressed asocial impulses.

reactive   In psychiatry, often used synonymously with EXOGENOUS to denote symptoms that arise in response to external circumstances or events. Contrast with ENDOGENOUS.

reactive attachment disorder   A disorder of infancy or early childhood, with onset before the child is 5 years old, characterized by markedly disturbed and developmentally inappropriate social RELAT-EDNESS. In the *inhibited* type of reactive attachment disorder, failure to respond predominates, and responses are hypervigilant, avoidant, or highly ambivalent and contradictory. In the *disinhibited* type, indiscriminate sociability is characteristic, such as excessive familiarity with relative strangers or lack of selectivity in choice of ATTACHMENT figures. Most children who develop this disorder are from a setting in which care has been grossly pathogenic. Typically, either the caregivers have neglected the child's basic physical and emotional needs or repeated changes of the primary caregiver have prevented the formation of stable attachments.

reading disorder   One of the LEARNING DISORDERS, characterized by impaired reading accuracy or comprehension that interferes significantly with academic performance or activities of living that require reading skills. Reading achievement is substantially below that expected, given the individual's age, measured INTELLIGENCE, and age-appropriate education.

reality principle   In psychoanalytic theory (see PSYCHOANALYSIS), the concept that the PLEASURE PRINCIPLE, which represents the claims of instinctual wishes, is modified by the demands and requirements of the external world. The reality principle reflects compromises and allows for the postponement of gratification to a more appropriate time. The reality principle usually becomes more prominent in the course of development but may be weak in certain psychiatric illnesses and undergo strengthening during treatment.

reality testing   The ability to evaluate the external world objectively and to differentiate adequately between it and the internal world. Falsification of reality, as with massive DENIAL or PROJECTION, indicates a severe disturbance of EGO functioning and/or of the perceptual and MEMORY processes on which it is partly based. See also PSYCHOSIS.

reality therapy   See EXPERIENTIAL THERAPY.

recall   The process of bringing a MEMORY into consciousness (see CONSCIOUS). Recall is often used to refer to the recollection of facts, events, and feelings that occurred in the immediate past.

receptive aphasia   See WERNICKE'S APHASIA.

receptive (communication)   The process of receiving and understanding a message. Contrast with EXPRESSIVE (communication/language).

receptive language disorder   See MIXED RECEPTIVE-EXPRESSIVE LANGUAGE DISORDER under COMMUNICATION DISORDERS.

receptor   A specialized area on a nerve membrane, a blood vessel, or a muscle that receives the chemical stimulation that activates or inhibits the nerve, blood vessel, or muscle.

reciprocal inhibition   In BEHAVIOR THERAPY, the hypothesis that if ANXIETY-provoking stimuli occur simultaneously with the INHIBITION of anxiety (e.g., relaxation), the bond between those stimuli and the anxiety will be weakened.

recovery   The process of overcoming a particular life problem, such as gambling, codependency, mental illness, or childhood ABUSE, through inner change and personal growth, usually through a self-help program or PSYCHOTHERAPY.

recurrent brief depressive disorder   A proposed disorder (listed in DSM-IV-TR Appendix B, "Criteria Sets and Axes Provided for Further Study") whose essential feature is the recurrence of brief depressive episodes that are identical to MAJOR DEPRESSIVE DISORDER in number and severity of symptoms but that do not meet the 2-week duration requirement. Contrast with MINOR DEPRESSIVE DISORDER.

reductionism   See EPIGENETICS.

refractory   In psychiatry, a term most frequently used to describe disorders or symptoms that do not respond to treatment (e.g., "treatment-refractory depression"). The term *resistant* is often used interchangeably with *refractory.*

regional cerebral blood flow (rCBF)   A measurement obtained by using a technique such as radioactive xenon to chart BRAIN blood flow. See also BRAIN IMAGING.

regression   Partial or symbolic return to earlier patterns of reacting or thinking. Manifested in a wide variety of circumstances such as normal SLEEP, play, physical illness, and many MENTAL DISORDERS. Also, a DEFENSE MECHANISM consisting of a return to some earlier level of ADAPTATION.

rehabilitation   In PSYCHIATRY, the methods and techniques used to achieve maximum functioning and optimum ADJUSTMENT for the patient and to prevent RELAPSES or recurrences of illness; sometimes termed *tertiary prevention* (see under PREVENTION).

reinforcement   The strengthening of a response by reward or avoidance of punishment. This process is central in OPERANT CONDITIONING.

relapse   The return of SYMPTOMS associated with the present episode of psychiatric illness after the symptoms had been reduced or eliminated for a brief period. In treatment of ALCOHOLISM and SUBSTANCE

USE DISORDERS, *relapse* refers to the reuse of the substance that produced the disorder.

relatedness   Sense of SYMPATHY and EMPATHY with others.

relational problems   Family and partner difficulties, not necessarily due to MENTAL DISORDER but often the focus of consultation or treatment. DSM-IV-TR specifies *parent-child relational problem* (with inadequate parental discipline, parental overprotection, or communication problems); *partner relational problem* (with negative or distorted communication); and *sibling relational problem.*

relaxation training   Use of relaxation techniques to help individuals control their physical and mental state in the treatment of psychiatric disorders, such as ANXIETY DISORDERS. Although there are many different techniques, most involve the alternate tensing and relaxing of different muscle groups, along with visualization of a pleasant scene or the use of a simple mantra to control distracting thoughts.

Relistor   Brand name for the injectable OPIOID ANTAGONIST drug METHYL-NALTREXONE.

REM   Rapid eye movement SLEEP.

Remeron   Brand name for the ATYPICAL ANTIDEPRESSANT drug MIRTAZA-PINE.

reminiscence   A normal, universal process of life review in an elderly person prompted in part by the realization of approaching death. The person reviews past life and CONFLICTS and possibilities for their resolution. DEPRESSION, ANXIETY, regret, and despair may be present.

Reminyl   Former brand name for the ACETYLCHOLINESTERASE INHIBITOR drug GALANTAMINE. In 2005, in response to reports of prescribing errors (resulting in two deaths) arising from the name's similarity to the diabetic drug Amaryl, the manufacturer began marketing Reminyl under a new product name, RAZADYNE.

remission   Abatement of an illness.

REM latency   The time lag between SLEEP onset (Stage II sleep) and the first REM period minus any awake time, often shortened during an episode of major DEPRESSION.

REM sleep   Rapid eye movement SLEEP. This is the time of vivid dreaming.

REM sleep behavior disorder   A sleep disorder characterized by loss of normal voluntary muscle atonia during REM SLEEP, associated with complex motor behavior while dreaming.

repetition compulsion   In psychoanalytic theory (see PSYCHOANALY-SIS), the IMPULSE to reenact earlier emotional experiences. Considered by Sigmund Freud (1856–1939) to be more fundamental than the PLEASURE PRINCIPLE.

repetitive self-mutilation   An IMPULSE-CONTROL DISORDER defined as repeated destruction of body tissue without suicidal intent. Examples include severe scratching, skin cutting or burning, and self-hitting.

repression   A DEFENSE MECHANISM, operating unconsciously, that banishes unacceptable ideas, FANTASIES, AFFECTS, or IMPULSES from consciousness or that keeps out of consciousness what has never been CONSCIOUS. The repressed material may sometimes emerge in disguised form. Often confused with the conscious mechanism of SUPPRESSION.

Requip   Brand name for the antiparkinsonian drug ROPINIROLE.

reserpine   An alkaloid (of *Rauwolfia serpentina*) used to treat hypertension and formerly used to treat PSYCHOSIS and other psychiatric disorders.

res gestae   See "Legal Terms."

resident   A physician who is in board-approved graduate training to qualify as a specialist in a particular field of medicine, such as PSYCHIATRY. The AMERICAN BOARD OF PSYCHIATRY AND NEUROLOGY (ABPN) requires 4 years of postgraduate training (after medical school) in an approved program to qualify to take the board examination in psychiatry.

residential treatment facility   See HALFWAY HOUSE.

residual   A term describing the phase of an illness that occurs after REMISSION of the florid SYMPTOMS or the full SYNDROME. The remaining symptoms are called *residua*.

residual schizophrenia   See SCHIZOPHRENIA.

res ipsa loquitur   See "Legal Terms."

resistance   One's CONSCIOUS or UNCONSCIOUS psychological defense against bringing repressed (unconscious) thoughts into conscious awareness.

respondeat superior   See "Legal Terms."

respondent conditioning (classical/Pavlovian conditioning)   Elicitation of a response by a stimulus that normally does not elicit that response. The response is one that is mediated primarily by the AUTONOMIC NERVOUS SYSTEM (ANS) (such as salivation or a change in heart rate). A previously neutral stimulus is repeatedly presented just before an unconditioned stimulus that normally elicits that response. When the response subsequently occurs in the presence of the previously neutral stimulus, it is called a *conditioned response,* and the previously neutral stimulus is called a *conditioned stimulus.*

restless legs syndrome (RLS) A SLEEP DISORDER that does not meet criteria for a specific DYSSOMNIA, characterized by an irresistible urge to move the legs accompanied by an uncomfortable crawling, creeping sensation. RLS is common in end-stage renal disease patients, during pregnancy, and in individuals with PARKINSON'S DISEASE or iron-deficiency anemia. Also known as *Wittmaack-Ekbom syndrome.*

Restoril Brand name for the BENZODIAZEPINE SEDATIVE-HYPNOTIC drug TEMAZEPAM.

restraint Any physical or mechanical device, material, or equipment, including drugs or medications, used to immobilize a patient for the purpose of preventing that patient from harming him-/herself or others. See also SECLUSION; SECLUSION AND RESTRAINT STATUTES.

restricted affect See AFFECT.

restricting type See ANOREXIA NERVOSA.

RET Rational-emotive psychotherapy. See EXPERIENTIAL THERAPY.

retardation See INTELLECTUAL DISABILITY; PSYCHOMOTOR RETARDATION.

retrograde amnesia See under AMNESIA.

retrospective falsification UNCONSCIOUS distortion of past experiences to conform to present emotional needs.

Rett's disorder A PERVASIVE DEVELOPMENTAL DISORDER and GENETIC condition characterized by the appearance, between ages 5 months and 48 months, of decelerated head growth, loss of previously acquired purposeful hand movements and development of stereotyped hand movements (hand wringing), loss of social engagement (social interaction may develop later), poorly coordinated gait or trunk movements, and impaired EXPRESSIVE and RECEPTIVE language with severe PSYCHOMOTOR RETARDATION.

reuptake inhibitor A drug that inhibits the reuptake of a NEUROTRANSMITTER from the synapse into the presynaptic neuron, leading to an increase in concentration of that neurotransmitter and therefore an increase in neurotransmission. Drugs that exert their psychological and physiological effects through reuptake inhibition include various ANTIDEPRESSANTS, ANXIOLYTICS, and STIMULANTS. Most known reuptake inhibitors affect SEROTONIN, NOREPINEPHRINE, and/or DOPAMINE.

ReVia Brand name for the OPIOID ANTAGONIST drug NALTREXONE.

rhinorrhea　Discharge from the nose; watery rhinorrhea may be a prominent SYMPTOM in OPIOID WITHDRAWAL.

rhythms　See BIOLOGICAL RHYTHMS.

ribonucleic acid (RNA)　A chemical substance involved in cellular protein synthesis, whose structure is coded for by DEOXYRIBONUCLEIC ACID (DNA).

right　See "Legal Terms."

rigidity　Resistance to change; inflexibility. Also, maintaining a physical stance or posture against all efforts to be moved. See CATATONIC BEHAVIOR; EXTRAPYRAMIDAL SYNDROME; PARKINSONISM.

risk behavior　See HIGH-RISK BEHAVIOR.

risk factor　A circumstance or condition that increases one's chances of developing a disease.

Risperdal　Brand name for the ATYPICAL ANTIPSYCHOTIC drug RISPERIDONE.

risperidone　An ATYPICAL ANTIPSYCHOTIC medication approved for the treatment of SCHIZOPHRENIA and for acute and maintenance treatment of BIPOLAR DISORDER. Marketed under the brand name RISPERDAL. See "Medications Used in Psychiatry."

Ritalin　Brand name for the CENTRAL NERVOUS SYSTEM (CNS) STIMULANT drug METHYLPHENIDATE.

ritual　A repetitive activity, usually a distorted or stereotyped ELABORATION of some routine of daily life, employed to relieve ANXIETY. Most commonly seen in OBSESSIVE-COMPULSIVE DISORDER.

rivastigmine　A reversible ACETYLCHOLINESTERASE INHIBITOR used to treat mild to moderate ALZHEIMER'S DISEASE. Marketed under the brand name EXELON. See "Medications Used in Psychiatry."

RLS　See RESTLESS LEGS SYNDROME (RLS).

RNA　See RIBONUCLEIC ACID (RNA).

Rohypnol　Brand name for the potent SEDATIVE-HYPNOTIC drug FLUNITRAZEPAM.

rok-joo　A CULTURE-SPECIFIC SYNDROME. See *KORO*.

role　A pattern of behavior a person acquires or adopts as influenced and expected by significant people in his or her milieu.

role responsiveness　As used by Joseph Sandler (1927–1998), a term referring to a COUNTERTRANSFERENCE response in the analyst in which he or she feels compelled to behave in a certain way so as to play out a role that the patient unconsciously has assigned to him or her.

rolfing　See EXPERIENTIAL THERAPY.

roofie　Street name for FLUNITRAZEPAM.

rootwork   A set of cultural interpretations that ascribe illness to witchcraft, hexing, sorcery, or the evil influence of another person. Symptoms may include generalized anxiety, gastrointestinal complaints, weakness, dizziness, fear of being poisoned, and sometimes fear of being killed. Rootwork is found in the southern United States among both African American and European American populations and in Caribbean societies, where it is known as MAL PUESTO or BRUJE-RIA. See CULTURE-SPECIFIC SYNDROMES.

ropinirole   A DOPAMINE AGONIST drug indicated for the treatment of the signs and symptoms of IDIOPATHIC PARKINSON'S DISEASE and of moderate to severe primary RESTLESS LEGS SYNDROME. Marketed under the brand name REQUIP.

Rorschach   The "ink blot" test—in which, by scoring the subject's responses to a set of 10 ambiguous forms on cards, inferences can be made about mental functioning and diagnosis, including psychological DEFENSES and major CONFLICTS. The test takes its name from its creator, Swiss Freudian psychiatrist and psychoanalyst Herman Rorschach (1884–1922).

Rozerem   Brand name for the nonbenzodiazepine SEDATIVE-HYPNOTIC drug RAMELTEON.

Rubenstein-Taybi syndrome   A syndrome characterized by short stature, moderate to severe learning difficulties, distinctive facial features, and broad thumbs and first toes. People with this condition have an increased risk of developing noncancerous and cancerous tumors, leukemia, and lymphoma. The syndrome is inherited in an autosomal dominant pattern and is uncommon, affecting an estimated 1 in 125,000 births.

rumination disorder   A feeding and EATING DISORDER of infancy consisting of the repeated regurgitation of food in the absence of associated gastrointestinal illness.

S

SAD   Seasonal affective disorder. See SEASONAL MOOD DISORDER.

S-adenosyl-L-methionine   See SAM-E (S-ADENOSYL-L-METHIONINE).

sadism   The seeking of pleasure in or the fantasy of inflicting pain or humiliation on another. The term also refers to a PARAPHILIA in which conscious sexual excitement is derived from inflicting pain or humiliation.

sadomasochistic relationship   Enjoyment of suffering by one person of an interacting couple with a complementary enjoyment in inflicting pain in the other.

SAM-e (*S*-adenosyl-L-methionine)   A natural substance made from the AMINO ACID methionine and the compound adenosine triphosphate, sometimes used by individuals to treat mild DEPRESSION. SAM-e has not been approved by the FOOD AND DRUG ADMINISTRATION (FDA) to treat DEPRESSIVE DISORDERS.

SAMHSA   See SUBSTANCE ABUSE AND MENTAL HEALTH SERVICES ADMINISTRATION (SAMHSA).

Sanfilippo syndrome   A fatal GENETIC condition due to enzyme deficiencies affecting the breakdown of heparan sulfate. The syndrome is characterized by progressive INTELLECTUAL DISABILITY, mild dwarfism, and other skeletal disorders. Severe neurological deterioration is accompanied by rapid deterioration of social and adaptive skills.

sangue dormido   A syndrome found among Portuguese Cape Verde Islanders and its immigrants, that includes pain, numbness, tremor, paralysis, convulsions, stroke, blindness, heart attack, infection, and miscarriage. See CULTURE-SPECIFIC SYNDROMES.

Saphris   Brand name for the ATYPICAL ANTIPSYCHOTIC drug ASENAPINE.

Sarafem   Brand name for a formulation of the SELECTIVE SEROTONIN REUPTAKE INHIBITOR (SSRI) ANTIDEPRESSANT drug FLUOXETINE marketed for treatment of PREMENSTRUAL DYSPHORIC DISORDER (PMDD).

SARIs   See SEROTONIN ANTAGONIST AND REUPTAKE INHIBITORS (SARIs).

satyriasis   Pathological or exaggerated SEXUAL DRIVE or excitement in a man; known as NYMPHOMANIA in women. May be of psychological or ORGANIC ETIOLOGY. See also HYPERSEXUALITY; –MANIA.

Savella   Brand name for the SEROTONIN-NOREPINEPHRINE REUPTAKE INHIBITOR (SNRI) ANTIDEPRESSANT drug MILNACIPRAN.

scatologia   See TELEPHONE SCATOLOGIA.

schema   The mental structure we use to organize and simplify our knowledge of the world around us. Schemas affect what we notice, how we interpret things, and how we make decisions and act.

Schilder's disease   See ADRENOLEUKODYSTROPHY.

schizoaffective disorder   A psychotic disorder in which either a MAJOR DEPRESSIVE or a MANIC EPISODE develops concurrently with the SYMP-

TOMS of SCHIZOPHRENIA. Although MOOD episodes are present for a substantial portion of the psychotic disturbance, there are also periods of DELUSIONS or HALLUCINATIONS in the absence of prominent mood symptoms.

schizoid personality disorder   See under PERSONALITY DISORDERS.

schizophrenia   A group of psychotic disorders characterized by both POSITIVE and NEGATIVE SYMPTOMS associated with disturbance in one or more major areas of functioning, such as work, academic development or achievement, interpersonal relations, and self-care. POSITIVE SYMPTOMS include DELUSIONS, which may be bizarre in nature; HALLUCINATIONS, especially auditory; disorganized speech; INAPPROPRIATE AFFECT; and disorganized behavior. NEGATIVE SYMPTOMS include flat AFFECT, AVOLITION, ALOGIA, and ANHEDONIA. Duration is variable: ICD-10 requires that continuous SIGNS of the disturbance persist for at least 1 month; DSM-IV-TR requires a minimum of 6 months. Some of the subtypes are as follows:

catatonic   Abnormal motor activity dominates the clinical picture. This may take the form of motor immobility, CATALEPSY, WAXY FLEXIBILITY, or STUPOR; extreme AGITATION with purposelessness and excessive motor activity; extreme NEGATIVISM and resistance or MUTISM; peculiar movements such as POSTURING, stereotyped movements, prominent mannerisms, or grimacing; and ECHOLALIA or ECHOPRAXIA.

disorganized   Formerly called *hebephrenic* schizophrenia. Disorganized speech and behavior and INAPPROPRIATE AFFECT dominate the clinical picture, if present at all, DELUSIONS and HALLUCINATIONS are fragmented.

paranoid   DELUSIONS or HALLUCINATIONS dominate the clinical picture.

undifferentiated   No one of the above clinical presentations predominates.

residual   Persistence of some SYMPTOMS but not of sufficient number or intensity to indicate that the patient is in an active phase. The existing symptoms may be only negative (e.g., social isolation, impaired grooming, blunted AFFECT, POVERTY OF SPEECH, lack of energy or initiative), but there also may be unusual behavior, vague and circumstantial speech, odd beliefs or MAGICAL THINKING, or unusual perceptual experiences. Patients who develop DEPRESSION (i.e., depressed MOOD plus other symptoms of a MAJOR DEPRESSIVE EPISODE) during the residual phase are labeled as having postpsychotic depression of schizophrenia.

schizophrenia and other psychotic disorders   In DSM-IV-TR, a group of MENTAL DISORDERS that includes SCHIZOPHRENIA, SCHIZOPHRENI-FORM DISORDER, SCHIZOAFFECTIVE DISORDER, DELUSIONAL DISORDER, BRIEF PSY-CHOTIC DISORDER, SHARED PSYCHOTIC DISORDER, PSYCHOTIC DISORDER DUE TO A GENERAL MEDICAL CONDITION, SUBSTANCE-INDUCED PSYCHOTIC DISORDER, and psychotic disorder not otherwise specified (see also SECONDARY DISORDER).

schizophreniform disorder   Clinical features are the same as those seen in SCHIZOPHRENIA, but the duration is less than that required for a DIAGNOSIS of schizophrenia (e.g., 6 months).

schizotaxia   A term first used in 1962 by Paul Meehl to describe a GE-NETIC predisposition to SCHIZOPHRENIA. The term has been used to de-scribe a variety of NEGATIVE SYMPTOMS and neuropsychological deficits present in 20%–50% of first-degree relatives of patients with schizo-phrenia.

schizotypal personality disorder   See under PERSONALITY DISORDERS.

school phobia   See SEPARATION ANXIETY DISORDER.

schools of psychiatry   The various theoretical frames of reference that influence and determine PSYCHIATRISTS' formulations of mental disorders and methods of treatment. Most commonly, the schools explain how psychiatric SYMPTOMS or disorders develop, how they in-terfere with functioning, and how and why they can be altered by therapeutic interventions.

SCID   See STRUCTURED CLINICAL INTERVIEW (SCID) FOR DSM.

SCN   See SUPRACHIASMATIC NUCLEUS.

scopophilia   Sexual pleasure derived from looking at another per-son's body or sexual organs.

scotophobia   The FEAR of darkness.

screen memory   A consciously tolerable MEMORY that serves as a cover for an associated memory that would be emotionally painful if recalled.

SDAs   See SEROTONIN-DOPAMINE ANTAGONISTS (SDAs).

SDAT   SENILE DEMENTIA of the ALZHEIMER'S type. See ALZHEIMER'S DISEASE.

seasonal mood disorder   Also called *seasonal affective disorder (SAD)*. A MOOD DISORDER (BIPOLAR, bipolar II, or recurrent MAJOR DEPRES-SIVE DISORDER) in which there has been a regular temporal relation-ship between onset or disappearance of the episode and a particular season. For example, a patient may develop DEPRESSION in the fall or winter, and REMISSION from the depression may occur in the spring.

seclusion   Involuntary confinement of a patient alone in a room or an area where the patient is physically prevented from leaving. See also RESTRAINT; SECLUSION AND RESTRAINT STATUTES.

seclusion and restraint statutes   Regulations governing SECLUSION and RESTRAINT interventions used in the treatment and management of disruptive, self-destructive, and violent behaviors in psychiatry. In the landmark 1982 case *Youngberg v. Romeo,* the Supreme Court recognized that the use of restraint is a drastic deprivation of personal liberty and that such use should reflect "the exercise of professional judgment."

secondary disorder   Symptomatic disorder; a MENTAL DISORDER that is due to a GENERAL MEDICAL CONDITION or induced by a substance.

secondary gain   The external gain derived from any illness, such as personal attention and service, monetary gains, DISABILITY benefits, and release from unpleasant responsibilities. See also PRIMARY GAIN.

secondary prevention   See PREVENTION.

secondary process   In psychoanalytic theory (see PSYCHOANALYSIS), mental activity and thinking characteristic of the EGO and influenced by the demands of the environment. Characterized by organization, systematization, INTELLECTUALIZATION, and similar processes leading to logical thought and action in adult life. See also PRIMARY PROCESS; REALITY PRINCIPLE.

second-generation antipsychotics (SGAs)   See ATYPICAL ANTIPSYCHOTICS.

sedative   A term broadly applied to any medication that quiets, calms, or allays EXCITEMENT in a person.

sedative-hypnotic   A term that denotes overlap in function of a drug with sedative and hypnotic effects. With sedation, a drug may also induce sleepiness, such as with the benzodiazepines.

sedative-, hypnotic-, or anxiolytic-related (or -induced) disorders   In DSM-IV-TR, a group of MENTAL DISORDERS that includes sedative, hypnotic, or anxiolytic DEPENDENCE; sedative, hypnotic, or anxiolytic ABUSE; sedative, hypnotic, or anxiolytic INTOXICATION; sedative, hypnotic, or anxiolytic WITHDRAWAL; sedative, hypnotic, or anxiolytic DELIRIUM; sedative-, hypnotic-, or anxiolytic-induced withdrawal DELIRIUM; sedative-, hypnotic-, or anxiolytic-induced persisting DEMENTIA; sedative-, hypnotic-, or anxiolytic-induced persisting AMNESTIC DISORDER; sedative-, hypnotic-, or anxiolytic-induced PSYCHOTIC DISORDER, with DELUSIONS or HALLUCINATIONS; sedative-, hypnotic-, or anxiolytic-induced MOOD DISORDER; sedative-, hypnotic-, or anxiolytic-induced

ANXIETY DISORDER; sedative-, hypnotic-, or anxiolytic-induced SLEEP DISORDER; and sedative-, hypnotic-, or anxiolytic-induced SEXUAL DYSFUNCTION.

seduction theory   Freud's early hypothesis, later abandoned, that the trauma of childhood sexual seduction by adults was the cause of CONVERSION symptoms.

seizure   A sudden misfire among nerve cells in the BRAIN that impairs normal brain function. Seizures are the most common SYMPTOM of EPILEPSY.

selective mutism   A disorder of infancy, childhood, or ADOLESCENCE characterized by persistent failure to speak in specific social situations by a child with demonstrated ability to speak. The mutism is not due to lack of fluency in the language being spoken or embarrassment about a speech problem. Also known as *elective* mutism.

selective serotonin reuptake inhibitors (SSRIs)   A class of ANTIDEPRESSANTS used primarily for the treatment of MAJOR DEPRESSIVE DISORDER and many of the ANXIETY DISORDERS, such as GENERALIZED ANXIETY DISORDER. PANIC DISORDER, SOCIAL PHOBIA, POSTTRAUMATIC STRESS DISORDER (PTSD), and OBSESSIVE-COMPULSIVE DISORDER. Clinical trials also have supported the use of SSRIs in the treatment of other MENTAL DISORDERS, including BULIMIA NERVOSA, and BORDERLINE PERSONALITY DISORDER. The principal pharmacological effect of the SSRIs is to increase the amount of SEROTONIN available in the SYNAPSE through inhibition of serotonin reuptake. The six SSRIs available in the United States are CITALOPRAM (CELEXA), FLUOXETINE (PROZAC), FLUVOXAMINE (LUVOX), PAROXETINE (PAXIL), SERTRALINE (ZOLOFT), and ESCITALOPRAM OXALATE (LEXAPRO). Also sometimes referred to as *serotonin reuptake inhibitors (SRIs)*. See "Medications Used in Psychiatry."

selegiline   A selective MONOAMINE OXIDASE (MAO) B inhibitor (also known as L-*deprenyl*) used as an ADJUVANT treatment in the management of PARKINSON'S DISEASE and, at higher doses (at which it is no longer selective), sometimes used to treat DEPRESSION REFRACTORY to more standard pharmacotherapies. Marketed under the brand name ELDEPRYL. See "Medications Used in Psychiatry."

selegiline transdermal system   A transdermal patch form of SELEGILINE, a selective MONOAMINE OXIDASE (MAO) B inhibitor approved for the treatment of MAJOR DEPRESSIVE DISORDER. Marketed under the brand name EMSAM. See "Medications Used in Psychiatry."

self   The psychophysical totality of a person, including both CONSCIOUS and UNCONSCIOUS attributes.

self-defeating personality disorder   Also known as *masochistic* PER-
SONALITY. Its major manifestations include choosing people and situations that lead to disappointment or mistreatment despite the
availability of other options; responding to positive personal events
with GUILT or pain-producing behavior; rejecting opportunities for
pleasure or enjoyment; or perceiving oneself as undeserving of being treated well.

self-fulfilling prophecy   A prediction or supposition of an event or
a situation that, with frequent repetition, influences a person, the
environment, or both to behave as expected by others in this social
setting.

self-help groups   People with a common problem who collectively
help one another by personal and group support. Examples are AL-
COHOLICS ANONYMOUS (AA), Gamblers Anonymous (GA), and Narcotics Anonymous (NA). See "Mental Health Resources."

self-injurious behavior   A behavior in which people intentionally
engage that causes physical bodily harm. Self-harm is often carried
out when individuals attempt to deal with difficult or overwhelming
emotions. Self-injury may take several forms, most commonly cutting, scraping, burning, biting, or hitting. Rationales for self-injury
include feeling anger toward oneself or others and relieving pain,
anger, and tension.

selfobject   In Heinz Kohut's (1913–1981) theory of SELF PSYCHOLOGY,
another person (or sometimes an inanimate object or abstract concept) who is experienced as part of the self because of the psychological functions that the other person provides. The SELFOBJECT
dimension of experience is usually UNCONSCIOUS but can be made
CONSCIOUS.

selfobject transference   In Heinz Kohut's (1913–1981) theory of SELF
PSYCHOLOGY, a TRANSFERENCE relationship in which the therapist serves
as a SELFOBJECT for the patient by providing needed self-enhancing
and self-regulatory functions and emotional stability, which can subsequently be internalized and transformed into the structure of the
patient's self. The therapist functions as a needed extension of the
patient's self rather than as a separate person. Three major types of
selfobject transference are recognized: MIRRORING, idealizing, and al-
ter-ego (twinship).

self psychology   A theory of psychoanalytic PSYCHOLOGY and a recon-
ceptualization of the psychoanalytic treatment process (see PSYCHO-
ANALYSIS) developed by Heinz Kohut (1913–1981) in an effort to

transcend the limitations of EGO PSYCHOLOGY that were highlighted by his experience in treating patients with NARCISSISTIC and BORDERLINE PERSONALITY DISORDERS. Self psychology is concerned not with the modulation of DRIVES and the avoidance of CONFLICT, but with the quest for affirmation and ACTUALIZATION in a healthy or an enfeebled SELF.

semantic dementia   One of three clinical syndromes associated with FRONTOTEMPORAL LOBAR DEGENERATION. A progressive neurodegenerative disorder characterized by loss of semantic memory in both the verbal and nonverbal domains. The most common presenting symptoms are in the verbal domain, with loss of word meaning.

senescence   A chronological period commonly referred to as old age; characterized by INTROSPECTION, awareness of death, sense of legacy, and the possibilities of frailty, DISABILITY, dependency, and abandonment.

senile dementia   A chronic, progressive DEMENTIA associated with generalized atrophy of the BRAIN involving the death of NEURONS from unknown causes. It is not due to AGING per se but may be a late form of ALZHEIMER'S DISEASE. Deterioration may range from minimal to severe.

sensitivity group   A group in which members strive to increase self-awareness and understanding of the group's dynamics, as distinct from treatments designed to ameliorate identified, individual, EGO-DYSTONIC emotional problems.

sensorimotor stage   See COGNITIVE DEVELOPMENT.

sensorium   Synonymous with consciousness. Includes the special sensory perceptive powers and their central correlation and integration in the BRAIN. A clear sensorium conveys the presence of a reasonably accurate MEMORY together with ORIENTATION for time, place, and person. See also MENTAL STATUS.

sensory deprivation   The experience of being cut off from usual external stimuli and the opportunity for PERCEPTION. This may occur experimentally or accidentally in various ways. For example, the loss of hearing or eyesight, physical isolation, or some hospital confinements may lead to disorganized thinking, DELIRIUM, DEPRESSION, PANIC, DELUSIONS, and HALLUCINATIONS.

sensory extinction   Failure to detect sensory stimuli from one region if another region is stimulated simultaneously, even though when the region in question is stimulated by itself, the stimulus is correctly reported.

sensory integration dysfunction   See SENSORY PROCESSING DISORDER (SPD).

sensory processing disorder (SPD)   A complex disorder of the BRAIN that affects the ability to process information brought in by the senses. People with SPD misinterpret everyday information, such as touch, sound, and movement, which gives them a different experience of the world from others. Also known as *sensory integration dysfunction*. SPD is not a recognized diagnosis in DSM-IV-TR.

separation anxiety   The sense of discomfort that a child feels when experiencing or being threatened by a separation from an ATTACHMENT figure. This is a normal stage of development that indicates a strong primary attachment. It typically develops between ages 10 and 15 months. These concerns may preoccupy children up to age 3 years. If the concerns persist or arise later and are of clinical significance, they may indicate a SEPARATION ANXIETY DISORDER.

separation anxiety disorder   A disorder with onset before age 18 years consisting of inappropriate ANXIETY concerning separation from home or from persons to whom the child is attached. Among the SYMPTOMS that may be seen are unrealistic concern about harm befalling to or loss of major ATTACHMENT figures; refusal to go to school (school PHOBIA) in order to stay at home and maintain contact with this figure; refusal to go to SLEEP unless close to this person; clinging; nightmares about the theme of separation; and development of physical symptoms or MOOD changes (APATHY, DEPRESSION) when separation occurs or in anticipated.

separation-individuation   Described by Margaret Mahler (1897–1985) as a phase in the mother-child relationship that follows the symbiotic stage. In the separation-individuation stage, the child begins to perceive himself or herself as distinct from the mother and develops a sense of individual IDENTITY. Mahler described four subphases of the process: DIFFERENTIATION, practicing, rapprochement (i.e., active approach toward the mother, which replaces the relative obliviousness to her that prevailed during the practicing period), and separation-individuation proper (i.e., awareness of discrete identity, separateness, and individuality). See also SYMBIOSIS.

Serax   Brand name (now discontinued) for the BENZODIAZEPINE ANXIOLYTIC drug OXAZEPAM.

Serentil   Former brand name for the withdrawn CONVENTIONAL ANTIPSYCHOTIC drug MESORIDAZINE.

Seroquel   Brand name for the ATYPICAL ANTIPSYCHOTIC drug QUETIAPINE.

serotonergic   Referring to the NEUROTRANSMITTER SEROTONIN (5-HYDROXY-TRYPTAMINE [5-HT]). See also BIOGENIC AMINES.

serotonin (5-hydroxytryptamine [5-HT])   A MONOAMINE NEURO-TRANSMITTER that, when decreased or deficient in the CENTRAL NERVOUS SYSTEM (CNS), may lead to DEPRESSION and ANXIETY. See also BIOGENIC AMINES.

serotonin agonists   Drugs that bind to SEROTONIN RECEPTORS in place of SEROTONIN and directly stimulate those receptors. Serotonin AGO-NISTS such as SUMATRIPTAN are used to reduce the pain of an acute MIGRAINE headache by increasing SEROTONIN levels.

serotonin antagonist and reuptake inhibitors (SARIs)   A class of ATYPICAL ANTIDEPRESSANT medications that block postsynaptic SERO-TONIN ($5\text{-}HT_2$) receptors and (to a lesser extent) inhibit presynaptic reuptake of serotonin. These medications are used primarily in the treatment of DEPRESSION and ANXIETY DISORDERS. Examples of SARIs include TRAZODONE and NEFAZODONE.

serotonin antagonists   Drugs that block or reverse the actions of SEROTONIN by preventing serotonin from attaching to SEROTONIN RECEP-TORS. See SEROTONIN ANTAGONIST AND REUPTAKE INHIBITORS (SARIs); SERO-TONIN-DOPAMINE ANTAGONISTS (SDAs).

serotonin-dopamine antagonists (SDAs)   A class of medications known as the ATYPICAL ANTIPSYCHOTICS. Both CONVENTIONAL ANTIPSY-CHOTICS and ATYPICAL ANTIPSYCHOTICS are ANTAGONISTS of DOPAMINE RECEP-TORS; however, the newer agents are also potent ANTAGONISTS of SEROTONIN RECEPTORS ($5\text{-}HT_{2A}$). As a result of this distinctive RECEPTOR profile, SDAs may be more effective than CONVENTIONAL ANTIPSYCHOT-ICS in reducing NEGATIVE SYMPTOMS of SCHIZOPHRENIA. They also may produce fewer EXTRAPYRAMIDAL SYMPTOMS (EPS) and decrease the risk for developing TARDIVE DYSKINESIA with long-term use; however, SDAs and CONVENTIONAL ANTIPSYCHOTICS are equally effective in treating the POSITIVE SYMPTOMS of SCHIZOPHRENIA. See ATYPICAL ANTIPSYCHOTICS.

serotonin-norepinephrine reuptake inhibitors (SNRIs)   A class of ATYPICAL ANTIDEPRESSANTS that exert their action by inhibiting pre-synaptic reuptake of the neurotransmitters SEROTONIN and NOREPI-NEPHRINE. They are used for the treatment of DEPRESSION and ANXIETY DISORDERS as well as in pain management of diabetic PERIPHERAL NEU-ROPATHY and FIBROMYALGIA. Examples of SNRIs include DULOXETINE (CYMBALTA), DESVENLAFAXINE (PRISTIQ), and VENLAFAXINE (EFFEXOR).

serotonin receptors   Sites located on the surface membranes of cells in the CENTRAL NERVOUS SYSTEM (CNS) and peripheral nervous system to which the NEUROTRANSMITTER SEROTONIN (5-HYDROXYTRYPTA-MINE [5-HT]) binds, thereby activating serotonin NEURONS and down-stream pathways. Serotonin receptors (seven classes [5-HT$_1$–5-HT$_7$] have been identified, many of which have multiple subtypes) are involved in many biological and neurological processes, including aggression, anxiety, appetite, cognition, learning, memory, mood, nausea, sleep, and thermoregulation.

serotonin syndrome   Excessive stimulation of SEROTONIN RECEPTORS. The SYNDROME may be caused by the concurrent consumption of two or more SEROTONERGIC drugs. SYMPTOMS include lethargy, mental con-fusion, flushing, diaphoresis, and TREMOR; in more severe cases, hy-perthermia, hypertonicity, renal failure, and death may occur.

sertraline   A SELECTIVE SEROTONIN REUPTAKE INHIBITOR (SSRI) ANTIDEPRES-SANT medication used to treat DEPRESSION and ANXIETY DISORDERS such as PANIC DISORDER, OBSESSIVE-COMPULSIVE DISORDER, and POSTTRAUMATIC STRESS DISORDER (PTSD). Marketed under the brand name ZOLOFT. See "Medications Used in Psychiatry."

serum levels   See BLOOD LEVELS.

Serzone   Brand name (now discontinued) for the ATYPICAL ANTIDEPRES-SANT drug NEFAZODONE.

sexual and gender identity disorders   A DSM-IV-TR class of disor-ders that includes SEXUAL DYSFUNCTIONS, PARAPHILIAS, and GENDER IDEN-TITY DISORDERS.

sexual arousal disorders   A subcategory of SEXUAL DYSFUNCTIONS that includes FEMALE SEXUAL AROUSAL DISORDER and MALE ERECTILE DISORDER.

>   **female sexual arousal disorder**   Refers to the inability to attain or maintain an adequate lubrication-swelling response of sexual excitement until completion of sexual activity.

>   **male erectile disorder**   Refers to the inability to attain or main-tain an erection until completion of sexual activity.

sexual aversion disorder   See under SEXUAL DESIRE DISORDERS.

sexual desire disorders   A subcategory of SEXUAL DYSFUNCTIONS that in-cludes HYPOACTIVE SEXUAL DESIRE DISORDER and SEXUAL AVERSION DISORDER.

>   **hypoactive sexual desire disorder**   Refers to absent or deficient sexual FANTASIES and sexual activity that causes the affected person marked distress or interpersonal difficulty.

>   **sexual aversion disorder**   Refers to avoidance of and CONSCIOUS aversion to genital sexual contact with a sexual partner that causes the affected person marked distress or interpersonal difficulty.

sexual deviation   See PARAPHILIAS.

sexual drive   One of the two primal DRIVES (the other is the aggressive drive) according to Freud's dual-instinct theory.

sexual dysfunctions   One of the major groups of SEXUAL AND GENDER IDENTITY DISORDERS; includes SEXUAL DESIRE DISORDERS, SEXUAL AROUSAL DISORDERS, ORGASMIC DISORDERS, SEXUAL PAIN DISORDERS, sexual dysfunction due to a GENERAL MEDICAL CONDITION, and substance-induced (INTOXICATION or WITHDRAWAL) sexual dysfunction.

sexual masochism   One of the PARAPHILIAS, characterized by marked distress over, or acting on, sexual urges to be humiliated, beaten, bound, or otherwise made to suffer by the sexual partner. Among the frequently reported masochistic acts are restraint (physical bondage), blindfolding, whipping or flagellation, electrical shocks, or being treated as a helpless infant and clothed in diapers (INFANTILISM).

sexual pain disorders   A subcategory of SEXUAL DYSFUNCTIONS that includes DYSPAREUNIA and VAGINISMUS.

dyspareunia   Refers to genital pain in either a male or a female before, during, or after sexual intercourse that is not due to a GENERAL MEDICAL CONDITION, drugs, or medication.

vaginismus   Refers to recurrent or persistent involuntary spasm of the musculature of the outer third of the vagina severe enough to interfere with coitus.

sexual sadism   One of the PARAPHILIAS, characterized by marked distress over, or acting on, desires to inflict physical or psychological suffering, including HUMILIATION, on the victim.

SGAs   Second-generation ANTIPSYCHOTICS; see ATYPICAL ANTIPSYCHOTICS.

shaman   A healer whose ability comes from trancelike or supernatural experiences.

shame   An EMOTION resulting from the failure to live up to self-expectations. See also GUILT; SUPEREGO.

shaping   REINFORCEMENT of responses in the patient's repertoire that increasingly approximate sought-after behavior.

shared psychotic disorder   Induced psychotic disorder; for example, person A develops a DELUSION in the context of a close relationship with person B, who has an already established delusion. The delusion in person A is similar in content to person B's delusion. One example is *FOLIE À DEUX*.

shell shock   Term used in World War I to designate a wide variety of MENTAL DISORDERS presumably due to combat experience. See also COMBAT FATIGUE.

shenjing shuairuo   In China, a condition characterized by physical and mental fatigue, concentration difficulties, sleep disturbances, and memory loss. In many cases, the symptoms would meet the criteria for a DSM-IV-TR mood or anxiety disorder. See CULTURE-SPECIFIC SYNDROMES.

shen-k'uei   A Chinese SYNDROME attributed to excessive semen loss from frequent intercourse, masturbation, nocturnal emission, or passing of "white turbid urine" believed to contain semen. This loss is feared because of the belief that it represents the loss of one's vital essence and can thereby be life threatening. Symptoms include dizziness, backache, general weakness, INSOMNIA, and complaints of SEXUAL DYSFUNCTION. Also known as *shenkui.* See also CULTURE-SPECIFIC SYNDROMES and *KHAT.*

shin-byung   A Korean syndrome characterized by anxiety and somatic complaints (general weakness, dizziness, fear, loss of appetite, INSOMNIA, and gastrointestinal problems), followed by DISSOCIATION and possession by ancestral spirits. See CULTURE-SPECIFIC SYNDROMES.

shock treatment   An inaccurate term often used to refer to ELECTROCONVULSIVE THERAPY (ECT). The term is inaccurate because the treatment produces a SEIZURE or a convulsion and does not shock the patient.

shook yong   A CULTURE-SPECIFIC SYNDROME. See *KORO.*

short-term memory   The recognition, RECALL, and reproduction of perceived material 10 seconds or longer after initial presentation. See also IMMEDIATE MEMORY.

Shprintzen syndrome   See VELOCARDIOFACIAL SYNDROME (VCFS).

shuk yang   A CULTURE-SPECIFIC SYNDROME. See *KORO.*

Shy-Drager syndrome   A degenerative neurological disorder affecting the CENTRAL NERVOUS SYSTEM and SYMPATHETIC NERVOUS SYSTEM; characterized by an abrupt decrease in blood pressure when moving from a supine to a sitting position or from a sitting to a standing position.

sibling relational problem   See RELATIONAL PROBLEMS.

sibling rivalry   The competition between siblings for the love of a parent or for other recognition or gain.

sibutramine   An appetite suppressant medication used in the management of OBESITY. Sibutramine (including all generic and brand [MERIDIA] products) was withdrawn from the U.S. market in 2010 because of its association with increased cardiovascular events and strokes.

sick role   An IDENTITY adopted by an individual as a "patient" that specifies a set of expected behaviors, usually dependent.

side effect   A secondary drug effect different from the principal effect for which the drug is taken. Most side effects are undesirable but cause only minor annoyances; others may cause serious problems.

sign   Objective evidence of disease or disorder. See also SYMPTOM.

signal anxiety   An EGO mechanism that results in activation of defensive operations to protect the ego from being overwhelmed by an excess of EXCITEMENT. The ANXIETY reaction that was originally experienced in a traumatic situation is reproduced in an attenuated form, allowing defenses to be mobilized before the current threat becomes overwhelming.

sildenafil   A phosphodiesterase inhibitor medication used for the treatment of erectile dysfunction (MALE ERECTILE DISORDER). Marketed under the brand name VIAGRA.

silok   A CULTURE-SPECIFIC SYNDROME. See *LATAH*.

simple phobia   See SPECIFIC PHOBIA under PHOBIA.

simultanagnosia   Inability to comprehend more than one element of a visual scene at the same time or to integrate the parts into a whole.

Sinemet   Brand name for the ANTIPARKINSONIAN MEDICATION CARBIDOPA-LEVODOPA.

Sinequan   Brand name (now discontinued) for the TRICYCLIC ANTIDEPRESSANT drug DOXEPIN.

single photon emission computed tomography (SPECT)   A nuclear medicine tomographic imaging technique using gamma rays that provides true three-dimensional information. SPECT scanning reveals how blood flows to tissues and organs. Studies have shown that it might be more sensitive to brain injury than either MAGNETIC RESONANCE IMAGING (MRI) or COMPUTED TOMOGRAPHY (CT) scanning because it can detect reduced blood flow to injured sites. Before a SPECT scan, the patient is injected with a chemical that is radiolabeled, meaning that it emits gamma rays that can be detected by the scanner.

sleep   The recurring period of relative physical and psychological disengagement from one's environment accompanied by characteristic ELECTROENCEPHALOGRAM (EEG) findings and divisible into two categories: non–rapid eye movement (NREM) sleep, also known as *orthodox* or *synchronized* (S) sleep; and rapid eye movement (REM) sleep, also referred to as paradoxical or desynchronized (D) sleep. *Dreaming sleep* is another, although less accurate, term for REM sleep. Four stages of NREM sleep based on EEG findings are Stage 1, occurring immediately after sleep begins, with a pattern of low amplitude and fast frequency; Stage 2, having characteristic waves of 12–16 cycles per second, known as *sleep spindles*; and Stages 3 and 4, having progressive further slowing of frequency and increase in amplitude of the wave forms.

Over a period of 90 minutes after the beginning of sleep, a person has progressed through the four stages of NREM sleep and emerges from them into the first period of REM sleep. REM sleep is associated with dreaming, and brief cycles (20–30 minutes) of this sleep recur about every 90 minutes throughout the night. Coordinated rapid eye movements give this type of sleep its name. See also SLEEP DISORDERS; SLEEP TERROR DISORDER; SOMNAMBULISM.

sleep apnea   Temporary cessation of breathing while asleep. The disorder is most commonly caused by obstruction of the airway from excessive tissue associated with OBESITY (i.e., OBSTRUCTIVE SLEEP APNEA), but it can also occur when the BRAIN does not send the signal to the muscles to take a breath, resulting in no muscular effort to take a breath (i.e., CENTRAL SLEEP APNEA). See BREATHING-RELATED SLEEP DISORDER.

sleep disorders   In DSM-IV-TR, this category includes Primary Sleep Disorders (DYSSOMNIAS and PARASOMNIAS), Sleep Disorders (INSOMNIA or HYPERSOMNIA) Related to Another Mental Disorder, and Other Sleep Disorders (including sleep disorders due to a GENERAL MEDICAL CONDITION or induced by substance INTOXICATION or WITHDRAWAL).

sleep terror disorder   One of the PARASOMNIAS, characterized by PANIC and confusion when abruptly awakening from SLEEP. This usually begins with a scream and is accompanied by intense ANXIETY. The person is often confused and disoriented after awakening. No detailed dream is recalled, and there is AMNESIA for the episode. Sleep terrors typically occur during the first third of sleep. Also known as *night terror (pavor nocturnus)*. Contrast with NIGHTMARE DISORDER.

sleep-wake transition disorder   See PARASOMNIAS.

sleepwalking disorder   One of the PARASOMNIAS, characterized by recurrent episodes of rising from bed during SLEEP and walking about. The sleepwalking person has a blank, staring face and is relatively unresponsive to attempts by others to awaken him or her. On awakening, either from the sleepwalking episode or the next morning, the person has AMNESIA for the episode. Sleepwalking typically occurs during the first third of the major sleep episode.

Smith-Lemli-Optiz syndrome   A metabolic DEVELOPMENTAL DISORDER characterized by distinctive facial features, small head size (microcephaly), INTELLECTUAL DISABILITY or LEARNING DISABILITY, behavioral problems such as self-stimulation and self-injury, and AUTISM SPECTRUM DISORDERS.

Smith-Magenis syndrome   A syndrome of abnormal physical, developmental, and behavioral features due to microdeletion of chromosome 17. Behavioral problems include affective lability, temper tantrums, impulsivity, anxiety, physical aggression, destruction, argumentativeness, and sleep difficulties.

smooth pursuit eye movements (SPEM)   A tracking system that enables the viewer to keep a moving target in focus. See EYE TRACKING.

SNRIs   See SEROTONIN-NOREPINEPHRINE REUPTAKE INHIBITORS (SNRIs).

social adaptation   The ability to live and express oneself according to society's restrictions and cultural demands.

social anthropology   The study of human society, with emphasis on the development of institutions, social ROLES, tribal organization, community structure, political systems, economic organization, and so forth. See CULTURAL ANTHROPOLOGY; ETHNOLOGY.

social breakdown syndrome   The concept that some psychiatric symptomatology is a result of treatment conditions and inadequate facilities and not a part of the primary illness. Factors bringing about the condition are social labeling, learning the ROLE of the chronically sick, atrophy of work and social skills, and IDENTIFICATION with the sick. See also REHABILITATION.

socialization   The process by which society integrates the person and the way he or she learns to become a functioning member of that society. See also SOCIOLOGY.

social phobia   See under PHOBIA.

social psychiatry   The field of PSYCHIATRY concerned with the cultural, ecological, and sociological factors that engender, precipitate, intensify, prolong, or otherwise complicate maladaptive patterns of behavior and their treatment.

social viscosity   See INTERICTAL BEHAVIOR SYNDROME.

social withdrawal   A pathological retreat from people or the world of reality, often seen in SCHIZOPHRENIA.

social work   A profession whose primary concern is how human needs—both of individuals and of groups—can be met within society. Social and BEHAVIORAL SCIENCES provide its educational base. The services provided include general social services, such as health and education, and welfare services to targeted groups such as the economically disadvantaged, the disabled, the elderly, or victims of disasters. See CLINICAL SOCIAL WORKER; PSYCHIATRIC SOCIAL WORK.

sociobiology The study of the evolution of social behavior. This field of study is rooted in evolutionary biology, ETHOLOGY, and comparative PSYCHOLOGY.

sociology The study of the governing principles and development of social organization and the group behavior of people, in contrast to individual behavior. It overlaps to some extent with anthropology. See also ALIENATION; SOCIALIZATION.

sociometry The science of assessing the interpersonal psychological structure of a group or society.

sociopath An unofficial term referring to a person with ANTISOCIAL PERSONALITY DISORDER (see under PERSONALITY DISORDERS).

sociotherapy Any treatment in which emphasis is on socioenvironmental and interpersonal rather than INTRAPSYCHIC factors, as in a THERAPEUTIC COMMUNITY. In most forms of sociotherapy, peer acceptance is an important element, typically achieved through CONFRONTATION by the group when peer expectations are not met.

sodomy Anal intercourse. See also PARAPHILIAS.

soma The body. Contrast with PSYCHE, the mind.

somatic compliance The participation of the body in the expression of UNCONSCIOUS INTRAPSYCHIC CONFLICT. Somatic compliance implies a readiness of specific organs or body parts to provide a somatic outlet for psychological processes, either because of their unconscious meanings or because a constitutional weakness predisposes them to be used in this way.

somatic delusion See DELUSIONAL DISORDER.

somatic therapy In PSYCHIATRY, the biological treatment of MENTAL DISORDERS (e.g., ELECTROCONVULSIVE THERAPY [ECT], psychopharmacological treatment). Contrast with PSYCHOTHERAPY.

somatization The use of the body to express psychological states.

somatization disorder One of the SOMATOFORM DISORDERS, characterized by multiple physical complaints not fully explained by any known medical condition yet severe enough to result in medical treatment or alteration in lifestyle. SYMPTOMS include pain in different sites, symptoms referable to the gastrointestinal tract and the sexual or reproductive system, and symptoms suggestive of a neurological disorder.

somatoform disorders A group of disorders with SYMPTOMS suggesting physical disorders but without demonstrable ORGANIC findings to explain the symptoms. There is positive evidence, or a strong presumption, that the symptoms are linked to psychological factors or CONFLICTS. In DSM-IV-TR, this diagnostic category includes BODY DYSMORPHIC DISORDER (BDD), CONVERSION DISORDER, HYPOCHONDRIASIS, PAIN DISORDER, SOMATIZATION DISORDER, undifferentiated somatoform disorder, and somatoform disorder not otherwise specified.

somnambulism   A form of SLEEP DISORDER in which the person gets out of bed and walks in an uncoordinated manner, usually during deep non–rapid eye movement (NREM) SLEEP. The person does not respond to communication by others and can be awakened only with great difficulty. On awakening, the person has AMNESIA for the event, although mental activity is not impaired.

Sonata   Brand name for the nonbenzodiazepine HYPNOTIC drug ZALEPLON.

Sotos syndrome   A rare GENETIC disorder characterized by excessive physical growth during the first 2 to 3 years of life. The disorder may be accompanied by mild INTELLECTUAL DISABILITY; delayed motor, cognitive, and social development; HYPOTONIA; and speech impairments. Children with Sotos syndrome tend to be large at birth and are often taller and heavier, and have larger heads, than is normal for their age. Also known as *cerebral gigantism*.

sovereign immunity   See "Legal Terms."

spatial agnosia   The inability to recognize spatial relations; disordered spatial ORIENTATION.

SPD   See SENSORY PROCESSING DISORDER (SPD).

specific phobia   See PHOBIA.

SPECT   See SINGLE PHOTON EMISSION COMPUTED TOMOGRAPHY (SPECT).

speech and language disorders   See COMMUNICATION DISORDERS.

speech disturbance   Any disorder of verbal communication that is not due to faulty innervation of speech muscles or organs of articulation. The term includes many language and LEARNING DISABILITIES. Contrast with AGRAPHIA, APHASIA, and APRAXIA. See also AMIMIA; DYSLEXIA.

SPEM   See SMOOTH PURSUIT EYE MOVEMENTS (SPEM).

splitting   A mental mechanism in which the SELF or others are viewed as all good or all bad, with failure to integrate the positive and negative qualities of the self and others into cohesive images. Often the person alternately idealizes and devalues the same person.

spongiform encephalopathies   A group of progressive conditions that affect the BRAIN and nervous system of many animals, including humans. According to the most widespread hypothesis, they are transmitted by PRIONS. Mental and physical abilities deteriorate and myriad tiny holes appear in the CEREBRAL CORTEX, causing it to look like a sponge when brain tissue obtained at autopsy is examined under a microscope. The disorders cause impairment of brain function, including memory changes, PERSONALITY CHANGES, and problems with movement that worsen over time. Prion diseases of humans include CREUTZFELDT-JAKOB DISEASE.

SSRI   See SELECTIVE SEROTONIN REUPTAKE INHIBITORS (SSRIs).

Stadol NS   Brand name for a nasal spray formulation of the OPIOID AGONIST-ANTAGONIST ANALGESIC drug BUTORPHANOL TARTRATE.

standard of care   See "Legal Terms."

stare decisis   See "Legal Terms."

status epilepticus   Continuous epileptic SEIZURES. See EPILEPSY.

statute   See "Legal Terms."

Stavzor   Brand name for the ANTICONVULSANT drug VALPROIC ACID.

Steele-Richardson-Olszewski syndrome   See PROGRESSIVE SUPRANU-CLEAR PALSY.

Stelazine   Brand name (now discontinued) for the CONVENTIONAL ANTI-PSYCHOTIC drug TRIFLUOPERAZINE.

12-step program   See TWELVE-STEP PROGRAM.

stereotypic movement disorder   A disorder of infancy, childhood, or ADOLESCENCE characterized by repetitive, driven, nonfunctional, and potentially self-injurious motor behavior such as head banging, self-biting, or picking at the skin. The behavior may be associated with INTELLECTUAL DISABILITY or a PERVASIVE DEVELOPMENTAL DISORDER.

stereotypy   A repetitive or ritualistic movement, posture, or utterance, that can be found in patients with AUTISM SPECTRUM DISORDERS, INTELLECTUAL DISABILITY, TARDIVE DYSKINESIA, or STEREOTYPIC MOVEMENT DISORDER. Stereotypies may be simple movements such as body rocking, or complex, such as self-caressing, crossing and uncrossing of legs, and marching in place.

Stevens-Johnson syndrome   A severe rash characterized by weeping lesions in the mouth, trunk, anogenital region, and conjunctiva, which can be a serious side effect of LAMOTRIGINE and (less commonly) of CARBAMAZEPINE.

stigma   The damaging labeling of a person or group to indicate that something is abnormal or evil. The stigma of mental illness is still strong enough that many individuals are reluctant or refuse to seek treatment. In some CULTURES, such as Asian or Hispanic, the stigma of mental illness is much more marked than in non-Western societies, leading to underutilization of MENTAL HEALTH services.

stimulants PSYCHOTROPIC medications (also called *psychostimulants*) that increase or enhance CENTRAL NERVOUS SYSTEM (CNS) activity. See "Medications Used in Psychiatry."

St. John's wort An herbal medication not approved by the FOOD AND DRUG ADMINISTRATION (FDA) but used by individuals to treat ANXIETY and DEPRESSION. The above-ground parts of the *Hypericum perforatum*, a perennial plant found throughout Europe, Asia, northern Africa, Australia, and New Zealand. At the start of the flowering season, the plant is cut and dried quickly, to extract hypericin, the active ingredient. Controlled clinical trials in the United States have not found St. John's wort to be effective in treating depression.

Stockholm syndrome A form of bonding in which a kidnapping or terrorist hostage identifies with and has SYMPATHY for his or her captors on whom he or she is dependent for survival.

stranger anxiety The sense of distress that a child feels at seeing a stranger. This is part of normal development. It begins at 26 weeks and is usually well established between 8 and 10 months.

Strattera Brand name for the nonstimulant selective NOREPINEPHRINE REUPTAKE INHIBITOR drug ATOMOXETINE.

strephosymbolia A tendency to reverse letters and words in reading and writing. Seen in LEARNING DISABILITY.

stress disorder/reaction, posttraumatic See POSTTRAUMATIC STRESS DISORDER (PTSD).

stress reaction An acute, maladaptive emotional response to industrial, domestic, civilian, or military disasters and other calamitous life situations. It also may be chronic, as seen in some combat veterans. See POSTTRAUMATIC STRESS DISORDER (PTSD).

stroke Gross cerebral hemorrhage or softening of the BRAIN following hemorrhage, thrombosis, or embolism of the cerebral arteries. SYMPTOMS may include COMA, paralysis (particularly on one side of the body), convulsions, APHASIA, and other neurological SIGNS determined by the location of the lesion.

Stroop test Named after John Ridley Stroop, this cognitive test emphasizes the interference that automatic processing of words has on the task of naming colors. The task of making an appropriate response when presented with two conflicting signals has tentatively been located in a part of the BRAIN called the anterior cingulate. The mechanism involved in this task is called *directed attention*; it requires one to inhibit or stop a response in order to say or do something else.

structural model   Sigmund Freud's model of the mental apparatus, composed of the ID, the EGO, and the SUPEREGO. See also TOPOGRAPHIC MODEL.

Structured Clinical Interview (SCID) for DSM   A semistructured clinically based interview, designed to apply DSM criteria to individuals and identify the presence of psychiatric disorders.

stupor   Marked decrease in reactivity to and awareness of the environment, with reduced spontaneous movements and activity. It can be seen as a type of CATATONIC BEHAVIOR in SCHIZOPHRENIA, but it can also be observed in neurological disorders.

stuttering   See under COMMUNICATION DISORDERS.

sua sponte   See "Legal Terms."

subacute spongiform encephalopathy   See CREUTZFELDT-JAKOB DISEASE; SPONGIFORM ENCEPHALOPATHIES.

subconscious   An obsolete term that was formerly used to include the PRECONSCIOUS (what can be recalled with effort) and the UNCONSCIOUS.

sublimation   A DEFENSE MECHANISM, operating unconsciously, by which instinctual DRIVES, consciously unacceptable, are diverted into personally and socially acceptable channels.

subpoena   See "Legal Terms."

subpoena *ad testificandum*   See "Legal Terms."

subpoena *duces tecum*   See "Legal Terms."

substance abuse   See ABUSE (of psychoactive substances).

Substance Abuse and Mental Health Services Administration (SAMHSA)   An agency of the U.S. Department of HEALTH AND HUMAN SERVICES created in 1992 and made up of the Center for Mental Health Services, the Center for Substance Abuse Prevention, and the Center for Substance Abuse Treatment. These programs were formerly contained in the ALCOHOL, DRUG ABUSE, AND MENTAL HEALTH ADMINISTRATION (ADAMHA).

substance dependence   See DEPENDENCE (on psychoactive substances).

substance-induced disorders   Mental SYNDROMES SECONDARY to the use of drugs (including alcohol). In DSM-IV-TR, these disorders (except for INTOXICATION and WITHDRAWAL) are placed in the diagnostic categories with which they share PHENOMENOLOGY. For example, substance-induced MOOD DISORDER is listed under mood disorders, and substance-induced SLEEP DISORDER is listed under sleep disorders.

The classifications of substance-induced mental disorders include DELIRIUM; DEMENTIA; AMNESTIC DISORDER; PSYCHOTIC DISORDER with DELUSIONS or HALLUCINATIONS; mood disorder; ANXIETY DISORDER; sleep disorder; and SEXUAL DYSFUNCTION.

Substance-induced disorders have a three-part name in DSM-IV-TR: the name of the specific substance (e.g., alcohol, COCAINE); the context in which symptoms appeared (i.e., INTOXICATION, WITHDRAWAL, or persisting beyond these states); and the specific presentation (e.g., mood disorder, anxiety disorder). Examples are *alcohol-induced persisting amnestic disorder* and *cocaine-induced mood disorder with depressive features, with onset during withdrawal.*

In DSM-IV-TR, INTOXICATION is recognized for alcohol; AMPHETAMINE; caffeine; cannabis; COCAINE; HALLUCINOGENS; inhalants; OPIOIDS; PHENCYCLIDINE (PCP); SEDATIVE, HYPNOTIC, or ANXIOLYTIC drugs; and combinations of drugs (polysubstance); WITHDRAWAL is recognized for nicotine and all of the above-mentioned substances except caffeine, cannabis, hallucinogens, inhalants, and PCP.

substance-induced psychotic disorder   This DSM-IV-TR disorder has as its prominent feature HALLUCINATIONS or DELUSIONS that develop during use of a substance or within 6 weeks of stopping its use. Such symptoms have been described during alcohol INTOXICATION and WITHDRAWAL; INTOXICATION with and WITHDRAWAL from SEDATIVE, HYPNOTIC, or ANXIOLYTIC drugs; and INTOXICATION with AMPHETAMINES, cannabis, COCAINE, HALLUCINOGENS, inhalants, OPIOIDS, and PHENCYCLIDINE (PCP).

substance intoxication   See INTOXICATION.

substance-related disorders   DEPENDENCE, ABUSE, INTOXICATION, and WITHDRAWAL syndromes associated with regular or episodic use of chemical substances. In DSM-IV-TR, this category includes SUBSTANCE USE DISORDERS and SUBSTANCE-INDUCED DISORDERS.

substance use disorders   DEPENDENCE or ABUSE SYNDROMES associated with regular or episodic use of chemical substances. Substance use disorders are recognized for alcohol; AMPHETAMINE; caffeine; cannabis; COCAINE; HALLUCINOGENS; inhalants; nicotine; OPIOIDS; PHENCYCLIDINE (PCP); SEDATIVE, HYPNOTIC, or ANXIOLYTIC drugs; and combinations of drugs (polysubstance). Specific disorders include DEPENDENCE (for all of the above-mentioned substances except caffeine) and ABUSE (for all except caffeine and nicotine). See also SUBSTANCE-RELATED DISORDERS and SUBSTANCE-INDUCED DISORDERS.

substance withdrawal See WITHDRAWAL SYMPTOMS.

substantia nigra A structure that is a part of the BASAL GANGLIA located in the MIDBRAIN that plays an important role in reward, addiction, movement, and mood.

substitution A DEFENSE MECHANISM, operating unconsciously, by which an unattainable or unacceptable goal, EMOTION, or OBJECT is replaced by one that is more attainable or acceptable.

subthalamic nucleus A small lens-shaped nucleus in the BRAIN where it is a part of the BASAL GANGLIA system, located ventral to the THALAMUS and dorsal to the SUBSTANTIA NIGRA. Chronic stimulation of the subthalamic nucleus, called DEEP BRAIN STIMULATION (DBS), is used to treat patients with PARKINSON'S DISEASE.

succinylcholine A short-acting depolarizing-type skeletal muscle relaxant used intravenously in ANESTHESIA. Also used in conjunction with ELECTROCONVULSIVE THERAPY (ECT) to minimize the possibility of complications.

suggestibility Uncritical compliance or acceptance of an idea, a belief, or an attribute.

suggestion The process of influencing a patient to accept an idea, a belief, or an attitude suggested by the therapist. See also HYPNOSIS.

suicidal ideation The presence of suicidal thoughts or plans. Many people with major DEPRESSION or PANIC DISORDER may have such SYMPTOMS, even if only transiently, or in a vague, nonspecific way.

suicide Deliberate taking of one's own life.

sukra prameha A CULTURE-SPECIFIC SYNDROME. See *DHAT*.

suk-yeong A CULTURE-SPECIFIC SYNDROME. See *KORO*.

sumatriptan A SEROTONIN AGONIST used to reduce the pain of an acute MIGRAINE headache. Marketed under the brand name IMITREX.

sundowning A state of increased agitation, activity, confusion, and negative behaviors that occurs at the end of the day and may continue into the night. Sundowning is a common symptom in people with DEMENTIA or PSYCHOSIS.

suo yang A CULTURE-SPECIFIC SYNDROME. See *KORO*.

superego In psychoanalytic theory (see PSYCHOANALYSIS), that part of the PERSONALITY structure associated with ethics, standards, and self-criticism. It is formed by IDENTIFICATION with important and esteemed persons in early life, particularly parents. The supposed or actual wishes of these significant persons are taken over as part of the child's own standards to help form the CONSCIENCE. See also EGO; GUILT; ID; SHAME.

support groups   A network of individuals who give courage, confidence, and help to one another through EMPATHY, INSIGHT, and constructive feedback. In PSYCHIATRY, these groups are especially helpful for patients with SUBSTANCE USE DISORDERS and for family members of patients with a psychiatric disorder.

supportive psychotherapy   A type of therapy in which the therapist-patient relationship is used to help patients cope with specific crises or difficulties that they are currently facing. Supportive therapy avoids, rather than encourages, the development of a TRANSFERENCE NEUROSIS. It employs a range of techniques, depending on the patient's strengths and weaknesses and the particular problems that are currently distressing. These techniques include listening in a sympathetic, concerned, understanding, and nonjudgmental fashion; providing factual information that may counter a patient's unrealistic FEARS; setting limits and encouraging the patient to control or relinquish self-destructive behavior and to give ATTENTION to more constructive action; and facilitating discharge of and relief from painful feelings within the controlled environment of the consultation room. See also PSYCHOTHERAPY.

suppression   The CONSCIOUS effort to control and conceal unacceptable IMPULSES, thoughts, feelings, or acts.

suprachiasmatic nucleus (SCN)   A tiny region on the brain's midline, situated directly above the optic chiasm, that receives photic input from the retina and is responsible for controlling BIOLOGICAL RHYTHMS. The neuronal and hormonal activities it generates regulate many different body functions in a 24-hour sleep-wake cycle.

Surmontil   Brand name for the TRICYCLIC ANTIDEPRESSANT drug TRIMIPRAMINE.

susto   A SYNDROME prevalent among Latinos in the United States and Latin America, *susto* is attributed to a frightening experience that causes the soul to leave the body and results in unhappiness and sickness. It is believed that in extreme cases, *susto* may result in death. Symptoms include appetite disturbances, inadequate or excessive sleep, and feelings of sadness and low self-worth (ANHEDONIA). It may be diagnosed as MAJOR DEPRESSIVE DISORDER, POSTTRAUMATIC STRESS DISORDER (PTSD), or SOMATOFORM DISORDER. See CULTURE-SPECIFIC SYNDROMES.

Sydenham's chorea   A disorder of the CENTRAL NERVOUS SYSTEM (CNS) characterized by emotional instability, purposeless movement, and muscular weakness. It is a major manifestation of acute rheumatic fever, occurring between ages 7 and 14, and caused by the CNS effects of streptococcus bacteria.

symbiosis   A mutually reinforcing and often beneficial relationship between two persons who are dependent on each other. It is a normal characteristic of the relationship between the mother and infant child. See SEPARATION-INDIVIDUATION.

symbiotic psychosis   As described by Margaret Mahler (1897–1985), a condition observed in 2- to 4-year-old children who had an abnormal relationship with a mothering figure. The PSYCHOSIS was characterized by intense SEPARATION ANXIETY, severe REGRESSION, abandonment of useful speech, and AUTISM. See EXOGENOUS PSYCHOSES.

symbolization   A general mechanism in all human thinking by which some mental representation comes to stand for some other thing, class of things, or attribute of something. This mechanism underlies dream formation and some SYMPTOMS, such as CONVERSION reactions. The link between the latent meaning of the symptom and the symbol is usually UNCONSCIOUS.

Symbyax   Brand name for OLANZAPINE–FLUOXETINE COMBINATION.

Symmetrel   Brand name (now discontinued) for the ANTIPARKINSONIAN MEDICATION AMANTADINE.

sympathetic nervous system   The part of the AUTONOMIC NERVOUS SYSTEM (ANS) that responds to dangerous or threatening situations by physiologically preparing a person for "fight or flight" (see FIGHT-OR-FLIGHT RESPONSE). EPINEPHRINE and NOREPINEPHRINE are the NEUROTRANSMITTERS chiefly involved with this system. Contrast with PARASYMPATHETIC NERVOUS SYSTEM.

sympathomimetic   Refers to a substance that produces a physiological effect similar to that produced by stimulation of the SYMPATHETIC NERVOUS SYSTEM.

sympathy   A feeling or capacity for sharing in the interests or concerns of another. May arise when there is no emotional ATTACHMENT to the person toward whom one is sympathetic because the feelings of the sympathetic person remain essentially internal. Contrast with EMPATHY.

symptom   A specific manifestation of a patient's condition indicative of an abnormal physical or mental state; a subjective PERCEPTION of illness.

synapse   The gap between the membrane of one nerve cell and the membrane of another. The synapse is the space through which the nerve impulse is passed, chemically or electrically, from one nerve to another.

synaptic transmission   Also called *neurotransmission*; an electrical movement within synapses caused by a propagation of nerve impulses.

syndrome   A configuration of SYMPTOMS that occur together and constitute a recognizable condition.

syntaxic mode   The mode of PERCEPTION that forms whole, logical, coherent pictures of reality that can be validated by others.

synucleinopathies   A class of neurodegenerative diseases characterized by fibrillary aggregates of alpha-synuclein protein in the cytoplasm of selective populations of neurons and glia. Examples of synucleinopathies include PARKINSON'S DISEASE, DEMENTIA WITH LEWY BODIES, and MULTIPLE SYSTEM ATROPHY. Compare with TAUOPATHIES; see also "PARKINSON'S PLUS" SYNDROMES.

syphilis   A sexually transmitted venereal disease, caused by the spirochetal bacterium *Treponema pallidum,* which, if untreated, may lead to CENTRAL NERVOUS SYSTEM (CNS) deterioration with psychotic manifestations in its later stages. See also GENERAL PARALYSIS.

systematic desensitization   A BEHAVIOR THERAPY procedure widely used to modify behaviors associated with PHOBIAS. The procedure involves the construction of a hierarchy of ANXIETY-producing stimuli by the subject and gradual presentation of the stimuli until they no longer produce anxiety. Also called *desensitization.* See also RECIPROCAL INHIBITION.

T

taboo   Prohibition or restriction interwoven in the CULTURE.

tacrine   A reversible ACETYLCHOLINESTERASE INHIBITOR used in the treatment of ALZHEIMER'S DISEASE. Marketed under the brand name COGNEX. See "Medications Used in Psychiatry."

taijin kyofusho   A culturally distinctive phobia in Japan, that resembles SOCIAL PHOBIA. The term refers to an individual's intense fear that his or her body, its parts, or its functions displease, embarrass, or are offensive to other people. See CULTURE-SPECIFIC SYNDROMES.

talion law or principle A primitive, unrealistic belief, usually UN-CONSCIOUS, conforming to the Biblical injunction of "an eye for an eye and a tooth for a tooth." In PSYCHOANALYSIS, the concept and FEAR that all injury, actual or intended, will be punished in kind.

Talwin Brand name for the NARCOTIC drug PENTAZOCINE.

tangentiality Replying to a question in an oblique or irrelevant way. Compare with CIRCUMSTANTIALITY.

***Tarasoff* case** A California court decision that imposes a duty on the therapist to warn the appropriate person or persons when the therapist becomes aware that the patient may present a risk of harm to a specific person or persons. See also "Legal Terms."

tardive dyskinesia A serious adverse effect associated mainly with CONVENTIONAL ANTIPSYCHOTIC medications that consists of abnormal, involuntary movements usually involving the tongue and mouth and sometimes involving the arms and trunk. The treatment is to stop the ANTIPSYCHOTIC medication, but many patients choose to continue taking the medication because their life may be intolerable without it. African Americans are at greater risk for developing tardive dyskinesia. The risk of this disorder is much lower with ATYPICAL ANTIPSYCHOTIC medications.

tardive dystonia A significant adverse effect consisting of sustained, involuntary muscle contractions that develop following treatment with CONVENTIONAL ANTIPSYCHOTIC medications.

Tasmar Brand name for the ANTIPARKINSONIAN MEDICATION TOLCAPONE.

tauopathies A class of neurodegenerative diseases resulting from the pathological aggregation of TAU PROTEIN in the NEUROFIBRILLARY TANGLES of the human brain. Examples of tauopathies include FRONTOTEMPORAL DEMENTIA, ALZHEIMER'S DISEASE, PROGRESSIVE SUPRANUCLEAR PALSY, CORTICOBASAL GANGLIONIC DEGENERATION, and FRONTOTEMPORAL LOBAR DEGENERATION (also known as PICK'S DISEASE). Compare with SYNUCLEINOPATHIES; see also "PARKINSON'S PLUS" SYNDROMES.

tau protein A protein, first identified in the 1970s, found in neurons, primarily in the CENTRAL NERVOUS SYSTEM (CNS). Several different versions of tau protein can be found in the body, and all are critical to the healthy functioning of the CNS. See also ALZHEIMER'S DISEASE; NEUROFIBRILLARY TANGLES.

TBI See TRAUMATIC BRAIN INJURY (TBI).

Tegretol   Brand name for the ANTICONVULSANT/MOOD STABILIZER drug
CARBAMAZEPINE.

telepathy   Communication of thought from one person to another
without the intervention of physical means. See also EXTRASENSORY
PERCEPTION (ESP); PARAPSYCHOLOGY.

telephone scatologia   One of the PARAPHILIAS, characterized by
marked distress over, or acting on, sexual urges that involve telephone calls to a nonconsenting listener in order to verbalize EROTIC
or obscene language (lewdness).

telepsychiatry   The application of telemedicine to the field of psychiatry, telepsychiatry is currently one of the most effective ways to
increase access to psychiatric care for individuals living in under-
served areas. In addition to offering an array of services including
diagnosis and assessment, medication management, and individual
and group therapy, telepsychiatry provides an opportunity for consultation among psychiatrists, primary care physicians, and other
health care providers.

temazepam   A BENZODIAZEPINE SEDATIVE-HYPNOTIC medication used in
the treatment of INSOMNIA. Marketed under the brand name RESTORIL.
See "Medications Used in Psychiatry."

temperament   Constitutional predisposition to react in a particular
way to stimuli. A component of one's PERSONALITY.

temporal lobe   One of the four major subdivisions in each hemisphere of the CEREBRAL CORTEX. The temporal lobe is involved with
speech, auditory, and memory functions as well as complex visual
PERCEPTIONS.

temporal lobe epilepsy   Also called *complex partial* SEIZURES, or PSY-
CHOMOTOR epilepsy. See EPILEPSY.

temporal lobe syndromes   Mental and behavioral disturbances asso-
ciated with TEMPORAL LOBE EPILEPSY or other TEMPORAL LOBE pathology.
Lesions in the dominant temporal lobe may produce auditory HALLUCI-
NATIONS, DELUSIONS, and impaired verbal and reading comprehension.
Lesions in the nondominant temporal lobe may produce DEPRESSION, IN-
APPROPRIATE AFFECT, and impaired visual and auditory MEMORY.

Tenex   Brand name for the alpha$_{2A}$-ADRENERGIC RECEPTOR AGONIST drug
GUANFACINE.

termination   In PSYCHOTHERAPY, *termination* refers to the mutual
agreement between patient and therapist to bring therapy to an end.
The idea of termination often occurs to both, but usually it is the

therapist who introduces the subject into the session as a possibility to be considered. In psychoanalytic treatment (see PSYCHOANALYSIS), the patient's reactions are worked through to completion before the treatment ends. The early termination that is characteristic of forms of BRIEF PSYCHOTHERAPY often requires more extensive work with the feelings of loss and separation.

terrorism   Actual or threatened violence to gain attention and to cause people to exaggerate the strength of the terrorists and the importance of their cause.

tertiary prevention   See PREVENTION.

testamentary capacity   See "Legal Terms."

tetrabenazine   An agent indicated for the treatment of chorea associated with HUNTINGTON'S DISEASE. Marketed under the brand name XENAZINE.

tetracyclic antidepressants   A class of drugs used primarily as ANTIDEPRESSANTS that were first introduced in the 1970s. They are named after their chemical structure, which contains four rings of atoms, and are closely related to the TRICYCLIC ANTIDEPRESSANTS, which contain three rings of atoms. See "Medications Used in Psychiatry."

thalamus   Two egg-shaped masses of nerve tissue deep within the BRAIN. It is an important relay station, which seems to act as a filter for sensory information flowing into the brain. The thalamus also may play a part in SHORT- and LONG-TERM MEMORY.

thanatology   The study of death and dying, emphasizing therapeutic interventions with dying persons and their survivors.

The Joint Commission (TJC)   Formerly Joint Commission on Accreditation of Healthcare Organizations (JCAHO); the agency that surveys hospitals and other health facilities and programs and certifies that they have met the standards set by The Joint Commission. See ACCREDITATION.

theophobia   The FEAR of God.

therapeutic alliance   A term that refers to the collaborative aspect of the relationship between therapist and client in the context of PSYCHOTHERAPY.

therapeutic community   A term of British origin, now widely used, for a specially structured mental hospital milieu that encourages patients to function within the range of social norms.

therapeutic window   A well-defined range of BLOOD LEVELS or medication dosage ranges associated with optimal clinical response to

ANTIDEPRESSANT medications. Levels above or below that range are associated with diminished therapeutic response.

thioridazine   An older CONVENTIONAL ANTIPSYCHOTIC medication (a PHENOTHIAZINE of the piperidine class) that is infrequently prescribed today because of its association with increased risk of cardiac arrhythmias and retinitis pigmentosa at higher doses. Now available only as generic but may still be known by the discontinued brand name MELLARIL. See "Medications Used in Psychiatry."

thiothixene   A CONVENTIONAL ANTIPSYCHOTIC medication (a THIOXANTHENE) used in the treatment of SCHIZOPHRENIA AND OTHER PSYCHOTIC DISORDERS. Marketed under the brand name NAVANE. See "Medications Used in Psychiatry."

thioxanthenes   A subgroup of CONVENTIONAL ANTIPSYCHOTIC drugs that includes THIOTHIXENE.

third ear (the)   The clinician's use of intuition, sensitivity, and awareness of subliminal cues to interpret clinical observations of patients in therapy.

third-party payer   Any organization (public or private) that pays or insures health or medical expenses on behalf of beneficiaries or recipients. Examples are MEDICARE, MEDICAID, Blue Cross, Blue Shield, and other commercial insurance companies.

Thorazine   Brand name (now discontinued) for CHLORPROMAZINE.

thought disorder   A disturbance of speech, communication, or content of thought, such as DELUSIONS, IDEAS OF REFERENCE, poverty of thought, FLIGHT OF IDEAS, PERSEVERATION, and LOOSENING OF ASSOCIATIONS. *Thought disorder* is often used synonymously with the term PSYCHOSIS.

thrombocytopenia   A decrease in the number of platelets in the blood leading to bleeding in the mouth and scattered bruises. This condition is sometimes caused by certain ANTICONVULSANT medications (MOOD STABILIZERS), such as CARBAMAZEPINE and VALPROATE, as well as by ANTIPSYCHOTICS such as CLOZAPINE.

tic   An involuntary, sudden, rapid, recurrent, nonrhythmic, stereotyped motor movement or vocalization. A tic may be an expression of an emotional CONFLICT, the result of neurological disease, the effect of a drug (especially a STIMULANT or other DOPAMINE AGONIST), or a combination of these.

tic disorders   In DSM-IV-TR, this category includes TOURETTE'S DISORDER, chronic motor or VOCAL TIC DISORDER, TRANSIENT TIC DISORDER, and tic disorder not otherwise specified; all but the last type begin before age 18 years. Chronic tics may occur many times a day, nearly every day, or intermittently over a period of more than a year. Transient tics do not persist for longer than 12 consecutive months.

TM   Transcendental meditation. See EXPERIENTIAL THERAPY.

TMS   See TRANSCRANIAL MAGNETIC STIMULATION (TMS).

Tofranil   Brand name for the TRICYCLIC ANTIDEPRESSANT drug IMIPRAMINE.

token economy   A system involving the application of the principles and procedures of OPERANT CONDITIONING to the management of a social setting such as a ward, classroom, or HALFWAY HOUSE. Tokens are given contingent on completion of specified activities and are exchangeable for goods or privileges desired by the patient.

tolcapone   An ADJUNCTIVE medication used in combination with CARBIDOPA-LEVODOPA therapy for patients with severe PARKINSON'S DISEASE. Tolcapone inhibits the metabolism of levodopa by CATECHOL-O-METHYLTRANSFERASE (COMT), allowing greater levels of levodopa to penetrate the brain, where it can be converted to DOPAMINE. Marketed under the brand name TASMAR.

tolerance   A characteristic of substance DEPENDENCE that may be shown by the need for markedly increased amounts of the substance to achieve INTOXICATION or the desired effect, by markedly diminished effect with continued use of the same amount of the substance, or by adequate functioning despite doses or BLOOD LEVELS of the substance that would be expected to produce significant impairment in a casual user.

tomography   Radiological imaging of serial planes ("cuts") through an anatomical structure. See also BRAIN IMAGING.

Topamax   Brand name for the ANTICONVULSANT drug TOPIRAMATE.

topiramate   An ANTICONVULSANT medication sometimes used as a MOOD STABILIZER to treat BIPOLAR DISORDER. Marketed under the brand name TOPAMAX. See "Medications Used in Psychiatry."

topographic model   Freud's model of the topography of the mind, first described in terms of the CONSCIOUS-PRECONSCIOUS-UNCONSCIOUS and a simple CONFLICT theory of the conscious opposing the unconscious. The more complex STRUCTURAL MODEL of ID, EGO, and SUPEREGO, and its correlated concept of intersystemic conflicts, replaced the topographic model, leading to a shift in clinical focus from discovery of unconscious DRIVE-related wishes to a systematic analysis of the ego's unconscious defensive operations.

topophobia   The FEAR of specific places or situations.

torsade de pointes   A ventricular tachyarrhythmia that can be induced by certain ANTIPSYCHOTIC and ANTIDEPRESSANT medications.

tort   See "Legal Terms."

torture   The deliberate, systematic infliction of physical and mental suffering for the purpose of forcing people to conform or to reveal information.

toucherism   See FROTTEURISM.

Tourette's disorder   A TIC DISORDER consisting of multiple motor and vocal TICS that occur in bouts, either concurrently or separately, almost every day or intermittently over a period of more than 12 months. Also known as GILLES DE LA TOURETTE'S SYNDROME.

toxicity   The capacity of a drug to damage body tissue or seriously impair body functions.

toxicology testing   Testing of urine and blood performed to determine the presence and level of drugs of ABUSE.

toxic psychosis   Psychosis caused by the poisonous effect of chemicals or drugs.

training analysis   The personal analysis that is required of prospective psychoanalysts and intended to help them become aware of their own psychological processes and to master UNCONSCIOUS CONFLICTS that might otherwise lead to interference with participation in the analytic treatment.

trance   A state of focused ATTENTION and diminished sensory and motor activity seen in HYPNOSIS, certain DISSOCIATIVE DISORDERS, and ecstatic religious states.

tranquilizer   A medication that decreases ANXIETY and AGITATION. Preferred terms are ANXIOLYTICS and ANTIPSYCHOTICS.

transactional analysis   A PSYCHODYNAMIC PSYCHOTHERAPY based on ROLE theory that attempts to understand the interplay between therapist and patient and ultimately between the patient and external reality.

transcendental meditation   See EXPERIENTIAL THERAPY.

transcranial magnetic stimulation (TMS)   Refers to the use of a magnetic field to stimulate or inhibit cortical NEURONS in treatment-resistant DEPRESSION. TMS is not intended to produce a SEIZURE, so anesthesia is not required.

transcultural psychiatry   See CROSS-CULTURAL PSYCHIATRY.

transference   The UNCONSCIOUS assignment to others of feelings and attitudes that were originally associated with important figures (e.g., parents, siblings) in one's early life. The PSYCHIATRIST uses this phenomenon as a therapeutic tool to help the patient understand emotional problems and their origins. In the patient-physician relationship, the transference may be negative (hostile) or positive (affectionate). See also COUNTERTRANSFERENCE; PARATAXIC DISTORTION.

transference cure   A term used to describe when a patient flees from further treatment in order to avoid dealing with repressed material. The patient is not cured but is in temporary REMISSION. RELAPSES are almost certain when the patient encounters further stress.

transference neurosis   In clinical PSYCHOANALYSIS, the analysand's re-experiencing of his or her characteristic INTRAPSYCHIC CONFLICTS and modes of DEFENSE, which are expressed in fantasies about the analyst.

transient tic disorder   See TIC DISORDERS.

transinstitutionalization   A term used to describe the shift of mentally ill individuals from the mental health care system into the criminal justice system. This phenomenon has also been described as "the criminalization of mentally disordered behavior."

transitional object   An object, other than the mother, selected by an infant between ages 4 and 18 months for self-soothing and ANXIETY reduction. Examples are a "security blanket" or a toy that helps the infant go to SLEEP. The transitional object provides an opportunity to master external objects and promotes DIFFERENTIATION of the SELF from the outer world.

transphobia   The FEAR of TRANSSEXUALISM or of transgender people.

transsexualism   See GENDER IDENTITY DISORDER.

transvestic fetishism   One of the PARAPHILIAS, characterized by marked distress over, or acting on, sexual urges involving cross-dressing, most frequently in a heterosexual male. The condition may occur with gender DYSPHORIA as part of a GENDER IDENTITY DISORDER, but more commonly the transvestite has no desire to change his sex but wants only, at a particular time, to appear to be a female.

transvestism   Sexual pleasure derived from dressing or masquerading in the clothing of the opposite sex, with the strong wish to appear as a member of the opposite sex. The sexual origins of transvestism may be UNCONSCIOUS.

Tranxene   Brand name for the BENZODIAZEPINE ANXIOLYTIC drug CLORAZEPATE.

tranylcypromine   A nonselective and irreversible MONOAMINE OXIDASE INHIBITOR (MAOI) ANTIDEPRESSANT medication used principally to treat DEPRESSION in patients who have failed to respond to more standard treatments. Marketed under the brand name PARNATE. See "Medications Used in Psychiatry."

traumatic brain injury (TBI)   A form of acquired BRAIN injury, that occurs when a sudden trauma causes damage to the brain. Symptoms of a TBI can be mild, moderate, or severe, depending on the extent and location of the damage. A person with a mild TBI may remain conscious or may experience a loss of consciousness for a few seconds or minutes. Other symptoms of mild TBI may include headache, confusion, light-headedness, dizziness, a change in sleep patterns, behavioral or mood changes, and trouble with memory, concentration, attention, or thinking. A person with a moderate or severe TBI may show these same symptoms, but may also have a headache that gets worse or does not go away, repeated vomiting or nausea, convulsions or seizures, an inability to awaken from sleep, and increased confusion, restlessness, or agitation.

trazodone   An ATYPICAL ANTIDEPRESSANT medication (characterized as a SEROTONIN ANTAGONIST AND REUPTAKE INHIBITOR [SARI]) indicated for the treatment of DEPRESSION but today used mainly to treat INSOMNIA. Although available only as generic, it may still be known by the discontinued brand name DESYREL. See "Medications Used in Psychiatry."

treatment resistance   Lack of response to a specific therapy that ordinarily would be expected to be effective.

tremor   A trembling or shaking of the body or any of its parts. It may be induced by medication.

Triavil   Brand name (now discontinued) for PERPHENAZINE–AMITRIPTYLINE COMBINATION.

triazolam   A BENZODIAZEPINE SEDATIVE-HYPNOTIC medication used for the short-term treatment of INSOMNIA. It is infrequently prescribed because of its propensity to produce AMNESIA and MEMORY disturbance, especially at high doses. Marketed under the brand name HALCION. See "Medications Used in Psychiatry."

trichotillomania   Pathological hair pulling that results in noticeable hair loss. As in other IMPULSE-CONTROL DISORDERS, an increasing sense of tension or affective AROUSAL immediately precedes an episode of hair pulling, which is then followed by a sense of pleasure, gratification, or relief. See also –MANIA.

tricyclic antidepressants   An older class of ANTIDEPRESSANTS that enhance the concentration of NOREPINEPHRINE and SEROTONIN in the CENTRAL NERVOUS SYSTEM (CNS). They are named after their chemical structure, which contains three rings of atoms, and are closely related to the TETRACYCLIC ANTIDEPRESSANTS, which contain four rings of atoms. See "Medications Used in Psychiatry."

trifluoperazine A CONVENTIONAL ANTIPSYCHOTIC medication (a PHENOTHIAZINE of the piperazine class) used to treat SCHIZOPHRENIA AND OTHER PSYCHOTIC DISORDERS. Now available only as generic but may still be known by the discontinued brand name STELAZINE. See "Medications Used in Psychiatry."

trihexyphenidyl An ANTICHOLINERGIC medication used to treat muscle stiffness and other motor SIDE EFFECTS from PARKINSON'S DISEASE or as a result of treatment with CONVENTIONAL ANTIPSYCHOTICS such as HALOPERIDOL (HALDOL). Now available only as generic but may still be known by the discontinued brand name ARTANE. See "Medications Used in Psychiatry."

Trilafon Brand name (now discontinued) for the CONVENTIONAL ANTIPSYCHOTIC drug PERPHENAZINE.

Trileptal Brand name for the ANTICONVULSANT drug OXCARBAZEPINE.

trimipramine A TRICYCLIC ANTIDEPRESSANT medication infrequently prescribed today. Marketed under the brand name SURMONTIL. See "Medications Used in Psychiatry."

tripa ida A CULTURE-SPECIFIC SYNDROME. See *SUSTO*.

triskaidekaphobia The FEAR of number 13.

trisomy The presence of three CHROMOSOMES instead of the two that normally represent each potential set of chromosomes. This can result in a developmental DISABILITY. An example of trisomy is DOWN SYNDROME, in which three number 21 chromosomes are present.

tuberous sclerosis complex A rare, multisystemic GENETIC disease that causes tumors to grow in the brain and on other vital organs such as the kidneys, heart, eyes, lungs, and skin. Symptoms may include seizures, DEVELOPMENTAL DELAY, attention deficits, hyperactivity, impulsivity, LEARNING DISABILITIES, cognitive deficits, skin abnormalities, and lung and kidney disease.

Turner's syndrome A chromosomal defect in women with a 45,X karyotype (45 CHROMOSOMES rather than 46). Clinical features include short stature, webbed neck, abnormal ovarian development, infertility, specific social and COGNITIVE DEFICITS such as nonverbal LEARNING DISABILITIES, and sometimes INTELLECTUAL DISABILITY.

twelve-step program A therapeutic process that uses 12 steps to combat alcohol or substance ABUSE, PATHOLOGICAL GAMBLING, and

PARAPHILIAS. Twelve-step programs are usually run by laypeople rather than professionals.

twin research   A powerful method of investigating the relative degree of phenotypic variance that can be attributed to GENETIC factors and to transmissible and nontransmissible environmental factors. For example, behavioral variations occurring in MONOZYGOTIC TWINS are compared with those occurring in nontwin siblings or DIZYGOTIC TWINS.

twinship transference   See SELFOBJECT TRANSFERENCE.

type A personality   A TEMPERAMENT characterized by excessive DRIVE, competitiveness, a sense of time urgency, impatience, unrealistic ambition, and need for control. Believed to be associated with a high INCIDENCE of coronary artery disease.

type B personality   A TEMPERAMENT characterized by a relaxed, easygoing demeanor; less time-bound and competitive than the TYPE A PERSONALITY.

type D personality   (*D* stands for "distressed.") Term used in PSYCHOSOMATIC MEDICINE to refer to a joint tendency toward negative affectivity (e.g., worry, irritability, pessimism) and social inhibition (e.g., reticence, lack of self-confidence). Research indicates that presence of type D personality may predict a worse prognosis for cardiac patients.

tyramine   A SYMPATHOMIMETIC AMINE that acts by displacing stored transmitter from ADRENERGIC axonal terminals. Tyramine is a constituent of many foods, such as green beans, cheese, and red wine, and the amine is normally degraded by MONOAMINE OXIDASE enzymes in the gastrointestinal tract when these foods are ingested. Patients taking MONOAMINE OXIDASE INHIBITORS (MAOIs) must restrict their intake of foods high in tyramine content because of the risk of a life-threatening HYPERTENSIVE CRISIS.

U

ultradian rhythms   See BIOLOGICAL RHYTHMS.

unconscious   That part of MEMORY and mental functioning that is rarely subject to awareness. It is a repository for data that have never been CONSCIOUS (primary REPRESSION) or that may have been conscious and are later repressed (secondary repression).

undifferentiated schizophrenia   See SCHIZOPHRENIA.

undoing   A DEFENSE MECHANISM consisting of behavior that symbolically atones for, makes amends for, or reverses previous thoughts, feelings, or actions.

United States Code (U.S.C.)   See "Legal Terms."

urophilia   One of the PARAPHILIAS, characterized by marked distress over, or acting on, sexual urges that involve urine.

use disorders   See SUBSTANCE USE DISORDERS.

utilization review committee   A committee of physicians and other clinical staff formed in a hospital to review the quality of services rendered, the length of hospital stay for inpatients, and the effective and appropriate use of various clinical services. See also PEER REVIEW ORGANIZATION (PRO); PROFESSIONAL STANDARDS REVIEW ORGANIZATION (PSRO).

V

vaginismus   See under SEXUAL PAIN DISORDERS.

vagus nerve stimulation (VNS)   Stimulation of the vagus nerve for the treatment of REFRACTORY SEIZURE disorders or treatment-resistant DEPRESSION.

valerian   The common name for *Valeriana officinalis.* The root and other underground parts of this plant, grown in Europe and in the warmer climates of Asia, are used by individuals to treat ANXIETY and mild INSOMNIA. It is believed to work by stimulating GABA (GAMMA-AMINOBUTYRIC ACID) RECEPTORS, which may reduce anxiety—the same mechanism of action produced by the BENZODIAZEPINES. Valerian's effectiveness has not been supported by controlled clinical trials in the United States.

Valium   Brand name for the BENZODIAZEPINE ANXIOLYTIC drug DIAZEPAM.

valproate   An ANTICONVULSANT medication used in NEUROLOGY in the treatment of complex partial SEIZURES and in PSYCHIATRY as a MOOD STA-

BILIZER to treat BIPOLAR DISORDER. Marketed under the brand name DEPACON. See "Medications Used in Psychiatry."

valproic acid   An ANTICONVULSANT medication used in NEUROLOGY in the treatment of complex partial SEIZURES and in PSYCHIATRY as a MOOD STABILIZER to treat BIPOLAR DISORDER. Marketed under the brand names DEPAKENE and STAVZOR. See "Medications Used in Psychiatry."

varenicline   A medication used to treat nicotine ADDICTION. A NICO- TINIC RECEPTOR partial AGONIST, it reduces cravings for and decreases the pleasurable effects of cigarettes and other tobacco products. Mar- keted under the brand name CHANTIX. See "Medications Used in Psy- chiatry."

vascular dementia   Formerly known as *multi-infarct dementia*; it is the result of multiple cerebral infarcts in persons with atheroscle- rotic disease. Typically, the course is one of a period of clinical sta- bility punctuated by sudden significant COGNITIVE and FUNCTIONAL losses (stepwise deterioration).

VCFS   See VELOCARDIOFACIAL SYNDROME (VCFS).

vegetative nervous system   Obsolete term for the AUTONOMIC NER- VOUS SYSTEM (ANS).

velocardiofacial syndrome (VCFS)   Highly variable presentation that may include midline defects such as cleft palate, cardiac anom- alies such as ventroseptal defect, LEARNING DISABILITIES or DEVELOPMEN- TAL DELAY, unusual FACIES, and PSYCHOSIS in ADOLESCENCE. Associated with CHROMOSOME arm 22q11 deletion. Also known as SHPRINTZEN SYN- DROME or DIGEORGE SYNDROME.

venlafaxine   An ANTIDEPRESSANT of the SEROTONIN-NOREPINEPHRINE RE- UPTAKE INHIBITOR (SNRI) class used to treat DEPRESSION and GENERALIZED ANXIETY DISORDER. Marketed under the brand name EFFEXOR. See "Medications Used in Psychiatry."

verbigeration   Stereotyped and seemingly meaningless repetition of words or sentences. See also PERSEVERATION.

vertical split   In SELF PSYCHOLOGY, a process by which conscious but unwanted qualities of the SELF are warded off and separated from conscious desirable self elements. The defenses associated with ver- tical split are DENIAL, DISSOCIATION, and disavowal. Contrast with HORI- ZONTAL SPLIT.

vertigo   A sensation that the external world is spinning around. It may be a SYMPTOM of vestibular dysfunction.

Viagra   Brand name for the phosphodiesterase inhibitor SILDENAFIL.

vicarious liability   See "Legal Terms."

Vistaril   Brand name for the ANTIHISTAMINE drug HYDROXYZINE.

Vivactil   Brand name for the TRICYCLIC ANTIDEPRESSANT drug PROTRIP-TYLINE.

Vivitrol   Brand name for an injectable form of the OPIOID ANTAGONIST drug NALTREXONE. Vivitrol must be administered by a health care professional. Administration is via INTRAMUSCULAR injection once a month. Patients should not be actively drinking at the time of initial administration.

VNS   See VAGUS NERVE STIMULATION (VNS).

vocal tic disorder   See TIC DISORDERS.

voice disorder   A COMMUNICATION DISORDER characterized by abnormal vocal pitch, loudness, quality, tone, or resonance of enough severity to interfere with educational or occupational achievement or with social communication. Unlike other communication disorders, voice disorder may not appear until adulthood.

voluntary admission   See COMMITMENT.

voyeurism   Peeping; one of the PARAPHILIAS, characterized by marked distress over, or acting on, urges to observe unsuspecting people, usually strangers, who are naked or in the process of disrobing or who are engaging in sexual activity.

Vyvanse   Brand name for the CENTRAL NERVOUS SYSTEM (CNS) STIMULANT drug LISDEXAMFETAMINE.

W

waxy flexibility   A SYMPTOM often present in catatonic SCHIZOPHRENIA, in which the patient's arm or leg remains in the position in which it is placed. Also known as *CEREA FLEXIBILITAS*.

weekend hospitalization   See PARTIAL HOSPITALIZATION.

Wellbutrin   Brand name for the ATYPICAL ANTIDEPRESSANT drug BUPROPION.

Wernicke-Korsakoff syndrome   A disease of CENTRAL NERVOUS SYSTEM (CNS) metabolism due to a lack of vitamin B$_1$ (thiamine) seen in chronic ALCOHOLISM. WERNICKE'S ENCEPHALOPATHY is the acute phase of the disease; KORSAKOFF'S SYNDROME is the CHRONIC phase. Wernicke's encephalopathy features irregularities of eye movements, incoordination, impaired thinking, and often sensorimotor DEFICITS. Korsakoff's syndrome is characterized by CONFABULATION and, more importantly, by a short-term, but not immediate, disturbance that leads to gross impairment in MEMORY and learning. Wernicke's encephalopathy and Korsakoff's syndrome begin suddenly and are often found in the same person simultaneously. See also SUBSTANCE-INDUCED PSYCHOTIC DISORDER.

Wernicke's aphasia   Loss of the ability to comprehend language coupled with production of inappropriate language. Also known as RECEPTIVE APHASIA. See also BROCA'S APHASIA.

Wernicke's encephalopathy   A disease due to a nutritional deficiency of vitamin B_1 (thiamine), which provokes acute mental confusion, ATAXIA, and ophthalmoplegia (paralysis of some or all the muscles of the eye).

Williams syndrome   An autosomal dominant disorder associated with a deletion on CHROMOSOME 7. Individuals with this SYNDROME have an "elfin" facial appearance, mild to moderate INTELLECTUAL DISABILITY, delayed acquisition of motor milestones, and persistent gross and fine motor clumsiness. In contrast, they often possess extraordinary talents in music and verbal fluency.

Wilson's disease   A autosomal recessive GENETIC disorder that causes excessive copper accumulation in the liver or BRAIN. Patients may develop a range of psychiatric SYMPTOMS, including homicidal or suicidal behavior, DEPRESSION, and AGGRESSION.

windigo   An idiom of distress often associated with the idea of the mystery and great concerns over a lost person. It is often cited in the literature as referring to the idea of cannibal compulsion among Algonkian Indians. See CULTURE-SPECIFIC SYNDROMES.

withdrawal (from psychoactive substances)   The cessation or significant reduction of use of a chemical substance in a person with a pattern of heavy or prolonged use of that substance, often accompanied by WITHDRAWAL SYMPTOMS.

withdrawal (social)   See SOCIAL WITHDRAWAL.

withdrawal symptoms   The constellation of SYMPTOMS and SIGNS that develops within a short period (usually hours) after cessation or significant reduction of use of a substance in a person with a pattern of heavy or prolonged use of that substance. The withdrawal symptoms tend to be specific for each substance.

alcohol Within hours of cessation of, or significant reduction in, alcohol use in a person with a pattern of heavy and prolonged drinking, the subject develops hand TREMOR and a variety of associated SYMPTOMS that may include nausea and vomiting; ANXIETY; perceptual disturbances such as transient visual, tactile, or auditory HALLUCINATIONS or ILLUSIONS with intact REALITY TESTING; sweating or increased pulse rate; PSYCHOMOTOR AGITATION; INSOMNIA; and grand mal SEIZURES. The most severe form is DELIRIUM TREMENS, which can be life-threatening. See also DELIRIUM.

amphetamine Cessation of prolonged heavy use of amphetamine or a related substance produces a dysphoric MOOD and physiological changes such as fatigue, vivid and unpleasant dreams, INSOMNIA or HYPERSOMNIA, and increased appetite.

cocaine SYMPTOMS and SIGNS are the same as in AMPHETAMINE withdrawal (see above).

nicotine Abrupt cessation of, or reduction in, nicotine use induces any combination of the following: dysphoric or depressed MOOD, INSOMNIA, irritability or anger, ANXIETY, difficulty in concentrating, restlessness, decreased heart rate, and increased appetite or weight gain.

opioid The SYNDROME follows cessation of prolonged moderate or heavy use of an OPIOID or reduction in the amount of opioid used, or administration of an opioid ANTAGONIST. SYMPTOMS include dysphoric MOOD, nausea or vomiting, muscle aches, LACRIMATION or RHINORRHEA, pupillary dilation, PILOERECTION, sweating, diarrhea, yawning, fever, and INSOMNIA.

sedative, hypnotic, or anxiolytic SYMPTOMS and SIGNS are the same as described for alcohol withdrawal (see above).

wool-hwa-byung A CULTURE-SPECIFIC SYNDROME. See *HWA-BYUNG*.

word blindness See LEARNING DISABILITY.

word salad A mixture of words and phrases that lack comprehensive meaning or logical coherence. It may be seen in patients with SCHIZOPHRENIA, especially the disorganized type.

working through Exploration of a problem by patient and therapist until a satisfactory solution has been found or until a SYMPTOM has been traced to its UNCONSCIOUS sources. This process aims at transforming intellectual understanding into emotional knowledge, resolving unconscious CONFLICTS and thus leading to an increase in adaptive functioning and a decrease in symptoms.

World Psychiatric Association (WPA)   A nongovernmental organization composed of about 120 member societies worldwide. Its headquarters are based in the home country of its secretariat.

WPA   See WORLD PSYCHIATRIC ASSOCIATION (WPA).

wraparound services   A network of community services and natural supports individualized to the needs of the child and family.

X

Xanax   Brand name for the BENZODIAZEPINE ANXIOLYTIC drug ALPRAZOLAM.

Xenazine   Brand name for the antichoreic drug TETRABENAZINE.

xenophobia   The FEAR of strangers.

X-linkage   Mode of GENETIC transmission in which a trait or GENE is linked to the X CHROMOSOME. X-linkage has been implicated in some cases of BIPOLAR DISORDER.

Y

yi-ping   A common form of psychoneurosis with characteristics of suggestibility, exaggeration, emotionality, and egocentricity commonly related to adverse mental suggestions. It manifests as sensory or motor impairment, organic and vegetative imbalance, and abnormal mental symptoms. A Chinese CULTURE-SPECIFIC SYNDROME.

yoga   See EXPERIENTIAL THERAPY.

Z

zaleplon   A nonbenzodiazepine HYPNOTIC medication used in the short-term treatment of INSOMNIA. Marketed under the brand name SONATA. See "Medications Used in Psychiatry."

zar   A general term applied in Ethiopia, Somalia, Egypt, Sudan, Iran and other North African and Middle Eastern societies to the experience of spirits possessing an individual. Persons may experience dissociative episodes, show apathy and SOCIAL WITHDRAWAL, or develop a long-term relationship with the possessing spirit. Such behavior is not considered to be pathological in these cultures. See CULTURE-SPECIFIC SYNDROMES.

zeitgeist   The general intellectual and cultural climate of taste characteristic of an era.

ziprasidone   An ATYPICAL ANTIPSYCHOTIC medication used to treat SCHIZOPHRENIA. Marketed under the brand name GEODON. See "Medications Used in Psychiatry."

Zoloft   Brand name for the SELECTIVE SEROTONIN REUPTAKE INHIBITOR (SSRI) ANTIDEPRESSANT drug SERTRALINE.

zolpidem   A nonbenzodiazepine HYPNOTIC medication used in the short-term treatment of INSOMNIA. Marketed under the brand name AMBIEN. See "Medications Used in Psychiatry."

zoophilia   One of the PARAPHILIAS, characterized by marked distress over, or acting on, urges to indulge in sexual activity that involves animals.

Zyban   Brand name for a formulation of the ATYPICAL ANTIDEPRESSANT drug BUPROPION marketed for treatment of nicotine addiction.

Zyprexa   Brand name for the ATYPICAL ANTIPSYCHOTIC drug OLANZAPINE

Bibliography

American Psychiatric Association: Diagnostic and Statistical Manual of Mental Disorders, 4th Edition, Text Revision. Washington, DC, American Psychiatric Association, 2000

American Psychiatric Association Task Force on Electroconvulsive Therapy: The Practice of Electroconvulsive Therapy: Recommendations for Treatment, Training, and Privileging, 2nd Edition. Washington, DC, American Psychiatric Association, 2001

Andreasen NC, Black DW (eds): Introductory Textbook of Psychiatry, 5th Edition. Washington, DC, American Psychiatric Publishing, 2011

Benedek EP, Ash P, Scott CL (eds): Principles and Practice of Child and Adolescent Forensic Mental Health. Washington, DC, American Psychiatric Publishing, 2010

Benjamin J, Ebstein RP, Belmaker RH (eds): Molecular Genetics and the Human Personality. Washington, DC, American Psychiatric Publishing, 2002

Berkow R (editor-in-chief): The Merck Manual of Diagnosis and Therapy, 16th Edition. Rahway, NJ, Merck Research Laboratories, 1992

Blazer DG, Steffens DC (eds): The American Psychiatric Publishing Textbook of Geriatric Psychiatry, 4th Edition. Washington, DC, American Psychiatric Publishing, 2009

Bourgeois JA, Hales RE, Young JS, et al. (eds): The American Psychiatric Publishing Board Review Guide for Psychiatry. Washington, DC, American Psychiatric Publishing, 2009

Brown JS: Environmental and Chemical Toxins and Psychiatric Illness. Washington, DC, American Psychiatric Publishing, 2002

Brown TE: ADHD Comorbidities: Handbook for ADHD Complications in Children and Adults. Washington, DC, American Psychiatric Publishing, 2009

Cabaj RP, Stein TS (eds): Textbook of Homosexuality and Mental Health. Washington, DC, American Psychiatric Press, 1996

Cepeda C: Concise Guide to the Psychiatric Interview of Children and Adolescents. Washington, DC, American Psychiatric Press, 2000

Chew RH, Hales RE, Yudofsky SC: What Your Patients Need to Know About Psychiatric Medications, 2nd Edition. Washington, DC, American Psychiatric Publishing, 2009

Coffey EC, Brumback RA (eds): Textbook of Pediatric Neuropsychiatry. Washington, DC, American Psychiatric Press, 1998

Coffey EC, Cummings JL (eds): The American Psychiatric Press Text-
    book of Geriatric Neuropsychiatry, 2nd Edition. Washington, DC,
    American Psychiatric Press, 2000
Cross T, Bazron B, Dennis K, et al (eds): Toward a Culturally Compe-
    tent System of Care, Vol 1. Washington, DC, Georgetown Univer-
    sity and Child Development Center CASSP Technical Assistance
    Center, 1989
Dougherty DD, Rauch SL (eds): Psychiatric Neuroimaging Research:
    Contemporary Strategies. Washington, DC, American Psychiatric
    Publishing, 2001
Drugs@FDA: Searchable on-line database for official information about
    FDA-approved brand name and generic drugs and therapeutic bio-
    logical products. Available at: http://www.accessdata.fda.gov/
    scripts/cder/drugsatfda/index.cfm.
Dulcan MK (ed): Dulcan's Textbook of Child and Adolescent Psychia-
    try. Washington, DC, American Psychiatric Publishing, 2010
Gabbard GO (editor-in-chief): Treatments of Psychiatric Disorders, 3rd
    Edition, Vols 1 and 2. Washington, DC, American Psychiatric Press,
    2001
Gabbard GO: Psychodynamic Psychiatry in Clinical Practice, 4th Edi-
    tion. Washington, DC, American Psychiatric Publishing, 2005
Gabbard GO (ed): Gabbard's Treatments of Psychiatric Disorders, 4th
    Edition. Washington, DC, American Psychiatric Press, 2007
Gabbard GO (ed): Textbook of Psychotherapeutic Treatments. Wash-
    ington, DC, American Psychiatric Press, 2009
Galanter M, Kleber HD (eds): The American Psychiatric Press Text-
    book of Substance Abuse Treatment, 4th Edition. Washington, DC,
    American Psychiatric Publishing, 2008
Gaw AC: Concise Guide to Cross-Cultural Psychiatry. Washington, DC,
    American Psychiatric Publishing, 2001
Glick ID, Berman EM, Clarkin JF, et al (eds): Marital and Family Ther-
    apy, 4th Edition. Washington, DC, American Psychiatric Press,
    2000
Gunderson JG: Borderline Personality Disorder: A Clinical Guide.
    Washington, DC, American Psychiatric Publishing, 2001
Halbreich U, Montgomery SA (eds): Pharmacotherapy for Mood, Anx-
    iety, and Cognitive Disorders. Washington, DC, American Psychi-
    atric Press, 2000
Hales RE, Yudofsky SC, Gabbard GO (eds): The American Psychiatric
    Press Textbook of Psychiatry, 5th Edition. Washington, DC, Amer-
    ican Psychiatric Publishing, 2008
Helzer JE, Hudziak JJ (eds): Defining Psychopathology in the 21st
    Century—DSM-V and Beyond. Washington, DC, American Psychi-
    atric Publishing, 2002

Jacobson SA, Pies RW, Greenblatt DJ (eds): Handbook of Geriatric Psychopharmacology. Washington, DC, American Psychiatric Publishing, 2002

Jenkins SC, Tinsley JA, Van Loon JA (eds): A Pocket Reference for Psychiatrists, 3rd Edition. Washington, DC, American Psychiatric Publishing, 2001

Kaplan GB, Hammer RP Jr: Brain Circuitry and Signaling in Psychiatry: Basic Science and Clinical Implications. Washington, DC, American Psychiatric Publishing, 2002

Levenson JL (ed): The American Psychiatric Publishing Textbook of Psychosomatic Medicine: Psychiatric Care of the Medically Ill, 2nd Edition. Washington, DC, American Psychiatric Publishing, 2010

Liberman RP: Recovery From Disability: Manual of Psychiatric Rehabilitation. Washington, DC, American Psychiatric Publishing, 2008

Lieberman JA, Stroup TS, Perkins DO (eds): The American Psychiatric Publishing Textbook of Schizophrenia. Washington, DC, American Psychiatric Publishing, 2006

Oldham JM, Skodol AE, Bender DS (eds): The American Psychiatric Publishing Textbook of Personality Disorders. Washington, DC, American Psychiatric Publishing, 2009

Person ES, Cooper AM, Gabbard GO (eds): The American Psychiatric Publishing Textbook of Psychoanalysis. Washington, DC, American Psychiatric Publishing, 2005

Reite M, Ruddy J, Nagel K: Concise Guide to Evaluation and Management of Sleep Disorders, 2nd Edition. Washington, DC, American Psychiatric Press, 1997

Rush AJ, First MB, Blacker D (eds): Handbook of Psychiatric Measures, 2nd Edition. Washington, DC, American Psychiatric Publishing, 2008

Schatzberg AF, Nemeroff CB (eds): The American Psychiatric Press Textbook of Psychopharmacology, 4th Edition. Washington, DC, American Psychiatric Publishing, 2009

Silver JM, McAllister TW, Yudofsky SC (eds): Textbook of Traumatic Brain Injury, 2nd Edition. Washington, DC, American Psychiatric Publishing, 2011

Simon RI, Shuman DW: Clinical Manual of Psychiatry and Law. Washington, DC, American Psychiatric Publishing, 2007

Stein DJ, Hollander E, Rothbaum BO (eds): Textbook of Anxiety Disorders, 2nd Edition. Washington, DC, American Psychiatric Publishing, 2010

Stein DJ, Kupfer DJ, Schatzberg AF (eds): The American Psychiatric Press Textbook of Mood Disorders. Washington, DC, American Psychiatric Publishing, 2006

Talbott JA, Hales RE (eds): Textbook of Administrative Psychiatry. Washington, DC, American Psychiatric Publishing, 2001

U.S. Public Health Service: Mental Health: Culture, Race, and Ethnicity: A Supplement to Mental Health: A Report of the Surgeon General. Rockville, MD, U.S. Public Health Service, Office of the Surgeon General, 2001

Weiner MF, Lipton AM (eds): The American Psychiatric Publishing Textbook of Alzheimer Disease and Other Dementias. Washington, DC, American Psychiatric Publishing, 2009

Wikipedia: The Free Encyclopedia. Encyclopedia on-line. Available at: http://en.wikipedia.org.

Wynn GH, Oesterheld JR, Cozza KL, et al: Clinical Manual of Drug Interaction Principles for Medical Practice. Washington, DC, American Psychiatric Publishing, 2008

Yudofsky SC, Hales RE (eds): The American Psychiatric Press Textbook of Neuropsychiatry and Clinical Neurosciences, 5th Edition. Washington, DC, American Psychiatric Publishing, 2008

Commonly Used Abbreviations

AA	Alcoholics Anonymous
AAAP	American Academy of Addiction Psychiatry
AAAS	American Association for the Advancement of Science
AABA	American Anorexia/Bulimia Association
AACAP	American Academy of Child and Adolescent Psychiatry
AACDP	American Association of Chairmen of Departments of Psychiatry
AACP	American Academy for Child Psychoanalysts
AACP	American Academy of Clinical Psychiatrists
AACP	American Association of Community Psychiatrists
AADPRT	American Association of Directors of Psychiatric Residency Training
AAFP	American Academy of Family Physicians
AAGHP	American Association of General Hospital Psychiatrists
AAGP	American Association for Geriatric Psychiatry
AAIDD	American Association on Intellectual Disability and Developmental Disabilities
AAMC	Association of American Medical Colleges
AAMD	American Association on Mental Deficiency
AAMFT	American Association for Marriage and Family Therapy
AAMI	age-associated memory impairment
AAMR	American Association on Mental Retardation (as of 2007, AAIDD)
AAN	American Academy of Neurology
AANP	American Association of Neuropathologists
AAP	Administrators in Academic Psychiatry
AAP	American Academy of Psychoanalysis
AAP	American Academy of Psychotherapists

AAP	Association for Academic Psychiatry
AAP	Association for the Advancement of Psychoanalysis
AAP	Association for the Advancement of Psychotherapy
AAPA	American Association of Psychiatric Administrators
AAPAA	American Association of Psychiatrists in Alcoholism and Addictions
AAPC	American Association of Pastoral Counselors
AAPH	American Association for Partial Hospitalization
AAPL	American Academy of Psychiatry and the Law
AAPT	Association for the Advancement of Psychotherapy
AAS	American Association of Suicidology
AASM	American Academy of Sleep Medicine
AASP	American Association for Social Psychiatry
AATA	American Art Therapy Association
ABFP	American Board of Forensic Psychiatry
ABMS	American Board of Medical Specialties
ABPN	American Board of Psychiatry and Neurology
ACMHA	American College of Mental Health Administration
ACMPD	American Council on Marijuana and Other Psychoactive Drugs
ACNP	American College of Neuropsychiatrists
ACNPP	American College of Neuropsychopharmacology
ACP	American College of Physicians
ACP	American College of Psychiatrists
ACP	Association for Child Psychoanalysis
ACPA	American College of Psychoanalysts
ACT	assertive community treatment
ACTH	adrenocorticotropic hormone
ADA	American with Disabilities Act of 1990
ADAMHA	Alcohol, Drug Abuse, and Mental Health Administration (as of 1992, SAMHSA)
ADD	attention-deficit disorder
ADDA	Attention Deficit Disorder Association
ADH	alcohol dehydrogenase

ADHD	attention-deficit/hyperactivity disorder
ADLs	activities of daily living
ADMSEP	Association of Directors of Medical Student Education in Psychiatry
ADPA	Alcohol and Drug Problems Association of North America
ADR	acute dystonic reaction
ADRDA	Alzheimer's Disease and Related Disorders Association
AFCR	American Federation for Clinical Research
AFSP	American Foundation for Suicide Prevention
AFTA	American Family Therapy Association
AGPA	American Group Psychotherapy Association
AGS	American Geriatrics Society
AHA	American Heart Association
AHA	American Hospital Association
AHCA	American Health Care Association
AHCPR	Agency for Health Care Policy and Research (as of 1999, AHRQ)
AHRQ	Agency for Healthcare Research and Quality
AI	artificial intelligence
AIBS	American Institute of Biological Sciences
AIDS	acquired immunodeficiency syndrome
AIMS	Abnormal Involuntary Movement Scale
AIPP	American Institute for Psychotherapy and Psychoanalysis
AIS	American Institute of Stress
AIS	androgen insensitivity syndrome
AJP	*American Journal of Psychiatry*
ALS	amyotrophic lateral sclerosis
ALT	alanine aminotransferase (alanine transaminase)
AMA	against medical advice
AMA	American Medical Association
AMERSA	Association of Medical Education and Research in Substance Abuse
AMHA	Association of Mental Health Administrators
AMHC	Association of Mental Health Clergy

AMHCA	American Mental Health Counselors Association
AMHF	American Mental Health Foundation
AMHF	American Mental Health Fund
AMHL	Association of Mental Health Librarians
AMSA	American Medical Student Association
AMSAODD	American Medical Society on Alcoholism and Other Drug Dependencies
AMTA	American Music Therapy Association
AMWA	American Medical Women's Association
ANA	American Neurological Association
ANA	American Nurses' Association
ANFMP	Association of Nervous and Former Mental Patients (Recovery, Inc.)
ANS	autonomic nervous system
AOA	American Orthopsychiatric Association
AOTA	American Occupational Therapy Association
APA	American Psychiatric Association
APA	American Psychological Association
APAL	Asociación Psiquiátrica de America Latina
APM	Academy of Psychosomatic Medicine
APPA	American Psychopathological Association
APPI	American Psychiatric Publishing, Inc.
APPM	Association for Psychoanalytic and Psychosomatic Medicine
APS	American Psychosomatic Society
APsaA	American Psychoanalytic Association
ARC	Association for Retarded Citizens of the United States (as of 1992, The Arc of the United States)
ARNMD	Association for Research in Nervous and Mental Disease
ASA	American Schizophrenia Association
ASAP	American Society for Adolescent Psychiatry
ASF	American Schizophrenia Foundation
ASGPP	American Society of Group Psychotherapy and Psychodrama
ASHP	American Society of Hispanic Psychiatry

ASLM	American Society of Law and Medicine
ASPD	antisocial personality disorder
ASPP	American Society of Psychoanalytic Physicians
ATP	adenosine triphosphate
AWA	away without authorization
BDD	body dysmorphic disorder
BDI	Beck Depression Inventory
BDNF	brain-derived neurotrophic factor
BEAM	brain electrical activity mapping
bid	twice a day
BIS	Brain Information Service
BMA	British Medical Association
BMI	body mass index
BN	bulimia nervosa
BPA	Black Psychiatrists of America
BPD	borderline personality disorder
BPH	benign prostatic hyperplasia
BPP	brief psychodynamic psychotherapy
BPRS	Brief Psychiatric Rating Scale
BRF	Brain Research Foundation
BSI	Brief Symptom Inventory
BTRS	Behavior Therapy and Research Society
BUN	blood urea nitrogen
CA	Cocaine Anonymous
CAD	coronary artery disease
CARPA	Caribbean Psychiatric Association
CAT	Children's Apperception Test
CAT	cognitive analytic therapy
CAT	computerized axial tomography
CATIE	Clinical Antipsychotic Trials of Intervention Effectiveness
CBASP	Cognitive Behavioral Analysis System of Psychotherapy
CBF	cerebral blood flow
CBT	cognitive-behavioral therapy
CCA	Crime Control Act of 1984

CD	conduct disorder
CDC	Centers for Disease Control and Prevention
CDD	childhood disintegrative disorder
CERAD	Consortium to Establish a Registry for Alzheimer's Disease
CHADD	Children and Adults With Attention-Deficit/Hyperactivity Disorder
CIDI	Composite International Diagnostic Interview
CISD	critical incident stress debriefing
CLIA	Clinical Laboratory Improvement Amendments
CMA	Canadian Medical Association
CME	continuing medical education
CMHA	Canadian Mental Health Association
CMHC	community mental health center
CMS	Centers for Medicare and Medicaid Services
CMSS	Council of Medical Specialty Societies
CNS	central nervous system
CoDA	Co-Dependents Anonymous
Cognistat	Neurobehavioral Cognitive Status Examination
CPA	Canadian Psychiatric Association
CPDD	Committee on Problems of Drug Dependence
CPT	Current Procedural Terminology (AMA)
CPT	cognitive processing therapy
CRF	corticotropin-releasing factor
CRSD	circadian rhythm sleep disorder
CSF	cerebrospinal fluid
CT	computed tomography
CVA	cerebrovascular accident; stroke
CWLA	Child Welfare League of America
DAT	dementia of the Alzheimer's type
DBD	disruptive behavior disorder
DBH	dopamine beta-hydroxylase
DBS	deep brain stimulation
DBSA	Depression and Bipolar Support Alliance

DBT	dialectical behavior therapy
DES	Dissociative Experiences Scale
DHHS	Department of Health and Human Services
DID	dissociative identity disorder
DIPD-IV	Diagnostic Interview for DSM-IV Axis II Personality Disorders
DIS	Diagnostic Interview Schedule
DLB	dementia with Lewy bodies
DMH	Department of Mental Health/Department of Mental Hygiene
DNA	deoxyribonucleic acid
DOV	discharged on visit
DPD	dependent personality disorder
DRG	diagnosis-related group
DRS	Delirium Rating Scale
DRS-R-98	Delirium Rating Scale—Revised—98
DSM	*Diagnostic and Statistical Manual of Mental Disorders*
DST	dexamethasone suppression test
DT	delirium tremens
DTI	diffusion tensor imaging
EAP	employee assistance program
ECA	Epidemiologic Catchment Area
ECFMG	Educational Commission for Foreign Medical Graduates
ECG	electrocardiogram
ECT	electroconvulsive therapy
EE	expressed emotion
EEG	electroencephalogram
EFA	Epilepsy Foundation of America
EKG	electrocardiogram
EMDR	eye movement desensitization and reprocessing
EMG	electromyogram
EPS	extrapyramidal symptoms
ESP	extrasensory perception
EST	electroshock treatment

FDA	Food and Drug Administration
FDMD	Foundation for Depression and Manic Depression
FEAST	focal electrical alternating current seizure therapy
FEAT	focal electrical alternating current therapy
FTD	frontotemporal dementia
GA	Gamblers Anonymous
GABA	gamma-aminobutyric acid
GAD	generalized anxiety disorder
GAF	Global Assessment of Functioning
GAP	Group for the Advancement of Psychiatry
GCS	Glasgow Coma Scale
GDS	Geriatric Depression Scale
GID	gender identity disorder
GOAT	Galveston Orientation and Amnesia Test
GSR	galvanic skin response
GTP	guanosine triphosphate
Ham-D	Hamilton Rating Scale for Depression (also HRSD)
HCFA	Health Care Financing Administration (as of 2001, CMS)
HIBR	Huxley Institute for Biosocial Research
HIPAA	Health Insurance Portability and Accountability Act of 1996
HIV	human immunodeficiency virus
HMO	health maintenance organization
HPA	hypothalamic-pituitary-adrenal
HPG	hypothalamic-pituitary-gonadal
HPT	hypothalamic-pituitary-thyroid
HRSD	Hamilton Rating Scale for Depression (also Ham-D)
HRT	hormone replacement therapy
IACPO	Inter-American Council of Psychiatric Organizations
IALMH	International Academy of Law and Mental Health
IASP	International Association for Suicide Prevention
IASSID	International Association for the Scientific Study of Intellectual Disabilities
IASSMD	International Association for the Scientific Study of

	Mental Deficiency
ICAMI	International Committee Against Mental Illness
ICD	impulse-control disorder
ICD	*International Classification of Diseases*
ICSD	*International Classification of Sleep Disorders*
ICSW	International Council on Social Welfare
IDEA	Individuals With Disabilities Education Act
IEP	individualized education plan
IFMP	International Federation for Medical Psychotherapy
IFPS	International Federation of Psychoanalytic Societies
im	intramuscular
IND	investigational new drug
IOM	Institute of Medicine
IPDE	International Personality Disorder Examination
IPO	Inventory of Personality Organization
IPT	interpersonal (psycho)therapy
IQ	intelligence quotient
IRB	Institutional Review Board
ITAA	International Transactional Analysis Association
iv	intravenous
JCAHO	Joint Commission on Accreditation of Healthcare Organizations (as of 2007, The Joint Commission)
JCMHC	Joint Commission on Mental Health of Children
JCMIH	Joint Commission on Mental Illness and Health
JCPA	Joint Commission on Public Affairs (APA)
LBD	Lewy body dementia
LBV	Lewy body variant of Alzheimer's disease
LD	learning disorder
LDA	Learning Disabilities Association of America
LOC	loss of consciousness
LOS	length of stay (in hospital)
LP	lumbar puncture
LSD	lysergic acid diethylamide
MA	mental age

MAO	monoamine oxidase
MAOI	monoamine oxidase inhibitor
MCI	mild cognitive impairment
MCMI-III	Millon Clinical Multiaxial Inventory–III
MDA	methylenedioxyamphetamine
MDAS	Memorial Delirium Assessment Scale
MDD	major depressive disorder
MDI	manic-depressive illness
MDMA	3,4-methylenedioxymethamphetamine (Ecstasy)
MET	motivational enhancement therapy
MHA	Mental Health America
MINI	Mini-International Neuropsychiatric Inventory
MMPI	Minnesota Multiphasic Personality Inventory
MMPI-2	Minnesota Multiphasic Personality Inventory–2
MMR	measles-mumps-rubella
MMSE	Mini-Mental State Examination
MPQ	Multidimensional Personality Questionnaire
MRAA	Mental Retardation Association of America
MRI	magnetic resonance imaging
MRS	magnetic resonance spectroscopy
MS	multiple sclerosis
MSLT	multiple sleep latency test
NA	Narcotics Anonymous
NADS	National Association for Down Syndrome
NAIL	Neurotics Anonymous International Liaison
NAMH	National Association for Mental Health
NAMI	National Alliance on Mental Illness
NANAD	National Association of Anorexia Nervosa and Associated Disorders
NAPHS	National Association of Psychiatric Health Care Systems
NARC	National Association for Retarded Citizens
NARSAD	National Alliance for Research on Schizophrenia and Depression
NAS	National Academy of Sciences

NASMHPD	National Association of State Mental Health Program Directors
NaSSA	noradrenergic and specific serotonergic antidepressant
NASW	National Association of Social Workers
NAVACP	National Association of Veterans Affairs Chiefs of Psychiatry
NBME	National Board of Medical Examiners
NCADD	National Council on Alcoholism and Drug Dependence
NCADI	National Clearinghouse for Alcohol and Drug Information
NCCMHC	National Council of Community Mental Health Centers
NCD	National Council on Drugs
NCI	National Cancer Institute
NCOA	National Council on Aging
NCS	National Comorbidity Survey
NCS-R	National Comorbidity Survey Replication
NCSE	Neurobehavioral Cognitive Status Examination
NDI	nephrogenic diabetes insipidus
NDMDA	National Depressive and Manic-Depressive Association (as of 2002, DBSA)
NDRI	norepinephrine-dopamine reuptake inhibitor
NE	norepinephrine
NEMESIS	Netherlands Mental Health Survey and Incidence Study
NESARC	National Epidemiologic Survey on Alcohol and Related Conditions
NGCP	National Guild of Catholic Psychiatrists
NGF	nerve growth factor
NGRI	not guilty by reason of insanity
NHC	National Health Council
NIA	National Institute on Aging
NIAAA	National Institute on Alcohol Abuse and Alcoholism
NIDA	National Institute on Drug Abuse
NIH	National Institutes of Health
NIMH	National Institute of Mental Health
NINDS	National Institute of Neurological Disorders and Stroke
NLN	National League for Nursing

NMA	National Medical Association
NMDA	N-methyl-D-aspartate
NMHA	National Mental Health Association (as of 2007, MHA)
NMR	nuclear magnetic resonance
NMS	neuroleptic malignant syndrome
NOMIC	National Organization for Mentally Ill Children
NOS	not otherwise specified
NPT	nocturnal penile tumescence
NRA	National Rehabilitation Association
NRC	National Research Council
NREM	non–rapid eye movement
NRG1	neuregulin 1
NRI	norepinephrine reuptake inhibitor
NSAC	National Society for Autistic Children
NSAID	nonsteroidal anti-inflammatory drug
NSF	National Science Foundation
OBD	organic brain disease
OBS	organic brain syndrome
OCD	obsessive-compulsive disorder
OCPD	obsessive-compulsive personality disorder
ODD	oppositional defiant disorder
OSA	obstructive sleep apnea
PAI	Personality Assessment Inventory
PANDAS	pediatric autoimmune neuropsychiatric disorders associated with streptococcal infections
PANSS	Positive and Negative Syndrome Scale
PCL-R	Psychopathy Checklist–Revised
PCP	phencyclidine
PDD	pervasive developmental disorder
PDI-IV	Personality Disorder Interview–IV
PDQ-4	Personality Diagnostic Questionnaire–4
PDR	*Physicians' Desk Reference*
PET	positron emission tomography
PET	process–experiential therapy

PFC	prefrontal cortex
PKU	phenylketonuria
PLMD	periodic limb movement disorder
PMDD	premenstrual dysphoric disorder
PMS	premenstrual syndrome
PPD	postpartum depression
PRIDE	Parents' Resource Institute for Drug Education
PRO	peer review organization
PSD	poststroke depression
PSR	Physicians for Social Responsibility
PSRO	professional standards review organization
PTSD	posttraumatic stress disorder
PVN	paraventricular nucleus
qid	four times a day
RAD	reactive attachment disorder
RANZCP	Royal Australian and New Zealand College of Psychiatrists
RBD	REM sleep behavior disorder
rCBF	regional cerebral blood flow
RCP	Royal College of Psychiatrists
RCPSC	Royal College of Physicians and Surgeons of Canada
REM	rapid eye movement
RLS	restless legs syndrome
RNA	ribonucleic acid
RSM	Royal Society of Medicine
SA	Schizophrenics Anonymous
SAD	seasonal affective disorder
SAD	separation anxiety disorder
SAMHSA	Substance Abuse and Mental Health Services Administration
SARI	serotonin antagonist and reuptake inhibitor
SBM	Society of Behavioral Medicine
SBP	Society of Biological Psychiatry
SCAN	Schedule for Clinical Assessment in Neuropsychiatry
SCHIP	State Children's Health Insurance Program

SCID	Structured Clinical Interview for DSM-IV
SCID-CV	Structured Clinical Interview for DSM-IV Axis I Disorders, Clinician Version
SCID-I	Structured Clinical Interview for DSM-IV Axis I Disorders
SCID-I/NP	Structured Clinical Interview for DSM-IV Axis I Disorders, Non-Patient Edition
SCID-II	Structured Clinical Interview for DSM-IV Axis II Personality Disorders
SCL-90-R	Symptom Checklist–90–Revised
SCN	suprachiasmatic nucleus
SDA	serotonin-dopamine antagonist
SDAT	senile dementia of the Alzheimer's type
SES	socioeconomic status
SIB	self-injurious behavior
SIECUS	Sexuality Information and Education Council of the United States
SMA	Southern Medical Association
SMD	stereotypic movement disorder
SNAP	Schedule for Nonadaptive and Adaptive Personality
SNP	single-nucleotide polymorphism
SNRI	serotonin-norepinephrine reuptake inhibitor
SNS	Society for Neuroscience
SPA	Southern Psychiatric Association
SPCP	Society of Professors of Child Psychiatry
SPECT	single photon emission computed tomography
SPEM	smooth pursuit eye movements
SRS	Sleep Research Society
SSI/SSDI	Social Security Insurance/Social Security Disability Insurance
SSRI	selective serotonin reuptake inhibitor
STAR*D	Sequenced Treatment Alternatives to Relieve Depression
SVZ	subventricular zone
TBI	traumatic brain injury
TCA	tricyclic antidepressant
TGA	transient global amnesia

TIA	transient ischemic attack
tid	three times a day
TLDP	time-limited dynamic psychotherapy
TM	transcendental meditation
TMS	transcranial magnetic stimulation
TRH	thyrotropin-releasing hormone
TSH	thyroid-stimulating hormone
USPHS	U.S. Public Health Service
VA	Veterans Affairs (formerly Veterans Administration)
VaD	vascular dementia
VCFS	velocardiofacial syndrome
VNS	vagus nerve stimulation
WAPR	World Association for Psychosocial Rehabilitation
WASP	World Association for Social Psychiatry
WBC	white blood cell
WCST	Wisconsin Card Sorting Test
WFMH	World Federation for Mental Health
WHO	World Health Organization
WIS	Wechsler Intelligence Scale
WMA	World Medical Association
WMS	Wechsler Memory Scale
WPA	World Psychiatric Association
WPI-IV	Wisconsin Personality Disorders Inventory–IV
Y-BOCS	Yale-Brown Obsessive-Compulsive Scale

Medications Used in Psychiatry

Generic name	Brand name*
ANTIANXIETY MEDICATIONS	
Benzodiazepines	
alprazolam	Xanax, Xanax XR
chlordiazepoxide	Librium
clonazepam	Klonopin
clorazepate	Tranxene
diazepam	Valium
lorazepam	Ativan
oxazepam	Serax (D)
Nonbenzodiazepine	
buspirone	BuSpar
MEDICATIONS FOR INSOMNIA	
Benzodiazepines	
estazolam	ProSom (D)
flurazepam	Dalmane
quazepam	Doral
temazepam	Restoril
triazolam	Halcion
Nonbenzodiazepines	
eszopiclone	Lunesta
meprobamate	Equanil (D); Miltown (D)
ramelteon	Rozerem
trazodone	Desyrel (D)
zaleplon	Sonata
zolpidem	Ambien, Ambien CR

*D = discontinued. Generic formulations are available for many of the medications listed.

Generic name	Brand name*
ANTIDEPRESSANTS	

Tricyclic Antidepressants (TCAs)

amitriptyline	Elavil (D); Endep (D)
amitriptyline/perphenazine combination	Etrafon (D); Triavil (D)
clomipramine	Anafranil
desipramine	Norpramin
doxepin	Adapin (D); Sinequan (D)
imipramine	Tofranil, Tofranil-PM
nortriptyline	Aventyl; Pamelor
protriptyline	Vivactil
trimipramine	Surmontil

Tetracyclic Antidepressants (TeCAs)

amoxapine	Asendin (D)
maprotiline	Ludiomil (D)

Monoamine Oxidase Inhibitors (MAOIs)

isocarboxazid	Marplan
phenelzine	Nardil
selegiline	Eldepryl
selegiline transdermal patch	EMSAM
tranylcypromine	Parnate

Selective Serotonin Reuptake Inhibitors (SSRIs)

citalopram	Celexa
escitalopram oxalate	Lexapro
fluoxetine	Prozac, Prozac Weekly
fluvoxamine	Luvox, Luvox CR
paroxetine hydrochloride	Paxil, Paxil CR
paroxetine mesylate	Pexeva
sertraline	Zoloft

Atypical Antipsychotic/SSRI Combination

olanzapine/fluoxetine combination	Symbyax

*D = discontinued. Generic formulations are available for many of the medications listed.

Generic name	Brand name*
Serotonin–Norepinephrine Reuptake Inhibitors (SNRIs)	
desvenlafaxine	Pristiq
duloxetine	Cymbalta
milnacipran	Savella
venlafaxine	Effexor, Effexor XR
Noradrenergic and Specific Serotonergic Antidepressant (NaSSA)	
mirtazapine	Remeron
Serotonin Antagonist and Reuptake Inhibitors (SARIs)	
nefazodone	Serzone (D)
trazodone	Desyrel (D)
Other	
bupropion	Wellbutrin, Wellbutrin SR, Wellbutrin XL; Zyban

MOOD STABILIZERS

Anticonvulsants

carbamazepine	Tegretol, Tegretol-XR
carbamazepine extended release	Equetro
divalproex sodium	Depakote, Depakote ER, Depakote Sprinkle
gabapentin	Neurontin
lamotrigine	Lamictal, Lamictal XR
oxcarbazepine	Trileptal
phenytoin/diphenylhydantoin	Dilantin
pregabalin (also used for neuropathic pain)	Lyrica
topiramate	Topamax, Topamax Sprinkle
valproic acid	Depakene
valproic acid delayed release	Stavzor
valproate sodium injection	Depacon

*D = discontinued. Generic formulations are available for many of the medications listed.

Generic name	Brand name*

Lithium Carbonate and Lithium Citrate

lithium carbonate	Eskalith (D), Eskalith CR (D)
lithium carbonate extended release	Lithobid
lithium citrate	—

ANTIPSYCHOTICS

First-Generation (Conventional) Antipsychotics

chlorpromazine	Thorazine (D)
fluphenazine	Prolixin (D)
fluphenazine decanoate	Prolixin Decanoate (D)
fluphenazine lactate injection	Prolixin Injection (D)
haloperidol	Haldol
haloperidol lactate injection	Haldol Injection
haloperidol decanoate	Haldol Decanoate
loxapine	Loxitane (D)
perphenazine	Trilafon (D)
perphenazine/amitriptyline combination	Etrafon (D); Triavil (D)
pimozide	Orap
thioridazine	Mellaril (D)
thiothixene	Navane
trifluoperazine	Stelazine (D)

Second-Generation (Atypical) Antipsychotics

aripiprazole	Abilify, Abilify DiscMelt
asenapine	Saphris
clozapine	Clozaril; FazaClo
iloperidone	Fanapt
olanzapine	Zyprexa, Zyprexa Zydis, Zyprexa IntraMuscular, Zyprexa Relprevv
paliperidone	Invega, Invega Sustenna
quetiapine	Seroquel, Seroquel XR
risperidone	Risperdal, Risperdal M-Tab, Risperdal Consta
ziprasidone	Geodon

*D = discontinued. Generic formulations are available for many of the medications listed.

Generic name	Brand name*

MEDICATIONS FOR ADHD AND NARCOLEPSY

Stimulants

amphetamine/dextroamphetamine combination	Adderall, Adderall XR
dextroamphetamine	Dexedrine (D), Dexedrine Spansules (D); DextroStat (D)
dexmethylphenidate immediate and extended release	Focalin, Focalin XR
lisdexamfetamine	Vyvanse
methamphetamine	Desoxyn
methylphenidate immediate release	Methylin; Ritalin
methylphenidate extended release	Concerta Metadate CD, Metadate ER; Methylin ER; Ritalin LA, Ritalin SR
methylphenidate transdermal patch	Daytrana

Nonstimulant Wakefulness-Promoting Agents

armodafinil	Nuvigil
atomoxetine	Strattera
modafinil	Provigil

MEDICATIONS TO IMPROVE COGNITION IN DEMENTIA

Acetylcholinesterase Inhibitors

donepezil	Aricept
galantamine	Razadyne, Razadyne ER
rivastigmine	Exelon
rivastigmine transdermal patch	Exelon Transdermal Patch
tacrine	Cognex

NMDA Receptor Antagonist

memantine	Namenda, Namenda XR

---

*D = discontinued. Generic formulations are available for many of the medications listed.

Generic name	Brand name*

MEDICATIONS FOR ALCOHOL/SUBSTANCE DEPENDENCE

Agents to Treat Opioid Addiction

buprenorphine injection	Buprenex
buprenorphine sublingual	Subutex
buprenorphine transdermal patch	Butrans
buprenorphine/naloxone combination sublingual	Suboxone
methylnaltrexone injection	Relistor
naloxone injection	Narcan (D)
naltrexone injection	Vivitrol
naltrexone oral	Depade (D), ReVia
pentazocine	Talwin

Agents to Promote Abstinence From Alcohol

acamprosate	Campral
disulfiram	Antabuse

Agents for Smoking Cessation

bupropion	Zyban
varenicline	Chantix

OTHER MEDICATIONS THAT PSYCHIATRISTS MAY PRESCRIBE

Agents to Treat Medication-Induced Parkinsonian and Acute Motor Symptoms

Anticholinergics

benztropine injection	Cogentin
biperiden	Akineton
trihexyphenidyl	Artane (D)

Antihistamines

diphenhydramine	Benadryl
hydroxyzine hydrochloride	Atarax (D)
hydroxyzine pamoate	Vistaril

NMDA receptor antagonist

amantadine	Symmetrel (D)

*D = discontinued. Generic formulations are available for many of the medications listed.

Generic name	Brand name*
Agents to Treat Erectile Dysfunction	
sildenafil	Viagra
tadalafil	Cialis
vardenafil	Levitra, Staxyn
Agent to Augment Antidepressant Treatment	
liothyronine (triiodothyronine [T₃]) (synthetic thyroid hormone)	Cytomel
Antihypertensive Agents With Psychiatric Uses	
clonidine (used in ADHD to treat insomnia secondary to stimulants)	Catapres, Catapres-TTS (transdermal patch)
guanfacine (used in ADHD as alternative to stimulants)	Intuniv (extended-release formulation)
prazosin (used to treat PTSD symptoms)	Minipress
propranolol (used to treat performance anxiety and agitation/aggression)	Inderal, Inderal LA

*D = discontinued. Generic formulations are available for many of the medications listed.

Psychiatric Measures

Diagnostic Measures for Adults

Composite International Diagnostic Interview (CIDI)
Diagnostic Interview Schedule (DIS)
Diagnostic Interview Schedule–IV (DIS-IV)
Mini International Neuropsychiatric Interview (MINI)
Patient Health Questionnaire (PHQ)
Psychiatric Diagnostic Screening Questionnaire (PDSQ)
Schedules for Clinical Assessment in Neuropsychiatry (SCAN)
Structured Clinical Interview for DSM-IV Axis I Disorders (SCID-I)

General Psychiatric Symptoms Measures

Behavior and Symptom Identification Scale (BASIS-32 and BASIS-24)
Brief Symptom Inventory (BSI)
General Health Questionnaire (GHQ)
Holden Psychological Screening Inventory (HPSI)
Mental Health Inventory (MHI)
Minnesota Multiphasic Personality Inventory (MMPI, MMPI-2, and MMPI-A)
Symptom Checklist–90—Revised (SCL-90-R)

This list of tests was obtained from Rush AJ, First MB, Blacker D (eds): *Handbook of Psychiatric Measures,* Second Edition. Washington, DC, American Psychiatric Publishing, 2008.

Mental Health Status, Functioning, and Disabilities Measures

Clinical Global Impression (CGI) Scale
Global Assessment Scale (GAS), Global Assessment of Functioning (GAF) Scale, Social and Occupational Functioning Assessment Scale (SOFAS)
Health of the Nation Outcome Scales (HoNOS)
Life Skills Profile (LSP)
Sheehan Disability Scale
Social Adjustment Scale (SAS)
World Health Organization Disability Assessment Schedule II (WHO-DAS II)

General Health Status, Functioning, and Disabilities Measures

Dartmouth Primary Care Cooperative Information Project Functional Assessment Charts (COOP Charts)
Duke Health Profile (DUKE)
Karnofsky Performance Status (KPS)
Katz Index of Independence in Activities of Daily Living (Katz ADL)
Lawton Instrumental Activities of Daily Living Scale (Lawton IADL)
Short-Form 36-Item Health Survey (SF-36)

Quality of Life Measures

Psychosocial Adjustment to Illness Scale (PAIS)
Quality of Life Enjoyment and Satisfaction Questionnaire (Q-LES-Q)
Quality of Life Index (QLI)
Quality of Life Interview
Quality of Life Inventory
Quality of Life Scale (QLS)
Spitzer Quality of Life Index (Spitzer QL-Index)
Wisconsin Quality of Life Index (W-QLI)
World Health Organization Quality of Life Scales (WHOQOL-100 and WHOQOL-BREF)

Adverse Effects Measures

Abnormal Involuntary Movement Scale (AIMS)

Arizona Sexual Experience Scale (ASEX)

Barnes Akathisia Rating Scale (BARS)

Frequency, Intensity, and Burden of Side Effects Rating (FIBSER)

MedWatch

Rating Scale for Extrapyramidal Side Effects or Simpson-Angus Extrapyramidal Side Effects (EPS) Scale

Systematic Assessment for Treatment Emergent Events—General Inquiry (SAFTEE-GI)

Udvalg for Kliniske Undersogelser (UKU) Side Effect Rating Scale

Patient Perceptions of Care Measures

Charleston Psychiatric Outpatient Satisfaction Scale (CPOSS)

Client Satisfaction Questionnaire–8 (CSQ-8)

Multidimensional Adolescent Satisfaction Scale (MASS)

Parent Satisfaction Scale (PSS)

Patient Satisfaction Questionnaire (PSQ-II; PSQ-III)

Perceptions of Care (PoC)

Working Alliance Inventory (WAI)

Stress and Life Events Measures

Coddington Life Events Scales (CLES)

Daily Hassles Scale

Derogatis Stress Profile (DSP)

Job Content Questionnaire (JCQ)

Life Events Scales for Children and Adolescents

Life Experiences Survey (LES)

Perceived Stress Scale (PSS)

Recent Life Changes Questionnaire (RLCQ)

Family Risk Factors Measures

Conflict Behavior Questionnaire (CBQ)
Conflict Tactics Scales (CTS)
Dyadic Adjustment Scale (DAS)
Family Assessment Device (FAD)
Family Assessment Measure III (FAM-III)
Parental Bonding Instrument (PBI)
Parenting Stress Index (PSI)
Perceived Criticism Measure (PCM)

Suicide Risk Measures

Beck Hopelessness Scale (BHS)
Beck Scale for Suicide Ideation (BSS); Scale for Suicide Ideation (SSI)
Columbia Suicide History Form (CSHF)
Harkavy Asnis Suicide Survey (HASS)
Suicide Intent Scale (SIS)

Child and Adolescent Measures for Diagnosis and Screening

Scales for Infants, Toddlers, and Preschool-Age Children

Bayley Scales of Infant Development—Second Edition (BSID II)
Infant-Toddler Social and Emotional Assessment (ITSEA); Brief ITSEA
    (BITSEA)
Denver Developmental Screening Test II (DDST-II)

Scales for School-Age Children and Adolescents

Anchored Brief Psychiatric Rating Scale for Children (BPRS-C)
Behavior Assessment System for Children, Second Edition (BASC-2)
Child and Adolescent Psychiatric Assessment (CAPA)
Child Behavior Checklists (CBCL/1.5–5 and CBCL/6–18), Teacher Report Form (TRF); Youth Self Report (YSR)

Diagnostic Interview for Children and Adolescents–IV (DICA-IV)

MacArthur Health and Behavior Questionnaire (HBQ)

National Institute of Mental Health Diagnostic Interview Schedule for Children (NIMH-DISC)

Patient Health Questionnaire for Adolescents (PHQ-A)

Preschool Age Psychiatric Assessment (PAPA)

Schedule for Affective Disorders and Schizophrenia for School-Aged Children: Present and Lifetime Version (K-SADS-PL)

Symptom-Specific Measures for Disorders Usually First Diagnosed in Infancy, Childhood, or Adolescence

Anxiety Disorders Interview Schedule for DSM-IV—Child Version (ADIS-IV-C)

Autism Diagnostic Interview—Revised (ADI-R)

Children's Depression Inventory (CDI)

Conners' Rating Scales—Revised (CRS-R)

Eyberg Child Behavior Inventory (ECBI)

Multidimensional Anxiety Scale for Children (MASC)

New York Teacher Rating Scale (NYTRS)

Reynolds Adolescent Depression Scale, 2nd Edition (RADS-2)

Screen for Child Anxiety Related Emotional Disorders (SCARED)

Yale Global Tic Severity Scale (YGTSS)

Child and Adolescent Measures of Functional Status

Global Measures of Functioning

Child and Adolescent Functional Assessment Scale (CAFAS)

Children's Global Assessment Scale (CGAS)

Columbia Impairment Scale (CIS)

Health of the Nation Outcome Scales for Children and Adolescents (HoNOSCA)

Youth Outcome Questionnaire (Y-OQ)

Unidimensional Measures of Functioning

Cognitive Functioning
Peabody Picture Vocabulary Test, Fourth Edition (PPVT-4)
Wechsler Individual Achievement Test—Second Edition (WIAT-II)
Wide Range Achievement Test 4 (WRAT4)

Social Functioning
Behavioral and Emotional Rating Scale, Second Edition (BERS-2)
Competence Scale of the Child Behavior Checklist (CBCL/6-18)
Social Skills Scale of the Social Skills Rating System (SSRS)

Self-Care and Independence
Vineland Adaptive Behavior Scales, Second Edition (Vineland-II)

Self-Concept and Self-Esteem
Self-Description Questionnaire (SDQ)

Measures for Delirium and the Behavioral Symptoms of Cognitive Disorders

Apathy Evaluation Scale (AES)
Behavior Pathology in Alzheimer's Disease Rating Scale (BEHAVE-AD)
Burden Interview (BI)
Confusion Assessment Method (CAM)
Cornell Scale for Depression in Dementia (CSDD)
Delirium Rating Scale (DRS)
Neuropsychiatric Inventory (NPI)
Psychogeriatric Dependency Rating Scale (PGDRS)
Screen for Caregiver Burden (SCB)

Neuropsychiatric Measures for Cognitive Disorders

Alzheimer's Disease Assessment Scale (ADAS)
Clinical Dementia Rating (CDR) Scale

Clock Drawing Test
Cognistat
CogState
Dementia Rating Scale (DRS)
Galveston Orientation and Amnesia Test (GOAT)
The GDS Staging System: Global Deterioration Scale (GDS), Brief Cognitive Rating Scale (BCRS), and Functional Assessment Staging (FAST)
Mini-Mental State Exam (MMSE)
National Institute on Aging (NIA) Alzheimer's Disease Center Uniform Data Set (UDS) cognitive test battery

Substance Use Disorders Measures

Screening and Case-Finding Measures

Alcohol Use Disorders Identification Test (AUDIT)
CAGE Questionnaire
CRAFFT Questionnaire
Drug Abuse Screening Test (DAST)
Fagerstrom Test for Nicotine Dependence (FTND)
Michigan Alcoholism Screening Test (MAST)
Personal Experience Screening Questionnaire (PESQ)
TWEAK Test

Treatment Planning and Monitoring Measures

Addiction Severity Index (ASI)
Alcohol Dependence Scale (ADS)
Alcohol Expectancy Questionnaire (AEQ)
Clinical Institute Withdrawal Assessment for Alcohol (CIWA-AD)
Drinker Inventory of Consequences (DrInC)
Obsessive Compulsive Drinking Scale (OCDS)
Stages of Change Readiness and Treatment Eagerness Scale (SOCRATES)
Timeline Followback (TLFB)
University of Rhode Island Change Assessment (URICA)

Psychotic Disorders Measures

Brief Psychiatric Rating Scale (BPRS)
Calgary Depression Scale for Schizophrenia (CDSS)
Clinician Alcohol Use Scale (AUS); Clinician Drug Use Scale (DUS)
Drug Attitude Inventory (DAI)
Insight and Treatment Attitudes Questionnaire (ITAQ)
Insight Scale (IS)
Positive and Negative Syndrome Scale (PANSS)
Scale for the Assessment of Positive Symptoms (SAPS); Scale for the
    Assessment of Negative Symptoms (SANS)
Schedule for the Deficit Syndrome (SDS)

Mood Disorders Measures

Depression Rating Scales for General Psychiatric or Community Populations

Beck Depression Inventory (BDI)
Center for Epidemiologic Studies Depression Scale (CES-D)
Hamilton Rating Scale for Depression (Ham-D)
Inventory of Depressive Symptomatology (IDS); Quick Inventory of
    Depressive Symptomatology (QIDS)
Montgomery-Åsberg Depression Rating Scale (MADRS)
Zung Self-Rating Depression Scale (Zung SDS)

Mania Rating Scales

Clinician-Administered Rating Scale for Mania (CARS-M)
Mood Disorder Questionnaire (MDQ)
Young Mania Rating Scale (YMRS)

Depression Rating Scales for Use in Special Populations

Edinburgh Postnatal Depression Scale (EPDS)
Geriatric Depression Scale (GDS)
Hospital Anxiety and Depression Scale (HADS)

Anxiety Disorders Measures

General Anxiety and Mixed Anxiety Disorder Measures

Beck Anxiety Inventory (BAI)
Fear Questionnaire (FQ)
Hamilton Anxiety Rating Scale (HARS)

Panic Disorder and Agoraphobia

Anxiety Sensitivity Index (ASI)
Mobility Inventory for Agoraphobia (MI)
Panic Disorder Severity Scale (PDSS)

Social Phobia

Brief Social Phobia Scale (BSPS)
Liebowitz Social Anxiety Scale (LSAS)
Social Phobia and Anxiety Inventory (SPAI)

Obsessive-Compulsive Disorder

Yale-Brown Obsessive Compulsive Scale (Y-BOCS)
Padua Inventory (PI)

Posttraumatic Stress Disorder

Clinician-Administered PTSD Scale (CAPS)
Impact of Event Scale (IES)
Posttraumatic Stress Diagnostic Scale (PDS)

Generalized Anxiety Disorder

Penn State Worry Questionnaire (PSWQ)

Somatoform and Fictitious Disorders and Malingering Measures

Body Dysmorphic Disorder Examination (BDDE)
Brief Pain Inventory (BPI)
Illness Attitude Scale (IAS)
McGill Pain Questionnaire (MPQ)
Somatoform Disorders Symptom Checklist; Screener for Somatoform Disorders; Somatoform Disorders Schedule (SDS)
Structured Interview of Reported Symptoms (SIRS)
Visual Analog Scales
West Haven–Yale Multidimensional Pain Inventory (WHYMPI)
Whiteley Index of Hypochondriasis
Wong-Baker FACES Pain Rating Scale
Yale-Brown Obsessive Compulsive Scale Modified for Body Dysmorphic Disorder (BDD-YBOCS)

Dissociative Disorders Measures

Child Dissociative Checklist (CDC)
Dissociative Disorders Interview Schedule (DDIS)
Dissociative Experiences Scale (DES)
Structured Clinical Interview for DSM-IV Dissociative Disorders—Revised (SCID-D-R)

Measures of Sexual Dysfunction and Disorders

Brief Male Sexual Function Inventory (BMSFI)
Center for Marital and Sexual Health Sexual Functioning Questionnaire (CMSH-SFQ)
Changes in Sexual Functioning Questionnaire (CSFQ)
Derogatis Interview for Sexual Functioning (DISF)
Derogatis Sexual Functioning Inventory (DSFI)
Female Sexual Distress Scale (FSDS)
Female Sexual Function Index (FSFI)
Golombok Rust Inventory of Sexual Satisfaction (GRISS)

International Index of Erectile Functioning (IIEF)
Profile of Female Sexual Function (PFSF)
Sexual Function Questionnaire (SFQ)

Eating Disorders Measures

Binge Eating Scale (BES)
Body Shape Questionnaire (BSQ)
Bulimia Test—Revised (BULIT-R)
Eating Attitudes Test (EAT)
Eating Disorder Examination (EDE)
Eating Disorder Inventory–3 (EDI-3)
Mizes Anorectic Cognitions (MAC) Questionnaire
Questionnaire on Eating and Weight Patterns—Revised (QEWP-R)
Three-Factor Eating Questionnaire (TFEQ) or Eating Inventory
Yale-Brown-Cornell Eating Disorder Scale (YBC-EDS)

Sleep Disorders Measures

Epworth Sleepiness Scale (ESS)
Insomnia Severity Index (ISI)
International Restless Legs Syndrome Study Group Rating Scale (IRLS)
Pittsburgh Sleep Quality Index (PSQI)
Sleep logs or diaries
Women's Health Initiative Insomnia Rating Scale (WHIIRS)

Impulse-Control Disorders Measures

Barratt Impulsiveness Scale, Version 11 (BIS-11)
Gambling Symptom Assessment Scale (G-SAS)
Kleptomania Symptom Assessment Scale (K-SAS)
Massachusetts General Hospital (MGH) Hairpulling Scale
Pathological Gambling Modification of the Yale-Brown Obsessive Com-
    pulsive Scale (PG-YBOCS)
Psychiatric Institute Trichotillomania Scale (PITS)
South Oaks Gambling Screen (SOGS)
State-Trait Anger Expression Inventory (STAXI)

Personality Disorders, Personality Traits, and Defense Mechanisms Measures

Semistructured Interviews for DSM-IV Personality Disorders

Diagnostic Interview for DSM-IV Personality Disorders (DIPD-IV)
International Personality Disorder Examination (IPDE)
Personality Disorder Interview–IV (PDI-IV)
Structured Clinical Interview for DSM-IV Axis II Personality Disorders (SCID-II)
Structured Interview for DSM-IV Personality (SIDP-IV)

Semistructured Interviews for Specific Personality Disorders

Diagnostic Interview for Borderline Patients (DIB); Revised Diagnostic Interview for Borderlines (DIB-R)
Hare Psychopathy Checklist—Revised (PCL-R)

Questionnaires for All Personality Disorders

Personality Diagnostic Questionnaire–4 (PDQ-4)
Millon Clinical Multiaxial Inventory–III (MCMI-III)
Minnesota Multiphasic Personality Inventory–2 Personality Disorder (MMPI-2 PD) Scales
Schedule for Nonadaptive and Adaptive Personality (SNAP)

Assessments for Personality Traits

Dimensional Assessment of Personality Pathology—Basic Questionnaire (DAPP-BQ)
Personality Assessment Inventory (PAI)
NEO Personality Inventory—Revised (NEO-PI-R)
Shedler-Westen Assessment Procedure–200 (SWAP-200)

Questionnaire for Defense Mechanisms

Defense Style Questionnaire (DSQ)

Aggression Measures

Aggression Questionnaire (AQ)
Life History of Aggression (LHA)
Overt-Aggression Scale—Modified (OAS-M)
State-Trait Anger Expression Inventory–2 (STAXI-2)

Legal Terms

action   A lawsuit brought by one or more parties. See CIVIL ACTION.

actus reus   The "bad act," which when proved beyond a reasonable doubt, produces criminal liability. The legal use of the phrase denotes one of the elements that must be proven by the prosecution before anyone can be liable for criminal punishment. The *actus reus* element is the act made criminal by some statute or other valid source of criminal law. Contrast with *MENS REA*.

adjudication   The formal pronouncement of a JUDGMENT or decree in a CAUSE OF ACTION.

advance directive   A method for individuals while competent to appoint PROXY health care decision makers in the event of future incompetency. A legal document that allows one to convey decisions about end-of-life care. See DURABLE POWER OF ATTORNEY; HEALTH CARE PROXY; LIVING WILL.

assault   Any willful attempt or threat to inflict injury.

battery   Intentional and wrongful physical contact with an individual without consent that causes some injury or offensive touching.

best interests of the child   General standard applied by courts to determine the "care and custody of minor children." Different states consider different factors relevant in defining what constitutes a "child's best interests." Some of the more common factors include the mental and physical health of all individuals involved (e.g., child, parents); the wishes of the child as to his or her choice of custodian; and the interaction and degree of "psychological connectedness" between the child and the proposed custodian.

beyond a reasonable doubt   The level of proof required to convict a person in a criminal trial. Of the three legal standards of proof, this is the highest level (90%–95% range of certainty) and the one required to establish the guilt of someone accused of a crime. See also CLEAR AND CONVINCING EVIDENCE; PREPONDERANCE OF THE EVIDENCE.

breach of contract   A violation of or failure to perform any or all of the terms of an agreement.

SMALL CAPS type indicates terms defined as main entries elsewhere in this glossary.

brief   A written statement prepared by legal counsel arguing a case.

burden of proof   The legal obligation to prove affirmatively a disputed fact related to an issue that is raised by the parties in a case.

capacity   The status or attributes necessary for a person so that his or her acts may be legally allowed and recognized.

case law   The aggregate of reported cases as forming a body of law on a particular subject.

cause in fact   The requirement of fact that without the defendant's wrongful conduct, the harm to the plaintiff would not have occurred.

cause of action   The grounds of an ACTION; that is, those facts that, if alleged and proved in a suit, would enable the PLAINTIFF to attain a JUDGMENT.

civil action   A lawsuit brought by a private individual or group to recover money or property, to enforce or protect a civil RIGHT, or to prevent or redress a civil wrong.

civil commitment   A process in which a judge decides whether a person who is alleged to be mentally ill should be required to go to a psychiatric hospital or accept other mental health treatment.

civil law   As contrasted with criminal law, a system for enforcement of private rights arising from sources such as torts and contracts.

clear and convincing evidence   The second-highest standard applied to determining whether alleged facts have been proven (75% range of certainty). This is the standard applied to civil commitment matters and similar circumstances in which there is the chance that valued civil liberty interests and freedoms are at stake. See also BEYOND A REASONABLE DOUBT; PREPONDERANCE OF THE EVIDENCE.

commitment   A legal process for admitting, usually involuntarily, a mentally ill person to a psychiatric treatment program. Although the legal definition and procedure vary from state to state, commitment usually requires a court or judicial procedure. Commitment also may be voluntary.

common law   A system of law based on customs, traditional usage, and prior CASE LAW rather than on codified written laws (STATUTES).

compensatory damages   DAMAGES awarded to a person as compensation, indemnity, or restitution for harm sustained.

competency   The mental CAPACITY to understand the nature of an act. See also COMPETENCY TO STAND TRIAL; INFORMED CONSENT; TESTAMENTARY CAPACITY.

competency to stand trial   Legal test applied to all criminal DEFEN-
DANTS regarding their cognitive ability at the time of trial to participate in the proceedings against them. As held in *Dusky v. United
States* (1960), a defendant is competent to stand trial if 1) he or she
possesses a factual understanding of the proceedings against him or
her, and 2) he or she has sufficient present ability to consult with his
or her lawyer with a reasonable degree of rational understanding.

confidentiality   The situation in which certain communications between persons who are in a FIDUCIARY or trust relationship to each
other (e.g., physician-patient) are generally not legally permitted to
be disclosed and are not admissible as evidence in court during a
trial. See also PRIVILEGED COMMUNICATION.

consent decree   Agreement by a DEFENDANT to cease activities as-
serted as illegal by the government without admitting fault or guilt.

conservatorship   The appointment of a person to manage and make
decisions on behalf of an incompetent person regarding the latter's
estate (e.g., authority to make CONTRACTS or sell property). See also
GUARDIANSHIP; INCOMPETENCE.

consortium   The RIGHT of a husband or wife to the care, affection,
company, and cooperation of the other spouse in every aspect of the
marital relationship.

contract   A legally enforceable agreement between two or more parties to do or not do a particular thing on sufficient consideration.

criminal law   The branch of the law that defines crimes and provides for their punishment. Unlike civil law, penalties include imprisonment.

damages   A sum of money awarded to a person injured by the unlawful act or NEGLIGENCE of another.

de facto   Something that is in fact, in deed, or actually in effect, especially without authority of law. Compare with *DE JURE*.

defendant   A person or legal entity against whom a claim or charge
is brought.

de jure   Something that is considered "lawful," "rightful," "legitimate,"
or "just." Compare with *DE FACTO*.

diminished capacity   Refers to insufficient cognitive ability to
achieve the state of mind (*MENS REA*) requisite for the commission of
a crime. Sometimes referred to as "partial INSANITY," this doctrine permits a court to consider the impaired mental state of the DEFENDANT

for purposes of reducing punishment or lowering the degree of the offense being charged.

doli incapax   Literally, "incapable of crime." The presumption, for instance, that children are incapable of committing criminal acts and as such, cannot be held legally responsible for their actions.

due process (of law)   The constitutional guarantee protecting individuals from arbitrary and unreasonable actions by the government that would deprive them of their basic RIGHTS to life, liberty, or property.

durable power of attorney   A person designated by another to act as his or her attorney-in-fact regardless of whether the principal eventually becomes incompetent. This is prescribed statutorily in all 50 states. See also ADVANCE DIRECTIVE; HEALTH CARE PROXY; LIVING WILL.

duress   Compulsion or constraint, as by force or threat, exercised to make a person do or say something against his or her will.

duty   Legal obligation that one person owes another. Whenever one person has a RIGHT, another person has a corresponding duty to preserve or not interfere with that right.

duty to warn   The responsibility of a counselor or therapist to breach confidentiality if a client or other identifiable person is in clear or imminent danger. See *TARASOFF* RULE.

emancipated minor   A person younger than 18 years who is considered totally self-supporting. Legal RIGHTS afforded at adulthood are typically extended to an emancipated minor.

entitlement program   In health law, legislatively defined rights to health care, such as Medicare and Medicaid programs.

expert testimony   Testimony about a scientific, technical, or professional issue given by a person qualified to testify because of familiarity with the subject or special training in the field.

expert witness   One who by reason of specialized education, experience, and/or training possesses superior knowledge about a subject that is beyond the understanding of an average or ordinary layperson. Expert witnesses are permitted to offer opinions about matters relevant to their expertise that will assist a jury in comprehending evidence that they would otherwise not understand or fully appreciate.

false imprisonment   The unlawful restraint or detention of one person by another.

fiduciary   A person who acts for another in a capacity that involves a confidence or trust.

forensic psychiatry   A subspecialty of psychiatry in which scientific and clinical expertise is applied to legal issues in legal contexts embracing civil, criminal, correctional, or legislative matters.

fraud   Any act of trickery, deceit, or misrepresentation designed to deprive someone of property or to do harm.

***Gault* decision**   A landmark Supreme Court decision in 1967 that found that juveniles were entitled to the same DUE PROCESS RIGHTS as adults—that is, the right to counsel, the right to notice of specific charges of the offense, the right to confront and cross-examine a witness, the right to remain silent, and the right to SUBPOENA witnesses in defense. The right to trial by jury was not included.

guardian *ad litem*   Literally, "guardian at law." A person who has the legal authority (and the corresponding duty) to care for the personal and property interests of another person, called a *ward*. Usually, a person has the status of guardian because the ward is incapable of caring for his or her own interests due to infancy, incapacity, or disability.

guardianship   The delegation, by the state, of authority over an individual's person or estate to another party. For example, a personal guardian for a mentally ill patient would have the legal RIGHT to make medical decisions on behalf of the patient.

habeas corpus   Latin for "you have the body." An order to bring a party before a judge or court; specifically, in regard to a person who is being retained within a hospital, to give the court the opportunity to examine that person and decide on the appropriateness of such retention.

health care proxy   A legal instrument akin to the DURABLE POWER OF ATTORNEY but specifically created for health care decision making. See also ADVANCE DIRECTIVE; LIVING WILL.

hold harmless   An agreement to protect a party from damages.

immunity   Freedom from DUTY or penalty.

incompetence   A lack of ability or fitness for some legal qualification necessary for the performance of an act (e.g., by being a minor, or by mental incompetence).

in forma pauperis   Latin for "in the manner of a pauper." The designation is given by both state and federal courts to someone who is without the funds to pursue the normal costs of a lawsuit or a criminal defense.

informed consent   A competent person's voluntary agreement to allow something to happen that is based on full disclosure of facts needed to make a knowing decision.

insanity   In law, the term denotes that degree of mental illness that negates an individual's legal responsibility or CAPACITY.

insanity defense   A legal concept that holds that a person cannot be held criminally responsible for his or her actions when, due to a mental illness, the person was unable to form the requisite intent for the crime he or she is charged with at the time the crime was committed. Historically, several standards or tests have been devised to define criminal INSANITY. Some of these include the following:

American Law Institute (ALI)/Model Penal Code test   A DEFENDANT would not be responsible for his or her criminal conduct if, as a result of mental disease or defect, he or she "lacked substantial CAPACITY either to appreciate the criminality of his or her conduct or to conform his or her conduct to the requirements of law."

Comprehensive Crime Control Act (CCCA) of 1984 standard   In 1984, as part of sweeping federal legislation, the CCCA altered the test for INSANITY in federal courts by holding that it was an affirmative defense to all federal crimes that at the time of the offense, "the DEFENDANT, as a result of a severe mental disease or defect, was unable to appreciate the nature and quality or the wrongfulness of his acts. Mental disease or defect does not otherwise constitute a defense."

Durham **rule**   A ruling by the U.S. Court of Appeals for the District of Columbia Circuit in 1954 that held that an accused person is not criminally responsible if his or her "unlawful act was the product of mental disease or mental defect." This decision was quite controversial, and within several years it was modified and then replaced altogether by the same court that originally formulated it.

irresistible impulse test   Acquittal of criminal responsibility is allowed if a DEFENDANT's mental disorder caused him or her to experience an "irresistible and uncontrollable impulse to commit the offense, even if he remained able to understand the nature of the offense and its wrongfulness."

M'Naghten **rule**   In 1843, the English House of Lords ruled that a person was not responsible for a crime if the accused "was laboring under such a defect of reason from a disease of mind as not to know the nature and quality of the act; or, if he knew it, that he did not know he was doing what was wrong." This rule, or some derivation of it, is still applied in many states today.

intentional tort A TORT in which the actor is expressly or implicitly judged to have possessed an intent or a purpose to cause injury.

inter alia Literally, "among other things." This phrase is often found in legal pleadings and writings to specify one example out of many possibilities.

judgment The final determination or ADJUDICATION by a court of the claims of parties in an ACTION.

jurisdiction Widely used to denote the legal RIGHT by which courts or judicial officers exercise their authority.

Lanterman-Petris-Short Act Coauthored by California State Assemblyman Frank Lanterman and California State Senators Nicholas C. Petris and Alan Short, and signed into law in 1967 by Governor Ronald Reagan, the Act went into full effect on July 1, 1972. It cited seven articles of intent: 1) to end the inappropriate, indefinite, and involuntary commitment of mentally disordered persons, people with developmental disabilities, and persons impaired by chronic alcoholism, and to eliminate legal disabilities; 2) to provide prompt evaluation and treatment of persons with serious mental disorders or impaired by chronic alcoholism; 3) to guarantee and protect public safety; 4) to safeguard individual rights through judicial review; 5) to provide individualized treatment, supervision, and placement services by a conservatorship program for gravely disabled persons; 6) to encourage the full use of all existing agencies, professional personnel and public funds to accomplish these objectives and to prevent duplication of services and unnecessary expenditures; and 7) to protect mentally disordered persons and developmentally disabled persons from criminal acts. The Act set the precedent for modern mental health commitment procedures in the United States.

lex talionis The principle or law of retaliation that a punishment inflicted should correspond in degree and kind to the offense of the wrongdoer, as "an eye for an eye, a tooth for a tooth."

living will Procedure by which competent persons can, under certain situations, direct their doctors to treat them in a prescribed way if they become incompetent (e.g., withdraw lifesaving medical care if in a vegetative state). See also ADVANCE DIRECTIVE; DURABLE POWER OF ATTORNEY; HEALTH CARE PROXY.

malitia supplet aetatem Latin for "malice supplies the age." The concept that children ages 7–14 years can be found guilty only if prosecutors can prove that the child defendants knew and understood the consequences of their acts.

medical malpractice Generally defined as "the failure to exercise the degree of skill in diagnosis or treatment that reasonably can be expected from one licensed and holding oneself out as a physician under the circumstances of a particular case" that directly causes harm to a patient. See also NEGLIGENCE; STANDARD OF CARE; TORT.

mens rea Literally, "guilty mind." One of two fundamental aspects of any crime. The other aspect is the act, or *ACTUS REUM*.

Miranda warning Refers to the *Miranda v. Arizona* decision (1966) that requires a four-part warning to be given prior to any custodial interrogation.

negligence In MEDICAL MALPRACTICE law, generally described as the failure to do something that a reasonable and prudent practitioner would have done (omission) or as doing something that a reasonable practitioner would not have done (commission) under particular circumstances. See also STANDARD OF CARE; TORT.

NGRI See NOT GUILTY BY REASON OF INSANITY.

nolle prosequi Literally, "unwilling to pursue." A declaration made by a prosecutor in a criminal case or by a plaintiff in a civil lawsuit either before or during trial, meaning the case against the defendant is being dropped. The declaration may be made because the charges cannot be proved, the evidence has demonstrated either innocence or a fatal flaw in the prosecution's claim, the prosecutor no longer thinks the accused is guilty, and/or the accused has passed away.

nolo contendere Literally, "I do not wish to contend." A plea made by a defendant who does not wish to contest the charges, but at the same time leaves it up to the judge to decide whether he or she is guilty.

nominal damages Generally, DAMAGES of a small monetary amount indicating a violation of a legal RIGHT without any important loss or damage to the PLAINTIFF.

non compos mentis Literally, "not of sound mind." Although typically used in law, this term can also be used metaphorically or figuratively (i.e., when one is in a confused state, intoxicated, or not of sound mind).

not guilty by reason of insanity (NGRI) A defendant attempting an INSANITY DEFENSE is often required to first undergo a mental examination by forensic professionals to ascertain whether the defendant was incapable of distinguishing between right and wrong at the time of the offense. Some jurisdictions require that the evaluation also address the issue of whether the defendant was able to control his or her behavior at the time of the offense. A defendant making the insanity argument might be said to be pleading "not guilty by reason of insanity" (NGRI). A successful NGRI defense can result in an indeterminate commitment to a psychiatric facility.

parens patriae   The authority of the state to exercise sovereignty and GUARDIANSHIP of a person of legal disability so as to act on his or her behalf in protecting health, comfort, and welfare interests.

plaintiff   The complaining party in an ACTION; the person who brings a CAUSE OF ACTION.

police power   The power of government to make and enforce all laws and regulations necessary for the welfare of the state and its citizens.

power of attorney   A document giving someone authority to act on behalf of the grantor.

preponderance of the evidence   The lowest of three levels or standards applied to determining whether alleged facts have been proven (51% range of certainty); more likely than not. This is the standard applied to civil lawsuits.

privilege   A statutorily based RIGHT of the patient to restrict or bar the disclosure of confidential information in a court of law in most circumstances. See also CONFIDENTIALITY.

privileged communication   Those statements made by certain persons within a protected relationship (e.g., doctor–patient) that the law protects from forced disclosure. See also CONFIDENTIALITY.

pro se   Literally, "for oneself." The right of a party to a legal action, as either a defendant or a plaintiff, to represent his or her own cause.

proximate cause   The direct, immediate cause to which an injury or loss can be attributed and without which the injury or loss would not have occurred.

proxy   A person empowered by another to represent, act, or vote for him or her.

punitive damages   DAMAGES awarded over and above those to which the PLAINTIFF is entitled, generally given to punish or make an example of the DEFENDANT.

res gestae Literally, "things done." Secondhand statements considered trustworthy for the purpose of admission as evidence in a lawsuit when repeated by a witness because they were made spontaneously and concurrently with an event.

res ipsa loquitur Literally, "the thing speaks for itself"; means that because the facts are so obvious, a party need explain no more.

respondeat superior The doctrine whereby the master (i.e., the employer) is liable in certain cases for the wrongful acts of his or her servants (i.e., the employees).

right A power, privilege, demand, or claim possessed by a particular person by virtue of law. Every legal right that one person has imposes corresponding legal DUTIES on other persons.

sovereign immunity The IMMUNITY of a government from being sued in court except with its consent.

standard of care In the law of medical negligence, that degree of care that a reasonably prudent medical practitioner having ordinary skill, training, and learning would exercise under the same or similar circumstances. Unless the practitioner is considered an expert or a specialist, the requisite degree of care is held to be only "ordinary" and "reasonable" care. If a physician's conduct falls below the standard of care, he or she may be liable in DAMAGES for any injuries resulting from such conduct.

stare decisis The duty to adhere to precedents and not to unsettle principles of law that are established.

statute An act of the legislature declaring, commanding, or prohibiting something.

sua sponte Literally, "on its own will." The term is usually applied to actions by a judge taken without a prior motion or request from the parties.

subpoena A command, typically at the request of a litigating party, to appear at a certain time and place to give testimony on a certain matter. Unless signed by a judge, a subpoena is not a court order compelling testimony but merely a court-issued order to show up.

subpoena *ad testificandum* A writ commanding a person to appear in court to give testimony.

subpoena *duces tecum* A writ commanding a person to produce specified records or documents at a certain time and place at trial.

***Tarasoff* rule**   Based on the 1976 California decision *Tarasoff v. The Regents of the University of California,* this landmark opinion held that when a patient presents a serious, imminent danger of violence to a foreseeable victim, the psychotherapist of that patient has a DUTY to use reasonable care to protect the intended victim against such danger. A number of JURISDICTIONS have issued a ruling or STATUTE involving some variation of the *Tarasoff* "duty to protect" doctrine.

testamentary capacity   Pertains to the state of mind of an individual at the time he or she writes or executes his or her will. Generally, to have sufficient testamentary capacity, testators must possess a certain level of understanding of the nature and extent of their property, of the persons who are the natural objects of their bounty, and of the disposition that they are making of their property and must appreciate these elements in relation to one another and form an orderly desire as to the disposition of their property.

tort   A civil wrong subject to lawsuit by private individuals, as distinguished from a criminal offense, which is only brought or prosecuted by the state on behalf of its citizens. See also CIVIL ACTION.

United States Code (U.S.C.)   The compilation of laws derived from federal legislation.

vicarious liability   Indirect legal responsibility for the actions or conduct of those over whom the principal has control. For example, a private physician is generally vicariously liable for the NEGLIGENCE of any assisting employees.

Mental Health Resources

General Resources

Mental Health Advocacy and Support

Assertive Community Treatment Association

P.O. Box 2428
Brighton, MI 48116
(810) 227-1859
www.actassociation.org
Organization that promotes, develops, and supports high-quality Assertive Community Treatment (ACT) services that improve the lives of people diagnosed with serious and persistent mental illness.

Association for Behavioral and Cognitive Therapies

305 7th Avenue, 16th Floor
New York, NY 10001
(212) 047-1090
www.abct.org
Interdisciplinary organization committed to advancement of a scientific approach to the understanding and amelioration of mental health problems through application of behavioral, cognitive, and other evidence-based principles to assessment, prevention, and treatment.

Mental Health America
(formerly National Mental Health Association)

2000 N. Beauregard Street, 6th floor
Alexandria, VA 22311
(703) 684-7722
(800) 969-6642
www.nmha.org
Oldest and largest nonprofit organization that addresses all aspects of mental health and mental illness.

National Alliance on Mental Illness

3803 N. Fairfax Drive, Suite 100
Arlington, VA 22203
(800) 950-NAMI (6264)
(703) 524-7600
www.nami.org
Self-help and advocacy organization for persons with mental disorders and their families.

National Mental Health Consumers' Self-Help Clearinghouse

1211 Chestnut Street, Suite 1207
Philadelphia, PA 19107
(800) 553-4539
(215) 751-1810
www.mhselfhelp.org
Consumer-run national technical assistance center serving the mental health consumer movement to help connect individuals to self-help and advocacy resources.

Recovery International/The Abraham Low Institute

105 W. Adams Street, Suite 2940
Chicago, IL 60603
(866) 221-0302
www.recovery-inc.com
Self-help group for people coping with psychiatric illness.

World Federation for Mental Health

12940 Harbor Drive, Suite 101
Woodbridge, VA 22192
(703) 494-6515
www.wfmh.org
International membership organization founded to advance, among all peoples and nations, the prevention of mental and emotional disorders, the proper treatment and care of those with such disorders, and the promotion of mental health.

Professional Organizations

Academy of Psychosomatic Medicine

5272 River Road, Suite 630
Bethesda, MD 20816-1453
(301) 718-6520
www.apm.org
Specialty organization dedicated to the advancement of medical science, education, and health care for persons with comorbid psychiatric and general medical conditions.

American Academy of Addiction Psychiatry

400 Massasoit Avenue, Suite 307, 2nd Floor
East Providence, RI 02914
(401) 524-3076
www.aaap.org
Specialty organization for addiction psychiatrists.

American Academy of Child and Adolescent Psychiatry

3615 Wisconsin Avenue, N.W.
Washington, DC 20016-3007
(202) 966-7300
www.aacap.org
Specialty organization for child and adolescent psychiatrists.

American Academy of Psychiatry and the Law

One Regency Drive
P.O. Box 30
Bloomfield, CT 06002
(860) 242-5450
(800) 331-1389
www.aapl.org
Specialty organization for forensic psychiatrists.

American Academy of Sleep Medicine

2510 North Frontage Road
Darien, IL 60561
(630) 737–9700
www.aasmnet.org
Professional society dedicated to the medical subspecialty of sleep medicine.

American Association for Geriatric Psychiatry

7910 Woodmont Avenue, Suite 1050
Bethesda, MD 20814-3004
(301) 654-7850
www.aagpgpa.org
Association that provides information and resources to help physicians and caregivers improve the quality of life for older people with mental disorders.

American College of Neuropsychopharmacology

545 Mainstream Drive, Suite 110
Nashville, TN 37228-1256
(615) 324-2360
www.acnp.org
Professional membership society in brain, behavior, and psychopharmacological research.

American College of Psychiatrists

122 South Michigan Avenue, Suite 1360
Chicago, IL 60603
(312) 662-1020
www.acpsych.org
Nonprofit honorary association dedicated to providing continuing education to its members, promoting the latest advances in the specialty, and supporting the highest standards in psychiatry.

American Group Psychotherapy Association

25 E. 21st Street, 6th Floor
New York, NY 10010
(212) 477-2677
(877) 668-2472
www.groupsinc.org
Association that seeks to enhance the practice, theory, and research of group therapy.

American Medical Association

515 N. State Street
Chicago, IL 60654
(312) 464–5000
www.ama-assn.org
Professional association of physicians.

American Mental Health Counselors Association

801 North Fairfax Street, Suite 304
Alexandria, VA 22314
(703) 548-6002
(800) 326-2642
www.amhca.org
Association that enhances the profession of mental health counseling through licensing, advocacy, education, and professional development.

American Neuropsychiatric Association

700 Ackerman Road, Suite 625
Columbus, OH 43202
(614) 447-2077
www.anpaonline.org
Specialty organization of professionals in neuropsychiatry, behavioral neurology, neuropsychology, and the clinical neurosciences.

American Psychiatric Association

1000 Wilson Boulevard, Suite 1825
Arlington, VA 22209-3901
(703) 907-7300
(888) 35-PSYCH
www.psych.org
World's largest specialty organization of psychiatrists.

American Psychoanalytic Association

309 East 49th Street
New York, NY 10017-1601
(212) 752-0450
www.apsa.org
Oldest national psychoanalytic organization in the United States.

American Psychological Association

750 First Street, N.E.
Washington, DC 20002-4242
(202) 336-5500
(800) 374-2721
www.apa.org
Largest association of psychologists worldwide.

Association for Psychological Science

1133 15th Street, NW, Suite 1000
Washington, DC 20005
(202) 293-9300
psychologicalscience.org
Professional organization for the advancement of scientifically oriented psychology.

National Association of Social Workers

750 First Street, N.E., Suite 700
Washington, DC 20002-4241
(202) 408-8600
(800) 638-8799
www.socialworkers.org
Largest membership organization of professional social workers in the world.

Governmental Agencies

Agency for Healthcare Research and Quality

Office of Communications and Knowledge Transfer
540 Gaither Road, Suite 2000
Rockville, MD 20850
(301) 427-1104
www.ahrq.gov
Lead Federal agency charged with improving the quality, safety, efficiency, and effectiveness of health care for all Americans.

Centers for Disease Control and Prevention

1600 Clifton Road
Atlanta, GA 30333
(800) 232-4636
www.cdc.gov
One of the major operating components of the U.S. Department of Health and Human Services; dedicated to collaboratively creating the expertise, information, and tools that people and communities need to protect their health.

National Institutes of Health

9000 Rockville Pike
Bethesda, MD 20892
(301) 496-4000
www.nih.gov
The principal medical research institution of the U.S. government, comprising 27 research institutes and centers and providing a focus for biomedical and behavioral research in the United States.

National Institute of Mental Health

Science Writing, Press, and Dissemination Branch
6001 Executive Boulevard, Room 8184, MSC 9663
Bethesda, MD 20892-9663
(301) 443-4513
(866) 615-6464
www.nimh.nih.gov
One of the component organizations of the National Institutes of Health and the largest research organization in the world specializing in mental illness.

National Library of Medicine

8600 Rockville Pike
Bethesda, MD 20894
(800) 735-2258
www.nlm.nih.gov
The world's largest medical library; collects materials and provides information and research services in all areas of biomedicine and health care.

Office of the Assistant Secretary for Health (formerly Office of Public Health and Science)

U.S. Department of Health and Human Services
200 Independence Avenue, S.W., Room 716-G
Washington, DC 20201
(202) 690-7694
(877) 696-6775
www.hhs.gov/ash
Office that oversees all matters pertaining to the Public Health Service, the main division of the U.S. Department of Health and Human Services.

SAMHSA's National Helpline

Substance Abuse and Mental Health Services Administration (SAMHSA)

(800) 662-HELP (4357)

(800) 66-AYUDA (27832) (Spanish-speaking callers)

(800) 487-4889 (TDD)

Toll-free, 24-hour information service for individuals and family members facing substance abuse or mental health issues. Callers can receive referrals to local treatment facilities, support groups, and community-based organizations and can also order free publications and other information in print on substance abuse and mental health issues.

Disorder-Based Advocacy Organizations

Alcohol, Drug, and Substance Abuse

Al-Anon/Alateen

Al-Anon Family Group Headquarters, Inc.

1600 Corporate Landing Parkway

Virginia Beach, VA 23454-5617

(888) 425-2666

www.al-anon.org

Fellowship of relatives and friends of alcoholics.

Alcoholics Anonymous

P.O. Box 459

New York, NY 10163

(212) 870-3400

www.aa.org

Voluntary, nonprofessional, self-help organization offering a 12-step fellowship program for recovering alcoholics.

American Council for Drug Education

50 Jay Street
Brooklyn, NY 11201
(718) 222-6641
www.acde.org
Substance abuse prevention and education agency.

Center for Substance Abuse Prevention, Substance Abuse and Mental Health Services Administration

5600 Fishers Lane
Rockwall II Building, Suite 900
Rockville, MD 20857
(301) 443-0365
www.samhsa.gov
Government agency that provides referrals and information for issues relating to substance abuse.

Center on Addiction and the Family

164 West 74th Street
New York, NY 10023
(212) 595-5810 Ext. 7760
www.coaf.org
National nonprofit organization that provides educational materials and services to help professionals, children, and adults break the intergenerational cycle of parental substance abuse.

Cocaine Anonymous World Services

21720 S. Wilmington Avenue, Suite 304
Long Beach, CA 90810-1641
(310) 559-5833
www.ca.org
Self-help, nonprofessional, 12-step fellowship program for men and women in recovery from cocaine addiction.

Co-Dependents Anonymous

P.O. Box 33577
Phoenix, AZ 85067-3577
(602) 277-7991
(888) 444-2359
www.coda.org
Fellowship of men and women whose common purpose is to develop healthy relationships.

Families Anonymous

World Service Office
P.O. Box 3475
Culver City, CA 90231-3475
(800) 736-9805
www.familiesanonymous.org
A 12-step, self-help, recovery, and fellowship program of support groups for relatives and friends of those who have alcohol, drug, or behavioral problems.

Narcotics Anonymous

World Service Office
P.O. Box 9999
Van Nuys, CA 91409
(818) 773-9999
www.na.org
Support organization for recovering narcotics addicts.

National Clearinghouse for Alcohol and Drug Information

P.O. Box 2345
Rockville, MD 20847-2345
(301) 468-2600
(800) 729-6686
www.health.org
Government agency that is one of the largest online repositories of science-based substance abuse prevention, education, and policy information.

National Families in Action

P.O. Box 133136
Atlanta, GA 30333-3136
(404) 248-9676
www.emory.edu/NFIA
National drug education, prevention, and policy center.

National Family Partnership

2490 Coral Way, Suite 501
Miami, FL 33145
(305) 856-4886
(800) 705-8997
www.nfp.org
Organization supporting families to nurture the potential of healthy, drug-free youth.

National Institute on Alcohol Abuse and Alcoholism

5635 Fishers Lane, MSC 9304
Bethesda, MD 20892-7003
(301) 443-3860
www.niaaa.nih.gov
Government agency that supports and conducts biomedical and behavioral research on the causes, consequences, treatment, and prevention of alcoholism and alcohol-related problems.

National Institute on Drug Abuse

6001 Executive Boulevard, Room 5213
Bethesda, MD 20892-9561
(301) 443-1124
www.nida.nih.gov
Government agency that supports and conducts research—and promotes the rapid and effective dissemination and use of research findings—to significantly improve prevention, treatment, and policy as they relate to drug abuse and addiction.

PRIDE Youth Programs
(formerly Parents' Resource Institute for Drug Education)

4 West Oak Street
Fremont, MI 49412
(231) 924-1662
(800) 668-9277
www.prideyouthprograms.org
Largest peer-to-peer organization in the nation devoted to prevention of drug abuse and violence through education.

Women for Sobriety, Inc.

109 W. Broad Street
P.O. Box 618
Quakertown, PA 18951-0618
(215) 536-8026
www.womenforsobriety.org
Nonprofit organization dedicated to helping women overcome alcoholism and other addictions.

Alzheimer's Disease

Alzheimer's Association

225 North Michigan Avenue, Floor 17
Chicago, IL 60601-7633
(312) 335-8700
(800) 272-3900
www.alz.org
Largest national voluntary health organization supporting Alzheimer's disease research and care.

Alzheimer's Foundation of America

322 8th Avenue, 7th Floor
New York, NY 10001
(866) 232-8484
www.alzfdn.org
Nonprofit organizational network dedicated to assuring quality of care and excellence in service to individuals with Alzheimer's disease and related illnesses, and to their caregivers and families.

Anxiety Disorders

Anxiety Disorders Association of America

8730 Georgia Avenue, Suite 600
Silver Spring, MD 20910
(240) 485-1001
www.adaa.org
Association dedicated to increasing public awareness about anxiety disorders, providing education resources, offering access to care, and supporting research.

International Society for Traumatic Stress

ISTSS Headquarters
111 Deer Lake Road, Suite 100
Deerfield, IL 60015
(847) 480-9028
istss@istss.org
International interdisciplinary professional organization promoting advancement and exchange of knowledge about traumatic stress.

Disorders Usually First Diagnosed in Infancy, Childhood, or Adolescence

American Association on Intellectual and Developmental Disabilities

501 3rd Street, N.W., Suite 200
Washington, DC 20001-2760
(202) 387-1968
(800) 424-3688
www.aamr.org
Organization promoting progressive policies, sound research, effective practices, and universal human rights for people with intellectual disabilities.

Attention Deficit Disorder Association

P.O. Box 7557
Wilmington, DE 19803-9997
(800) 939-1019
www.add.org
International nonprofit organization whose mission is to provide information, resources, and networking opportunities to help adults with attention-deficit/hyperactivity disorder lead better lives.

Children and Adults With Attention-Deficit/Hyperactivity Disorder

8181 Professional Place, Suite 150
Landover, MD 20785
(301) 306-7070
(800) 233-4050
www.chadd.org
Nonprofit charitable organization working to improve the lives of people with attention-deficit/hyperactivity disorder.

Learning Disabilities Association of America

4156 Library Road
Pittsburgh, PA 15234-1349
(412) 341-1515
www.ldanatl.org
Nonprofit organization dedicated to advancing the education and general welfare of children and adults of normal or potentially normal intelligence who manifest disabilities of a perceptual, conceptual, or coordinative nature.

The Arc (formerly National Association for Retarded Children)

1660 L Street, N.W., Suite 301
Washington, DC 20036
(202) 534-3700
(800) 433-5255
www.thearc.org
National organization dedicated to promoting and protecting the human rights of people with intellectual and developmental disabilities and actively supporting their full inclusion and participation in the community throughout their lifetimes.

Tourette Syndrome Association

42-40 Bell Boulevard
Bayside, NY 11361
(718) 224-2999
www.tsa-usa.org
National voluntary nonprofit membership organization devoted to identifying the cause of, finding the cure for, and controlling the effects of Tourette syndrome.

Eating Disorders

National Association of Anorexia Nervosa and Associated Disorders

P.O. Box 640
Naperville, IL 60566
(630) 577-1330 (hot line)
www.anad.org
Association that provides counseling and information for anorexic and bulimic patients, their families, and professionals.

National Eating Disorders Association

603 Stewart Street, Suite 803
Seattle, WA 98101
(206) 382-3587
(800) 931-2237
www.nationaleatingdisorders.org
Self-help group that provides information and referrals to physicians and therapists.

Overeaters Anonymous

P.O. Box 44020
Rio Rancho, NM 87174-4020
(505) 891-2664
www.overeatersanonymous.org
Self-help group for those who wish to stop eating compulsively.

Mood Disorders

Child and Adolescent Bipolar Foundation

820 Davis Street, Suite 520
Evanston IL 60201
(847) 492-8519
www.bpkids.org
Nonprofit organization of families raising children and teens affected by depression, bipolar disorder, and other mood disorders.

Depression and Bipolar Support Alliance

730 N. Franklin Street, Suite 501
Chicago, IL 60654-7225
(800) 826-3632
www.dbsalliance.org
Association that represents adults living with depression and bipolar disorder.

Lithium Information Center

Madison Institute of Medicine
6515 Grand Teton Plaza, Suite 100
Madison, WI 53719
(608) 827-2470
www.miminc.org
Resource for information on lithium treatment of bipolar disorders and on other medical and biological applications of lithium.

National Bipolar Foundation

111 S. Highland Street, Suite 129
Memphis, TN 38111-4640
www.nationalbipolarfoundation.org
Nonprofit organization devoted to reducing stigma, educating, and seeking affordable health care for people living with bipolar disorder.

Neurological Disorders

American Brain Coalition

6257 Quantico Lane North
Maple Grove, MN 55331
(763) 557-2913
www.americanbraincoalition.org
Nonprofit organization of professional neurological, psychological, and psychiatric associations and patient organizations dedicated to advancing understanding of the functions of the brain and to reducing the burden of brain disorders through public advocacy.

National Institute of Neurological Disorders and Stroke

P.O. Box 5801
Bethesda, MD 20824
(301) 496-5751
(800) 352-9424
www.ninds.nih.gov
The nation's leading biomedical research institute on disorders of the brain and nervous system.

Obsessive-Compulsive Disorder

International OCD Foundation

P.O. Box 961029

Boston, MA 02196

(617) 973-5801

www.ocfoundation.org

Voluntary organization dedicated to early intervention in controlling and finding cures for obsessive-compulsive disorder and for improving the welfare of people with this disorder.

Personality Disorders

National Education Alliance for Borderline Personality Disorder

P.O. Box 974

Rye, New York 10580

www.borderlinepersonalitydisorder.com

Nonprofit organization, staffed by volunteering consumers, family members, and professionals, that seeks to raise public awareness, provide education, promote research on borderline personality disorder, and enhance the quality of life of those affected by this serious mental illness.

Treatment and Research Advancements Association for Personality Disorder

23 Greene Street

New York, NY, 10013

(212) 966-6514

www.tara4bpd.org

Nonprofit organization whose mission is to foster education and research in the field of personality disorder, specifically but not exclusively borderline personality disorder (BPD); to support research into the causes, psychobiology, and treatment of personality disorders; to support and encourage educational programs and endeavors targeting mental health professionals, consumers of mental health services, families and/or the community at large in order to reduce stigma and increase awareness of personality disorder; to disseminate available information on etiology and treatment; and to lawfully advocate for accomplishment of these goals.

Schizophrenia

Schizophrenia Research Forum (Web site sponsored by NARSAD)

www.schizophreniaforum.org
Web site created to foster collaboration among researchers by providing an international online forum where ideas, research news, and data on schizophrenia and related diseases can be presented and discussed.

NARSAD (formerly National Alliance for Research on Schizophrenia and Depression)

60 Cutter Mill Road, Suite 404
Great Neck, NY 11021
(516) 829-0091
(800) 829-8289
www.narsad.org
National nonprofit organization that raises and distributes funds for scientific research into the causes, cures and treatments, and prevention of severe mental illness, primarily schizophrenia and depression.

Sleep and Sleep Disorders

American Sleep Apnea Association

6856 Eastern Avenue, N.W., Suite 203
Washington, DC 20012
(202) 293-3650
www.sleepapnea.org
Nonprofit organization dedicated to reducing injury, disability, and death from sleep apnea and to enhancing the well-being of those affected by this common disorder.

American Sleep Association

www.sleepassociation.org
National organization focused on improving public awareness about sleep disorders and sleep health, promoting sleep medicine research, and providing a portal for communication between patients, physicians/health care professionals, corporations, and scientists. The ASA is a member-driven public service project that depends on volunteer efforts.

Narcolepsy Network

110 Ripple Lane
North Kingston, RI 02852
(888) 292-6522
www.narcolepsynetwork.org
Nonprofit organization dedicated to individuals with narcolepsy and related sleep disorders, with a mission of providing services to educate, advocate, support, and improve awareness of this neurological sleep disorder.

Suicide

American Association of Suicidology

5221 Wisconsin Avenue, N.W.
Washington, DC 20015
(202) 237-2280
www.suicidology.org
Organization dedicated to the understanding and prevention of suicide; promotes research, public awareness programs, education, and training for professionals and volunteers.

American Foundation for Suicide Prevention

120 Wall Street, 22nd Floor
New York, New York 10005
(212) 363-3500
(888) 333 2377
www.afsp.org
Foundation dedicated to advancing knowledge of suicide and its prevention.

National Hopeline Network

Kristin Brooks Hope Center
1250 24th Street N.W., Suite 300
Washington, DC 20037
(202) 536-3200
www.hopeline.com
1-800-442-HOPE (4673)
1-800-SUICIDE (784-2433)
National hotline network created to help those in crisis find help and hope immediately.

National Suicide Prevention Lifeline

1-800-273-TALK (8255)

Free 24-hour hotline available to anyone in suicidal crisis or emotional distress. Lifeline is funded by the Substance Abuse and Mental Health Services Administration (SAMHSA).